Hospital Acquired Infections, Multidrug Resistant (MDR) Bacteria, Alternative Approaches to Antibiotic Therapy

Hospital Acquired Infections, Multidrug Resistant (MDR) Bacteria, Alternative Approaches to Antibiotic Therapy

Editors

Pavel Bostik
Milan Kolar

MDPI • Basel • Beijing • Wuhan • Barcelona • Belgrade • Manchester • Tokyo • Cluj • Tianjin

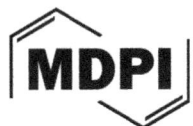

Editors

Pavel Bostik
Institute of Clinical Microbiology
Charles University
Faculty of Medicine in Hradec Kralove,
and Faculty Hospital Hradec Kralove
Czech Republic

Milan Kolar
Department of Microbiology
Faculty of Medicine and Dentistry
Palacky University,
and University Hospital Olomouc
Czech Republic

Editorial Office
MDPI
St. Alban-Anlage 66
4052 Basel, Switzerland

This is a reprint of articles from the Special Issue published online in the open access journal *Antibiotics* (ISSN 2079-6382) (available at: www.mdpi.com/journal/antibiotics/special_issues/Hospital_Acquired).

For citation purposes, cite each article independently as indicated on the article page online and as indicated below:

LastName, A.A.; LastName, B.B.; LastName, C.C. Article Title. *Journal Name* **Year**, *Volume Number*, Page Range.

ISBN 978-3-0365-4418-2 (Hbk)
ISBN 978-3-0365-4417-5 (PDF)

Cover image courtesy of Pavel Bostik

© 2022 by the authors. Articles in this book are Open Access and distributed under the Creative Commons Attribution (CC BY) license, which allows users to download, copy and build upon published articles, as long as the author and publisher are properly credited, which ensures maximum dissemination and a wider impact of our publications.

The book as a whole is distributed by MDPI under the terms and conditions of the Creative Commons license CC BY-NC-ND.

Contents

Preface to "Hospital Acquired Infections, Multidrug Resistant (MDR) Bacteria, Alternative Approaches to Antibiotic Therapy" vii

Milan Kolar, Miroslava Htoutou Sedlakova, Karel Urbanek, Patrik Mlynarcik, Magdalena Roderova and Kristyna Hricova et al.
Implementation of Antibiotic Stewardship in a University Hospital Setting
Reprinted from: *Antibiotics* **2021**, *10*, 93, doi:10.3390/antibiotics10010093 1

Patrik Mlynarcik, Hana Chudobova, Veronika Zdarska and Milan Kolar
In Silico Analysis of Extended-Spectrum β-Lactamases in Bacteria
Reprinted from: *Antibiotics* **2021**, *10*, 812, doi:10.3390/antibiotics10070812 17

Radek Sleha, Vera Radochova, Jiri Malis, Alexander Mikyska, Milan Houska and Karel Krofta et al.
Strong Antimicrobial and Healing Effects of Beta-Acids from Hops in Methicillin-Resistant *Staphylococcus aureus*-Infected External Wounds In Vivo
Reprinted from: *Antibiotics* **2021**, *10*, 708, doi:10.3390/antibiotics10060708 39

Radek Sleha, Vera Radochova, Alexander Mikyska, Milan Houska, Radka Bolehovska and Sylva Janovska et al.
Strong Antimicrobial Effects of Xanthohumol and Beta-Acids from Hops against *Clostridioides difficile* Infection In Vivo
Reprinted from: *Antibiotics* **2021**, *10*, 392, doi:10.3390/antibiotics10040392 53

Kristýna Hricová, Taťána Štosová, Pavla Kučová, Kateřina Fišerová, Jan Bardoň and Milan Kolář
Analysis of Vancomycin-Resistant Enterococci in Hemato-Oncological Patients
Reprinted from: *Antibiotics* **2020**, *9*, 785, doi:10.3390/antibiotics9110785 65

Katarina Pomorska, Vladislav Jakubu, Lucia Malisova, Marta Fridrichova, Martin Musilek and Helena Zemlickova
Antibiotic Resistance, *spa* Typing and Clonal Analysis of Methicillin-Resistant *Staphylococcus aureus* (MRSA) Isolates from Blood of Patients Hospitalized in the Czech Republic
Reprinted from: *Antibiotics* **2021**, *10*, 395, doi:10.3390/antibiotics10040395 75

Jan Papajk, Kristýna Mezerová, Radovan Uvízl, Taťána Štosová and Milan Kolář
Clonal Diversity of *Klebsiella* spp. and *Escherichia* spp. Strains Isolated from Patients with Ventilator-Associated Pneumonia
Reprinted from: *Antibiotics* **2021**, *10*, 674, doi:10.3390/antibiotics10060674 91

Pavla Kucova, Lumir Kantor, Katerina Fiserova, Jakub Lasak, Magdalena Röderova and Milan Kolar
Bacterial Pathogens and Evaluation of a Cut-Off for Defining Early and Late Neonatal Infection
Reprinted from: *Antibiotics* **2021**, *10*, 278, doi:10.3390/antibiotics10030278 101

Lucia Mališová, Vladislav Jakubů, Katarína Pomorská, Martin Musílek and Helena Žemličková
Spread of Linezolid-Resistant *Enterococcus* spp. in Human Clinical Isolates in the Czech Republic
Reprinted from: *Antibiotics* **2021**, *10*, 219, doi:10.3390/antibiotics10020219 113

Tomokazu Shoji, Natsu Sato, Haruhisa Fukuda, Yuichi Muraki, Keishi Kawata and Manabu Akazawa
Clinical Implication of the Relationship between Antimicrobial Resistance and Infection Control Activities in Japanese Hospitals: A Principal Component Analysis-Based Cluster Analysis
Reprinted from: *Antibiotics* **2022**, *11*, 229, doi:10.3390/antibiotics11020229 . . . . **121**

Bing-Mu Hsu, Jung-Sheng Chen, I-Ching Lin, Gwo-Jong Hsu, Suprokash Koner and Bashir Hussain et al.
Molecular and Anti-Microbial Resistance (AMR) Profiling of Methicillin-Resistant *Staphylococcus aureus* (MRSA) from Hospital and Long-Term Care Facilities (LTCF) Environment
Reprinted from: *Antibiotics* **2021**, *10*, 748, doi:10.3390/antibiotics10060748 . . . . **135**

Dawid Rozenkiewicz, Erika Esteve-Palau, Mar Arenas-Miras, Santiago Grau, Xavier Duran and Luisa Sorlí et al.
Clinical and Economic Impact of Community-Onset Urinary Tract Infections Caused by ESBL-Producing *Klebsiella pneumoniae* Requiring Hospitalization in Spain: An Observational Cohort Study
Reprinted from: *Antibiotics* **2021**, *10*, 585, doi:10.3390/antibiotics10050585 . . . . **149**

Răzvan-Cosmin Petca, Silvius Negoiță, Cristian Mareș, Aida Petca, Răzvan-Ionuț Popescu and Călin Bogdan Chibelean
Heterogeneity of Antibiotics Multidrug-Resistance Profile of Uropathogens in Romanian Population
Reprinted from: *Antibiotics* **2021**, *10*, 523, doi:10.3390/antibiotics10050523 . . . . **159**

Wasan Katip, Suriyon Uitrakul and Peninnah Oberdorfer
Short-Course Versus Long-Course Colistin for Treatment of Carbapenem-Resistant *A. baumannii* in Cancer Patient
Reprinted from: *Antibiotics* **2021**, *10*, 484, doi:10.3390/antibiotics10050484 . . . . **173**

Alessandra Oliva, Alessandro Bianchi, Alessandro Russo, Giancarlo Ceccarelli, Francesca Cancelli and Fulvio Aloj et al.
Effect of *N*-Acetylcysteine Administration on 30-Day Mortality in Critically Ill Patients with Septic Shock Caused by Carbapenem-Resistant *Klebsiella pneumoniae* and *Acinetobacter baumannii*: A Retrospective Case-Control Study
Reprinted from: *Antibiotics* **2021**, *10*, 271, doi:10.3390/antibiotics10030271 . . . . **185**

Preface to "Hospital Acquired Infections, Multidrug Resistant (MDR) Bacteria, Alternative Approaches to Antibiotic Therapy"

Bacterial resistance to known and currently used antibiotics represents a growing issue worldwide. It poses a major problem in the treatment of infectious diseases in general and hospital-acquired infections in particular. This is in part due to the overuse and misuse of antibiotics in past decades, which led to the selection of highly resistant bacteria and even so-called superbugs –multidrug-resistant (MDR) bacteria. Nosocomial infections, particularly, are often caused by MDR bacterial pathogens and the treatment of such infections is very complicated and extensive, often leading to various side effects, including adverse effects on the natural human microbiome. At the same time, the development of novel antibiotics is lagging with very few new ones in the pipeline. Finding viable alternatives to treat such infections may help to overcome these therapeutic issues.

Even though MDR bacteria are widespread globally, their epidemiology varies by region. Hospital-acquired infections caused by MDR bacteria remain an unresolved problem in the healthcare system. A very important part of the overall therapeutic approach is the microbiological examination of adequate clinical materials, including molecular typing that may identify epidemiologically related cases and reveal the source or route of transmission, including possible clonal spread of bacterial pathogens.

This publication thus focuses on the field of bacterial resistance, mainly in the hospital settings, adequate antibiotic therapy, and identification of compounds useful to battle this growing issue. We hope that it finds its readers among clinical microbiologists, infectious disease specialists and epidemiologists worldwide, bringing to them current developments useful for their future work.

Pavel Bostik and Milan Kolar
Editors

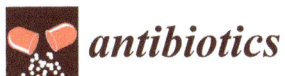

Article

Implementation of Antibiotic Stewardship in a University Hospital Setting

Milan Kolar [1], Miroslava Htoutou Sedlakova [1,*], Karel Urbanek [2], Patrik Mlynarcik [1], Magdalena Roderova [1], Kristyna Hricova [1], Kristyna Mezerova [1], Pavla Kucova [1], Jana Zapletalova [3], Katerina Fiserova [1] and Pavel Kurfurst [4]

1. Department of Microbiology, University Hospital Olomouc, Faculty of Medicine and Dentistry, Palacký University Olomouc, 779 00 Olomouc, Czech Republic; milan.kolar@fnol.cz (M.K.); patrik.mlynarcik@upol.cz (P.M.); magdalena.roderova@upol.cz (M.R.); kristyna.hricova@upol.cz (K.H.); kristyna.mezerova@upol.cz (K.M.); pavla.kucova@fnol.cz (P.K.); katerina.fiserova@fnol.cz (K.F.)
2. Department of Pharmacology, University Hospital Olomouc, Faculty of Medicine and Dentistry, Palacký University Olomouc, 779 00 Olomouc, Czech Republic; karel.urbanek@fnol.cz
3. Department of Medical Biophysics, Faculty of Medicine and Dentistry, Palacký University Olomouc, 779 00 Olomouc, Czech Republic; ja.zapletalova@upol.cz
4. Department of Foreign Languages, Faculty of Medicine and Dentistry, Palacký University Olomouc, 779 00 Olomouc, Czech Republic; pavel.kurfurst@upol.cz
* Correspondence: miroslava.htoutousedlakova@fnol.cz; Tel.: +420-585-639-511

Abstract: The article describes activities of an antibiotic center at a university hospital in the Czech Republic and presents the results of antibiotic stewardship program implementation over a period of 10 years. It provides data on the development of resistance of *Escherichia coli*, *Klebsiella pneumoniae*, *Pseudomonas aeruginosa* and *Staphylococcus aureus* to selected antibiotic agents as well as consumption data for various antibiotic classes. The genetic basis of resistance to beta-lactam antibiotics and its clonal spread were also assessed. The study showed significant correlations between aminoglycoside consumption and resistance of *Escherichia coli* and *Klebsiella pneumoniae* to gentamicin (r = 0.712, r = 0.869), fluoroquinolone consumption and resistance of *Klebsiella pneumoniae* to ciprofloxacin (r = 0.896), aminoglycoside consumption and resistance of *Pseudomonas aeruginosa* to amikacin (r = 0.716), as well as carbapenem consumption and resistance of *Pseudomonas aeruginosa* to meropenem (r = 0.855). Genotyping of ESBL-positive isolates of *Klebsiella pneumoniae* and *Escherichia coli* showed a predominance of CTX-M-type; in AmpC-positive strains, DHA, EBC and CIT enzymes prevailed. Of 19 meropenem-resistant strains of *Klebsiella pneumoniae*, two were identified as NDM-positive. Clonal spread of these strains was not detected. The results suggest that comprehensive antibiotic stewardship implementation in a healthcare facility may help to maintain the effectiveness of antibiotics against bacterial pathogens. Particularly beneficial is the work of clinical microbiologists who, among other things, approve administration of antibiotics to patients with bacterial infections and directly participate in their antibiotic therapy.

Keywords: antibiotic stewardship; resistance; consumption of antibiotics; clonal spread

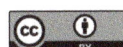

1. Introduction

Antibiotic stewardship may be defined as a set of measures leading to rational antibiotic therapy based on the adequate selection of antibacterial agents, appropriate duration of their administration and a suitable route of administration [1–4]. The need for antibiotic stewardship implementation stems from the likely prospect of antibiotics losing their effectiveness and thus their ability to treat bacterial infections [5–7]. The increasing prevalence of bacteria resistant to antibacterial drugs, mainly those producing extended-spectrum beta-lactamases including metallo-beta-lactamases and carbapenemases opens the possibility of a new non-antibiotic era in which adequate antibiotics will be unavailable to

treat infections caused by multidrug-resistant bacteria [8,9]. To prevent this, antibiotic stewardship programs have been developed as comprehensive systems comprising a range of activities that may be briefly characterized as follows:
- early and adequate microbiological diagnosis including the correct interpretation of microbiological results,
- early and reliable detection of the susceptibility/resistance of bacterial pathogens to antibiotics consistent with the European guidelines, namely those by the European Committee on Antimicrobial Susceptibility Testing (EUCAST) [10],
- immediate reporting of critical results (e.g., information on positive blood cultures),
- regular assessment of the prevalence of pathogenic bacteria and their antibiotic resistance and development of local guidelines for initial antibiotic therapy based on these data,
- adequate antibiotic prophylaxis.

It must be stressed, however, that the scope of antibiotic stewardship is much broader, involving numerous other activities that are also very important for adequate antibiotic therapy and preventing the spread of multidrug-resistant bacteria. These activities may be described as follows:
- analyzing the routes of spread of multidrug-resistant bacteria using modern molecular methods,
- providing antibiotic consultant service for clinical physicians and deciding on antibiotic administration based on microbiological results and the knowledge of primary resistance of bacterial pathogens in patients with bacterial infections,
- assessing the consumption of antibiotics in the relevant epidemiological units and, if needed, introducing necessary regulatory measures,
- close cooperation with hospital hygiene officers, epidemiologists and clinical pharmacologists.

At the University Hospital Olomouc, Czech Republic, antibiotic stewardship is coordinated by the Antibiotic Center, a section of the Department of Microbiology. Based on analyses of the development of bacterial resistance and antibiotic consumption, including the overall costs of this group of drugs, recommendations for initial antibiotic therapy and prophylaxis are formulated and quarterly presented to the hospital management who subsequently approve these recommendations and make them valid.

The article describes efforts of the Antibiotic Center and presents outcomes of its activity over a period of 10 years (2010–2019).

2. Materials and Methods

2.1. Characteristics of the Healthcare Facility

The University Hospital Olomouc is one of the largest inpatient healthcare facilities in the Czech Republic, dating back to 1896. It is part of a network of nine teaching hospitals directly controlled by the Ministry of Health of the Czech Republic. Basic data on the facility are shown in Table 1.

Table 1. Basic information on the University Hospital Olomouc in 2019.

No. of units	68
No. of beds	1198
No. of employees	4199
No. of outpatients per year	925,162
No. of inpatients per year	53,633
Mean length of stay (days)	5.6
No. of operations per year	22,715
No. of units	68

2.2. Process of Approving Antibiotic Administration

To better understand the study, it is reasonable to define the process of approving antibiotic administration at the University Hospital Olomouc. For a particular patient with a bacterial infection, the attending physician selects an antibiotic based on their own clinical reasoning and microbiological results (if available), while observing the hospital's guidelines for initial antibiotic therapy. Alternatively, an adequate antibiotic is recommended by a clinical microbiologist based on a consultation with the attending physician. If an antibiotic is selected to treat a particular bacterial infection, its administration must be approved by an Antibiotic Center member. The approval is granted electronically using the hospital information system. The clinical microbiologist (always holding a specialist qualification in medical microbiology) verifies the selection of the antibiotic focusing on all microbiological test results and, if adequate, approves its administration. The Antibiotic Center member has the right to disapprove administration of an antibiotic in case:

- some required data are missing (e.g., diagnosis of infection or antibiotic dosage),
- they reasonably doubt that the antibiotic has been adequately selected,
- ongoing microbiological tests have identified bacteria whose definitive susceptibility is yet to be determined but due to their primary resistance to the selected antibiotic, this cannot be approved.

In case of disapproval, the reason and a more adequate antibiotic or recommendations from a consultation with the Antibiotic Center clinical microbiologist are entered into the hospital information system. This takes place daily between 7 a.m. and 4 p.m. Outside these hours, antibiotic therapy is selected in line with the hospital's guidelines and the antibiotic therapy is scrutinized on the following day.

2.3. Assessing Antibiotic Consumption

A computerized database of the hospital's Department of Pharmacology was used to obtain data on antibiotic consumption during the study period. The data were processed according to the 2020 ATC/DDD system and expressed as numbers of defined daily doses for various antibiotic classes [11]. Antibiotic consumption was analyzed for both the entire hospital and its Department of Anesthesiology and Intensive Care Medicine with 25 intensive care beds.

2.4. Identification of Bacteria and Determination of Their Susceptibility/Resistance to Antibacterial Agents

Bacterial pathogens (*Escherichia coli*, *Klebsiella pneumoniae*, *Pseudomonas aeruginosa*, and *Staphylococcus aureus*) were isolated from clinical samples (tracheal secretion, bronchoalveolar lavage fluid, sputum, blood, urine, pus, puncture samples, wound secretion, bile, cerebrospinal fluid) obtained from hospitalized patients with a suspected bacterial infection. For each patient, only the first isolate from particular clinical samples was included.

The identification of bacteria was performed by MALDI-TOF MS (Biotyper Microflex, Bruker Daltonics, Bremen, Germany) [12].

The susceptibility/resistance to antibiotics was tested using a broth microdilution method according to the EUCAST [10]. The following reference strains were used as quality control organisms: *Escherichia coli* ATCC 25922, *Pseudomonas aeruginosa* ATCC 27853 and *Staphylococcus aureus* ATCC 29213. All strains of *Staphylococcus aureus* were also tested for the resistance to methicillin using selective diagnostic chromogenic media (Colorex/TM/MRSA, TRIOS, Prague, Czech Republic) and an immunochromatographic assay for the detection of PBP2a (PBP2a SA Culture Colony Test, Alere™, Abbott, Prague, Czech Republic). The production of beta-lactamases, such as ESBL and AmpC, was detected by phenotypic tests [13]. The production of carbapenemases was detected by the Carba NP test [14].

Additionally, methicillin-resistant *Staphylococcus aureus* (MRSA) strains isolated from the Department of Anesthesiology and Intensive Care Medicine patients were confirmed by the *mecA* gene detection [15]. The production of ESBL and AmpC beta-lactamases in *Escherichia coli* and *Klebsiella pneumoniae* was confirmed by PCR detection of the *bla* genes only in pre-defined groups of strains/patients from above mentioned department (from tracheal aspirates in patients with hospital-acquired pneumonia, from stool in hospitalized patients etc.) [13]. The search for potential production of carbapenemases in the meropenem-resistant *Klebsiella pneumoniae* strains at this department was carried out by simplex PCR with primers targeting bla_{FRI}, bla_{GES}, bla_{GIM}, bla_{IMI}, bla_{IMP}, bla_{KPC}, bla_{NDM}, bla_{VIM}, bla_{OXA-23} and bla_{OXA-48}. Detailed information on the primers is listed in Table 2. PCR assays were performed on Rotor-Gene TM 6000 (Corbett Research, Mortlake, Australia). PCR was run in a final volume of 25 µL using 100 ng of DNA template, 0.5 µM of forward and reverse primers, 200 µM of each dNTP, 2.5 mM of $MgCl_2$ and 1.25 U Combi Taq Polymerase (Top-Bio, Vestec, Czech Republic) in 1× Buffer (Top-Bio, Vestec, Czech Republic). The PCR conditions were as follows: initial denaturation at 94 °C for 3 min, followed by 30 cycles at 94 °C for 30 s, 72 °C for different times (45 s to 60 s) with a final extension at 72 °C for 10 min. PCR products were then separated on a 1% agarose gel containing SYBR Safe (Invitrogen) and visualized on a UV transilluminator. Bacterial isolates for genetic analysis were stored in cryotubes at −80 °C (Cryobank B, ITEST, Hradec Králové, Czech Republic).

Table 2. Primer sequences used to detect the carbapenemase genes by PCR.

Target (Subtypes)	Primer Name	Sequence (5' to 3' Direction) [a]	Amplicon Size (bp)	Tm (°C)	Reference
FRI (8)	FRI-F/R	ACAGACARGATGAGAGATTTCCT, CAGGTRCCTGTTTTATCGCC	538	58	This study
GES (42)	GES-F/R	ACGTTCAAGTTTCCGCTAG, GGCAACTAATTCGTCACGT	624	53	This study
GIM (2)	GIM-F/R	TCGACACACCTTGGTCTGAA, AACTTCCAACTTTGCCATGC	477	55	Ellington et al., 2007 [16]
IMI (11)	IMI-F/R	CTACGCTTTAGACACTGGC, AGGTTTCCTTTTCACGCTCA	482	54	Mlynarcik et al., 2016 [17]
IMP (69)	IMP-F1/R1	GAGTGGCTTAATTCTCRATC, CCAAACYACTASGTTATCT	183	52	Mlynarcik et al., 2016 [17]
IMP (2)	IMP-F2/R2	GCGGAATAGGGTGGCTTA, AGTTGCTTGGTTTTGATGGTT	435	52	This study
IMP (3)	IMP-F3/R3	TGACGGGGTTAGTTATTGGCT, CGGTTTCGCTATGACCTGAA	248	57	Mlynarcik et al., 2019 [18]
KPC (51)	KPC-F/R	GTTCTGCTGTCTTGTCTCTCA, CGGTCGTGTTTCCCTTTAG	625	56	This study
NDM (29)	NDM-F/R	GGGGATTGCGACTTATGC, AGATTGCCGAGCGACTTG	258	53	Mlynarcik et al., 2019 [18]
OXA-23-like (37)	OXA(23-like)-F/R	ACTTGCTATGTGGTTGCTTCTC, ACCTTTTCTCGCCCTTCCAT	310	56	Mlynarcik et al., 2016 [17]
OXA-48-like (31)	OXA(48-like)-F/R	AACGGGCGAACCAAGCATTTT, TGAGCACTTCTTTTGTGATGGCT	597	57	Mlynarcik et al., 2016 [17]
VIM (68)	VIM-F/R	CGCGGAGATTGARAAGCAAA, CGCAGCACCRGGATAGAARA	247	57	Mlynarcik et al., 2016 [17]

[a] For degenerate primers: R = A or G; S = G or C; Y = C or T.

2.5. Clonality

The clonality of MRSA and meropenem-resistant isolates of *Klebsiella pneumoniae* detected at the Department of Anesthesiology and Intensive Care Medicine was assessed with pulsed-field gel electrophoresis (PFGE). Bacterial DNA extracted with a technique described by Husičková et al. [19] was digested by the *Xba*I restriction endonuclease (New England Biolabs, Ipswitch, MA, USA) for 24 h at 37 °C in *Klebsiella pneumoniae* isolates and by the

SmaI restriction endonuclease (New England Biolabs, Ipswitch, MA, USA) for 24 h at 25 °C in *Staphylococcus aureus* strains. The obtained DNA fragments were separated by PFGE on 1.2% agarose gel for 24 h at 6 V/cm and pulse times of 2–35 s for both *Klebsiella pneumoniae* and *Staphylococcus aureus* strains. Subsequently, the gel was stained with ethidium bromide. The resulting restriction profiles were analyzed with the GelCompar II software (Applied Maths, Kortrijk, Belgium) using the Dice coefficient (1.2%) for comparing similarity and unweighted pair group method with arithmetic means for cluster analysis. The results were interpreted according to criteria described by Tenover et al. [20].

2.6. Statistical Analysis

Trends in the consumption of antibacterial agents, or antibiotic classes, bacterial resistance and their relationships were analyzed with Spearman's correlation. The data were processed with IBM SPSS Statistics 22 (Armonk, NY, USA).

3. Results

Tables 3–6 show the prevalence of *Escherichia coli*, *Klebsiella pneumoniae*, *Pseudomonas aeruginosa* and *Staphylococcus aureus* strains resistant to selected antibiotics over the 10-year period for the entire hospital. The results indicate an increase in resistance of *Escherichia coli* to piperacillin/tazobactam (r = 0.939), gentamicin (r = 0.826), ciprofloxacin (r = 0.816) and cefotaxime (r = 0.734). In *Klebsiella pneumoniae*, resistance to ciprofloxacin (r = 0.665) and cefotaxime increased (r = 0.644). *Pseudomonas aeruginosa* was shown to increase its resistance to colistin (r = 0.722) and amikacin (r = 0.691).

Table 3. Resistance of *Escherichia coli* to antibiotics at the University Hospital Olomouc in 2010–2019.

	2010	2011	2012	2013	2014	2015	2016	2017	2018	2019
AMS	28 (4118)	23 (3552)	28 (3558)	19 (3464)	22 (3529)	22 (3905)	25 (3998)	26 (4145)	24 (4133)	26 (4350)
PPT	10 (3121)	9 (2652)	11 (2624)	11 (2482)	13 (2525)	14 (2751)	16 (2953)	14 (3256)	15 (3078)	18 (3091)
CTX	9 (3143)	8 (2650)	13 (2624)	12 (2480)	14 (2522)	15 (2748)	16 (2950)	13 (3236)	14 (3084)	15 (3077)
MER	0 (3120)	0 (2651)	0 (2623)	0 (2482)	0 (2525)	0 (2750)	0 (2954)	0 (3257)	0 (3078)	0 (3091)
GEN	6 (4161)	6 (3552)	7 (3557)	6 (3464)	7 (3529)	8 (3908)	9 (3997)	8 (4144)	8 (4168)	8 (4378)
AMI	4 (3120)	3 (2651)	3 (2624)	3 (2480)	4 (2521)	3 (2751)	2 (2953)	2 (3255)	1 (3076)	1 (3091)
CIP	21 (3144)	18 (2651)	22 (2624)	20 (2481)	21 (2523)	21 (2754)	24 (2954)	23 (3257)	26 (3082)	27 (3093)
COL	0 (4129)	1 (3250)	0 (3558)	0 (3463)	1 (3529)	1 (3905)	0 (3999)	0 (4143)	0 (4147)	0 (4354)
TIG	1 (3080)	0 (2645)	1 (2623)	4 (2480)	2 (2520)	4 (2744)	1 (2948)	0 (3234)	1 (3079)	1 (3071)

Legend: Resistance percentages (total number of isolates tested), AMS—ampicillin/sulbactam, PPT—piperacillin/tazobactam, CTX—cefotaxime, MER—meropenem, GEN—gentamicin, AMI—amikacin, CIP—ciprofloxacin, COL—colistin, TIG—tigecycline.

Table 4. Resistance of *Klebsiella pneumoniae* to antibiotics at the University Hospital Olomouc in 2010–2019.

	2010	2011	2012	2013	2014	2015	2016	2017	2018	2019
AMS	55 (2534)	50 (1868)	46 (2017)	43 (2180)	52 (2341)	54 (2247)	52 (2189)	54 (2124)	49 (2104)	49 (2240)
PPT	42 (2270)	41 (1725)	39 (1821)	42 (1958)	51 (2147)	52 (2072)	52 (1986)	53 (1977)	48 (1927)	46 (2046)
CTX	38 (2275)	39 (1725)	37 (1821)	40 (1958)	50 (2152)	51 (2072)	51 (1988)	51 (1958)	46 (1930)	43 (2044)
MER	0 (2270)	<1 (1724)	<1 (1818)	<1 (1958)	<1 (2147)	0 (2069)	<1 (1986)	<1 (1975)	<1 (1926)	<1 (2047)
GEN	35 (2554)	36 (1867)	31 (2017)	35 (2180)	42 (2337)	45 (2247)	44 (2191)	45 (2123)	37 (2106)	36 (2243)
AMI	11 (2269)	7 (1725)	5 (1821)	5 (1954)	6 (2147)	4 (2070)	3 (1985)	2 (1976)	2 (1926)	1 (2044)
CIP	40 (2275)	42 (1725)	37 (1821)	40 (1958)	48 (2147)	52 (2072)	54 (1988)	54 (1978)	49 (1927)	46 (2048)
COL	1 (2538)	5 (1868)	5 (2017)	4 (2179)	3 (2337)	2 (2247)	2 (2187)	1 (2122)	3 (2102)	1 (2229)
TIG	4 (2254)	6 (1725)	9 (1821)	12 (1958)	8 (2150)	11 (2070)	8 (1985)	5 (1957)	7 (1929)	8 (2041)

Legend: Resistance percentages (total number of isolates tested).

Table 5. Resistance of *Pseudomonas aeruginosa* to antibiotics at the University Hospital Olomouc in 2010–2019.

	2010	2011	2012	2013	2014	2015	2016	2017	2018	2019
PPT	8 (1360)	23 (1353)	24 (1627)	30 (1677)	26 (1529)	28 (1664)	17 (1689)	13 (1541)	13 (1472)	14 (1725)
CTZ	18 (1367)	19 (1353)	15 (1625)	24 (1677)	18 (1529)	18 (1664)	12 (1689)	9 (1541)	13 (1472)	17 (1724)
MER	28 (1367)	39 (1353)	36 (1627)	40 (1677)	36 (1529)	39 (1664)	37 (1688)	32 (1541)	28 (1471)	34 (1724)
GEN	22 (1367)	23 (1350)	22 (1626)	26 (1678)	25 (1529)	25 (1664)	20 (1689)	16 (1540)	16 (1471)	11 (1722)
AMI	1 (1367)	5 (1352)	4 (1627)	4 (1677)	4 (1528)	5 (1664)	7 (1689)	5 (1541)	6 (1470)	5 (1725)
CIP	34 (1366)	35 (1353)	34 (1627)	38 (1675)	34 (1528)	32 (1664)	26 (1689)	24 (1540)	24 (1471)	23 (1725)
COL	0 (1043)	0 (1349)	0 (1625)	0 (1678)	0 (1529)	0 (1664)	1 (1689)	0 (1538)	1 (1469)	1 (1725)

Legend: Resistance percentages (total number of isolates tested), CTZ—ceftazidime.

Table 6. Resistance of *Staphylococcus aureus* to antibiotics at the University Hospital Olomouc in 2010–2019.

	2010	2011	2012	2013	2014	2015	2016	2017	2018	2019
OXA	3 (2129)	4 (1744)	3 (1794)	4 (1825)	3 (1860)	4 (2031)	4 (2111)	6 (2149)	4 (2559)	4 (2615)
CIP	5 (2125)	5 (1746)	5 (1794)	6 (1825)	7 (1860)	7 (2029)	7 (2110)	8 (2150)	7 (2560)	7 (2615)
GEN	4 (2106)	8 (1739)	11 (1792)	8 (1826)	10 (1858)	8 (2005)	6 (2100)	6 (2148)	6 (2560)	7 (2608)
VAN	0 (2127)	0 (1742)	0 (1793)	0 (1822)	0 (1856)	0 (2002)	0 (2072)	0 (2146)	0 (2556)	0 (2610)

Legend: Resistance percentages (total number of isolates tested), OXA—oxacillin, VAN—vancomycin.

Consumption of antibiotics or antibiotic classes at the University Hospital Olomouc is shown in Table 7. The data indicate increasing consumption of carbapenems ($r = 0.964$), tigecycline ($r = 0.879$), third- and fourth-generation cephalosporins ($r = 0.867$) and fluoroquinolones ($r = 0.733$). Conversely, consumption of penicillins combined with beta-lactamase inhibitors decreased ($r = -0.745$). Analysis of the relationship between antibiotic consumption and resistance in the entire hospital showed significant correlations between aminoglycoside consumption and resistance of *Escherichia coli* to gentamicin ($r = 0.712$), fluoroquinolone consumption and resistance of *Klebsiella pneumoniae* to ciprofloxacin ($r = 0.896$) and aminoglycoside consumption and resistance of *Pseudomonas aeruginosa* to amikacin ($r = 0.716$) (Figures 1–3).

Table 7. Antibiotic consumption in defined daily doses (DDDs) at the University Hospital Olomouc.

Antibiotic Class/Antibiotic	2010	2011	2012	2013	2014	2015	2016	2017	2018	2019
Penicillins combined with beta-lactamase inhibitors	89,977	80,212	77,168	76,803	76,937	81,889	70,248	71,774	74,446	76,427
3rd and 4th generation cephalosporins	4497	4056	3713	4018	4188	4601	4812	5553	6250	7716
Carbapenems	4518	5216	6223	6761	9956	10,242	10,910	12,322	13,196	11,900
Aminoglycosides	8433	10,636	10,695	10,657	9937	10,911	11,517	11,208	10,756	10,413
Fluoroquinolones	11,322	10,870	10,618	11,365	11,935	13,642	14,875	12,957	13,133	12,421
Colistin	714	1153	1261	1738	1905	2278	1648	1714	1832	1669
Glycopeptides	2921	2464	3026	3167	4578	4048	4012	3322	3152	3088
Tigecycline	554	572	426	499	1314	1302	2334	2683	3019	2824

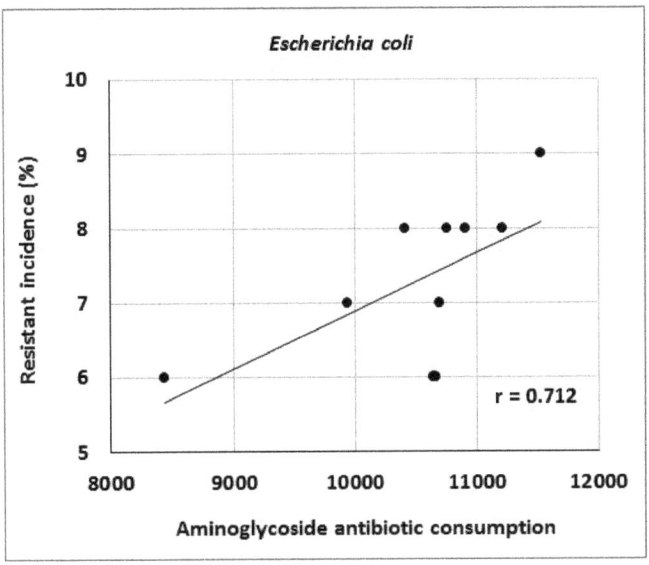

Figure 1. Correlation between aminoglycoside consumption (in numbers of defined daily doses) and resistance of *Escherichia coli* to gentamicin.

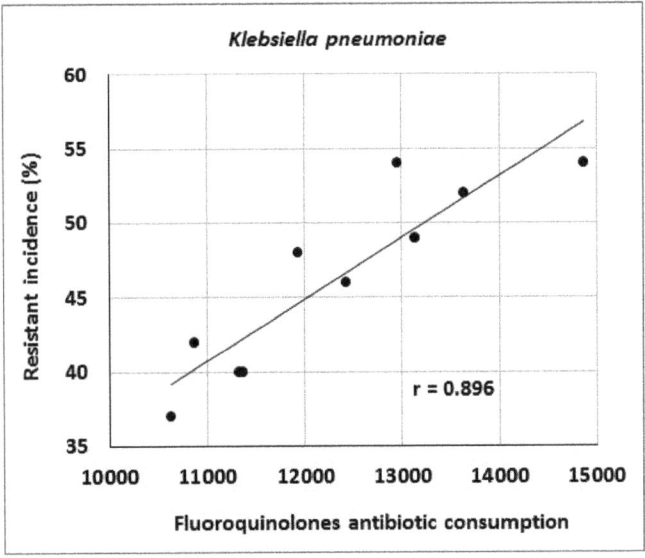

Figure 2. Correlation between fluoroquinolone consumption (in numbers of defined daily doses) and resistance of *Klebsiella pneumoniae* to ciprofloxacin.

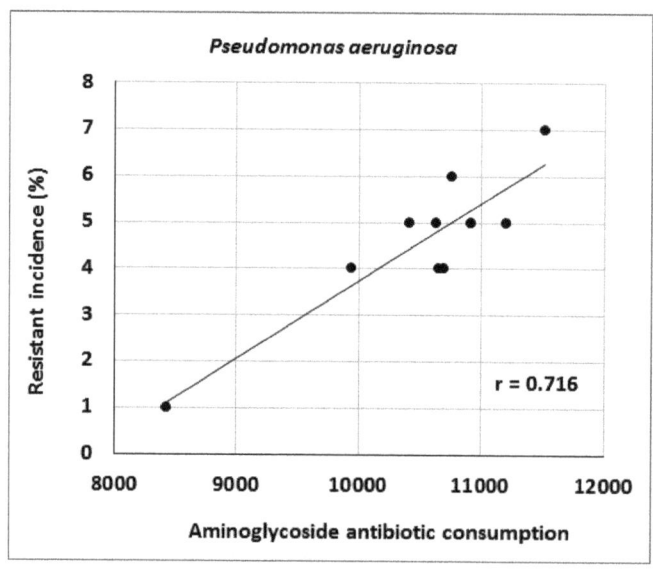

Figure 3. Correlation between aminoglycoside consumption (in numbers of defined daily doses) and resistance of *Pseudomonas aeruginosa* to amikacin.

Tables 8–11 document resistance of particular bacterial species at the Department of Anesthesiology and Intensive Care Medicine over the study period. The results show increasing resistance of *Escherichia coli* to piperacillin/tazobactam (r = 0.845) and cefotaxime (r = 0.729), resistance of *Klebsiella pneumoniae* to cefotaxime (r = 0.778) and resistance of *Pseudomonas aeruginosa* to meropenem (r = 0.988).

Table 8. Resistance of *Escherichia coli* to antibiotics at the Department of Anesthesiology and Intensive Care Medicine in 2010–2019.

	2010	2011	2012	2013	2014	2015	2016	2017	2018	2019
AMS	40 (115)	48 (143)	49 (140)	28 (129)	45 (110)	42 (103)	37 (97)	45 (102)	44 (116)	34 (182)
PPT	13 (116)	21 (141)	20 (138)	16 (125)	15 (107)	23 (100)	22 (98)	25 (102)	27 (117)	25 (182)
CTX	9 (116)	16 (141)	17 (138)	14 (125)	10 (107)	20 (100)	14 (97)	18 (102)	26 (117)	31 (182)
MER	0 (116)	0 (141)	0 (138)	0 (125)	0 (107)	0 (100)	0 (98)	0 (102)	0 (117)	0 (182)
GEN	6 (116)	20 (143)	16 (140)	13 (129)	12 (110)	11 (103)	12 (97)	13 (102)	18 (117)	23 (182)
AMI	7 (116)	6 (141)	9 (138)	2 (125)	8 (105)	3 (100)	5 (98)	5 (102)	1 (117)	2 (182)
CIP	35 (116)	30 (141)	27 (138)	27 (125)	29 (107)	24 (100)	30 (97)	34 (102)	36 (117)	29 (182)
COL	0 (116)	3 (142)	1 (140)	0 (129)	0 (110)	1 (103)	0 (98)	0 (102)	0 (116)	0 (182)
TIG	0 (115)	2 (140)	0 (138)	4 (125)	0 (107)	8 (100)	0 (97)	1 (102)	2 (117)	3 (182)

Legend: Resistance percentages (total number of isolates tested).

At the Department of Anesthesiology and Intensive Care Medicine, consumption of tigecycline (r = 0.939), carbapenems (r = 0.879), third- and fourth-generation cephalosporins (r = 0.867) and glycopeptides (r = 0.636) increased (Table 12). There were significant correlations between carbapenem consumption and resistance of *Pseudomonas aeruginosa* to meropenem (r = 0.855) as well as between aminoglycoside consumption and resistance of *Klebsiella pneumoniae* to gentamicin (r = 0.869) (Figures 4 and 5).

Table 9. Resistance of *Klebsiella pneumoniae* to antibiotics at the Department of Anesthesiology and Intensive Care Medicine in 2010–2019.

	2010	2011	2012	2013	2014	2015	2016	2017	2018	2019
AMS	72 (148)	78 (181)	75 (165)	66 (247)	70 (234)	77 (222)	77 (145)	76 (127)	80 (196)	76 (404)
PPT	58 (149)	67 (181)	61 (165)	65 (247)	62 (233)	73 (222)	71 (145)	65 (126)	67 (195)	69 (401)
CTX	49 (149)	64 (181)	58 (165)	62 (247)	60 (234)	74 (222)	71 (145)	63 (126)	74 (195)	78 (404)
MER	0 (149)	3 (181)	0 (165)	<1 (247)	<1 (233)	0 (222)	2 (145)	2 (125)	1 (195)	1 (402)
GEN	46 (149)	64 (181)	54 (165)	63 (247)	60 (233)	75 (222)	72 (145)	60 (127)	62 (195)	71 (402)
AMI	19 (149)	14 (181)	9 (165)	13 (246)	17 (233)	6 (222)	6 (145)	4 (126)	2 (195)	7 (402)
CIP	64 (149)	71 (181)	53 (165)	63 (247)	64 (233)	76 (222)	75 (145)	67 (126)	77 (195)	72 (402)
COL	3 (148)	13 (181)	10 (165)	8 (247)	9 (233)	2 (222)	7 (145)	2 (127)	6 (195)	1 (398)
TIG	7 (148)	9 (181)	13 (165)	12 (247)	7 (234)	8 (222)	17 (145)	6 (126)	12 (195)	7 (403)

Legend: Resistance percentages (total number of isolates tested).

Table 10. Resistance of *Pseudomonas aeruginosa* to antibiotics at the Department of Anesthesiology and Intensive Care Medicine in 2010–2019.

	2010	2011	2012	2013	2014	2015	2016	2017	2018	2019
PPT	29 (106)	32 (150)	39 (188)	41 (200)	45 (224)	42 (223)	46 (150)	44 (111)	39 (142)	43 (219)
CTZ	32 (106)	35 (150)	39 (188)	41 (200)	48 (224)	42 (223)	35 (150)	34 (111)	31 (142)	33 (218)
MER	22 (106)	31 (150)	33 (188)	38 (200)	36 (224)	44 (223)	52 (150)	53 (111)	56 (142)	59 (219)
GEN	31 (106)	42 (150)	44 (188)	37 (200)	36 (224)	43 (223)	36 (150)	26 (109)	33 (141)	32 (217)
AMI	0 (106)	5 (149)	5 (188)	2 (200)	5 (224)	7 (223)	9 (150)	12 (111)	16 (141)	3 (219)
CIP	29 (106)	33 (150)	48 (188)	47 (200)	41 (224)	43 (223)	40 (150)	35 (111)	37 (142)	35 (219)
COL	0 (83)	0 (150)	0 (188)	0 (200)	0 (224)	0 (223)	0 (150)	0 (109)	2 (142)	1 (217)

Legend: Resistance percentages (total number of isolates tested).

Table 11. Resistance of *Staphylococcus aureus* to antibiotics at the Department of Anesthesiology and Intensive Care Medicine in 2010–2019.

	2010	2011	2012	2013	2014	2015	2016	2017	2018	2019
OXA	9 (46)	5 (37)	9 (56)	14 (65)	6 (47)	16 (45)	5 (43)	6 (48)	12 (49)	5 (83)
CIP	11 (46)	8 (37)	7 (56)	20 (65)	4 (47)	18 (45)	7 (43)	6 (48)	16 (49)	11 (83)
GEN	0 (45)	0 (37)	13 (56)	5 (65)	6 (47)	5 (43)	2 (43)	6 (48)	4 (49)	11 (83)
VAN	2 (46)	0 (37)	0 (56)	0 (65)	0 (47)	0 (43)	0 (42)	0 (48)	0 (48)	0 (83)

Legend: Resistance percentages (total number of isolates tested).

Table 12. Antibiotic consumption in defined daily doses (DDD) at the Department of Anesthesiology and Intensive Care Medicine.

Antibiotic Class/Antibiotic	2010	2011	2012	2013	2014	2015	2016	2017	2018	2019
Penicillins combined with beta-lactamase inhibitors	1539	1463	1369	1376	1357	1288	1486	1519	1339	1473
3rd and 4th generation cephalosporins	125	130	234	144	428	241	260	325	394	556
Carbapenems	618	739	505	946	1290	1427	1298	1280	1498	1822
Aminoglycosides	209	691	629	667	682	806	812	589	677	841
Fluoroquinolones	589	460	514	576	501	639	670	484	398	510
Colistin	167	253	233	410	433	498	340	190	228	478
Glycopeptides	83	75	128	204	191	237	324	158	148	249
Tigecycline	55	85	80	70	185	230	245	275	450	415

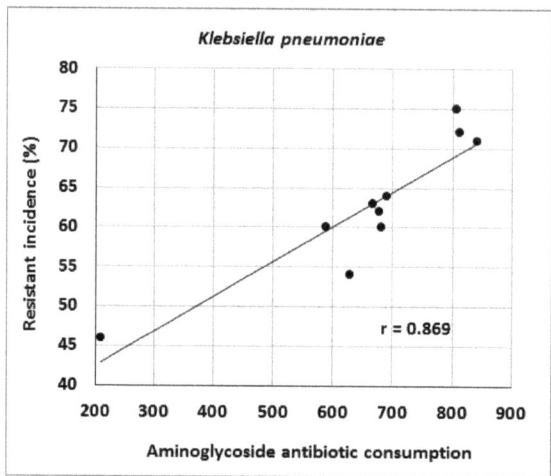

Figure 4. Correlation between aminoglycoside consumption (in numbers of defined daily doses) and resistance of *Klebsiella pneumoniae* to gentamicin.

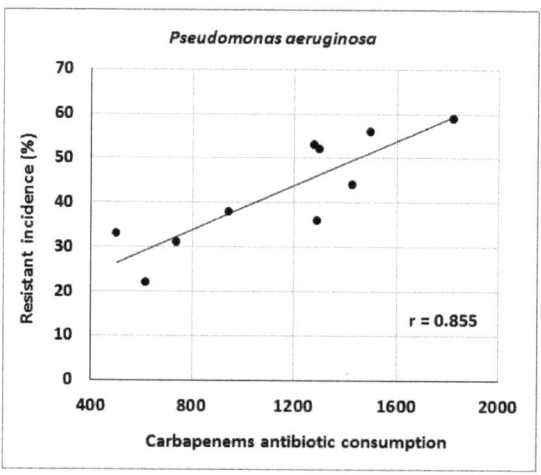

Figure 5. Correlation between carbapenem consumption (in numbers of defined daily doses) and resistance of *Pseudomonas aeruginosa* to meropenem.

Genotyping of ESBL- positive isolates of *Klebsiella pneumoniae* and *Escherichia coli* in particular patient groups (from tracheal aspirates in patients with hospital-acquired pneumonia, from stool in hospitalized patients etc.) at the Department of Anesthesiology and Intensive Care Medicine showed a predominance of CTX-M-type, namely of the CTX-M-15 and CTX-M-9 types (data not shown). In AmpC-positive strains, EBC and CIT enzymes prevailed in *Escherichia coli* and the DHA type in *Klebsiella pneumoniae* (data not shown).

Between 2010 and 2019, a total of 19 meropenem-resistant strains of *Klebsiella pneumoniae* were detected in patients staying at the Department of Anesthesiology and Intensive Care Medicine. Only 2 strains were NDM-positive (data not shown). However, no other carbapenemase genes were detected. The total number of isolated MRSA at the Department of Anesthesiology and Intensive Care Medicine was 45 strains. In case of meropenem-resistant *Klebsiella pneumoniae* strains and MRSA, no significant clonal spread was noted.

No identical clone was detected in meropenem-resistant *Klebsiella pneumoniae* isolates and only two pairs of identical MRSA strains were identified.

4. Discussion

Today's medicine is characterized by exponentially expanding knowledge in all specialties, resulting in considerable improvements of both diagnostic and therapeutic activities. Despite past achievements, however, there is one issue posing a serious therapeutic challenge. It is the role of bacterial infections that have continued to increase in recent years. One reason is rising resistance of bacteria to the effects of antibacterial drugs and the associated risk of treatment failure. Numerous studies have been published documenting higher mortality and shorter survival of patients with infections caused by multidrug-resistant bacteria compared to those due to susceptible strains of the same species [21–25]. The present study yielded interesting results when compared with the national and European resistance rates as reported by the European Antimicrobial Resistance Surveillance Network (EARS-Net). In 2019, the mean prevalence of MRSA in the Czech Republic and Europe was 13% and 15%, respectively; the University Hospital Olomouc rates ranged from 3% to 6% [26,27]. Similarly, very low prevalence was also noted for meropenem-resistant strains of *Klebsiella pneumoniae*. According to the ECDC's Annual Epidemiological Report for 2019, the mean prevalence of carbapenem-resistant strains of *Klebsiella pneumoniae* in Europe was 8%, with some European countries even reporting rates higher than 10% [26]. At the University Hospital Olomouc, however, the resistance of this species to meropenem did not exceed 1% or, in case of the Department of Anesthesiology and Intensive Care Medicine, 3%. Only two strains were found to produce NDM- carbapenemases. For meropenem-resistant isolates without the carbapenemase gene, we assume that the resistance is due to mechanisms such as loss or mutation of porins with AmpC beta-lactamase or ESBL hyperproduction or overexpression of the efflux pumps.

There were considerable differences in resistance of *Klebsiella pneumoniae* to third-generation cephalosporins in Europe (31%) and in the Czech Republic (50%) in 2019 [26,27]. The University Hospital Olomouc rate (43%) was below the mean rate for the entire country.

Resistance of *Escherichia coli* to cefotaxime and resistance of *Pseudomonas aeruginosa* to ceftazidime, aminoglycosides and fluoroquinolones at the University Hospital Olomouc do not greatly differ from the mean rates in Europe.

Of concern is the prevalence of *Pseudomonas aeruginosa* strains resistant to meropenem (34%), exceeding both the Czech (15%) and European (17%) mean rates [26,27]. However, carbapenems are mainly needed to treat infections caused by members of *Enterobacterales* producing ESBL and AmpC beta-lactamases; the resistance of these bacterial species to meropenem does not increase. Despite that, there will be efforts to reduce carbapenem consumption in the following years. It should be stated that carbapenems account for 6% of the overall antibiotic consumption at the University Hospital Olomouc (unpublished data).

With the exception of a higher prevalence of meropenem-resistant *Pseudomonas aeruginosa*, prevalence rates of other studied phenotypes are below the rates reported by the EUCAST [26,27]. The main causes of the development and spread of bacterial resistance are the administration of antibiotics and their selection pressure [28–34]. Therefore, the restriction of certain antibacterial agents and relevant antibiotic classes aimed to limit their selection pressure is a possible solution to the problem [35]. However, selection pressure is a more complex issue. Apparently, consumption of certain antibiotics may only be reduced if the consumption of others increases. Moreover, antibiotic resistance is often multiple, meaning that selection pressure of a particular antibiotic agent results in increased resistance to other antibiotics, for example, resistance of ESBL-positive enterobacteria to cephalosporins and fluoroquinolones or resistance of MRSA to clindamycin [36,37]. Another important aspect influencing the selective pressure is antibiotic concentration, that is the correct dosage of antibiotics and their distribution in the body. Clinical microbiologists and physicians care about the accurate dosage in terms of pharmacodynamic/pharmacokinetic parameters to achieve satisfactory outcomes in patients. However, the question is how the selected dosage and the final concentration of an antibiotic promotes the genesis of resistant mutants. The phenomenon of bacterial resistance represents a complex problem and the emergence of antibiotic-resistant mutants depends on different aspects such physiology, genetics, historical behavior of bacterial populations, antibiotic-bacterium dynamics and others [38,39].

Studies have shown that there may not be a direct relationship between the administration of selected antibiotics and bacterial resistance. Several studies failed to confirm correlations between bacterial resistance to particular antibiotic classes and their consumption [40–42]. Similarly, Htoutou Sedláková et al. reported decreasing consumption of third-generation cephalosporins and fluoroquinolones but increasing resistance of *Enterobacteriaceae* to these drugs [43]. This may be due to multiple mechanisms. Some authors claim that the relationship between antibiotic consumption and resistance disappears after a certain resistance threshold is exceeded, since mobile genetic elements (in particular plasmids and transposons) circulate in bacterial populations and a decrease in antibiotic selection pressure does not influence this phenomenon any more [44]. It is documented that transfer rates of ESBL-plasmids are highest in the absence of the antibiotic [45]. Another explanation could be the collateral effect of antibiotics, which means that not only subinhibitory concentrations of an antibiotic could stimulate the emergence and the dissemination of its corresponding resistant gene, but that collateral stimulation by other antibiotics is also possible. For example, the mobile genetic element carrying the gene for tetracycline resistance is able to exhibit a 1000-fold increase of its transfer frequency when exposed to subinhibitory concentrations of tetracyclines, but also macrolides, lincosamides and streptogramins [46].

Our findings suggest that the increasing bacterial resistance is mainly determined by the selection pressure of antibiotics. Neither significant horizontal clonal spread of multidrug-resistant bacteria nor increasing bacterial resistance to a particular antibiotic whose consumption decreases have been observed.

As part of antibiotic resistance surveillance, the Antibiotic Center not only controls the appropriate administration of antibiotics, that is the adequate indication and dosage in a particular patient, but also regularly monitors important bacterial resistance phenotypes and genotypes, in particular MRSA, vancomycin-resistant enterococci, ESBL- and AmpC-positive *Enterobacterales*, Gram-negative bacteria resistant to carbapenems, fluoroquinolones and others, as well as their clonal spread. For technical reasons, such surveillance is not performed in the entire hospital, but is mostly limited to selected departments and pre-defined patient groups and time periods. This approach to antibiotic stewardship has been reflected in numerous studies carried out at our department [47–50]. Based on their outcomes, certain conclusions have been drawn and relevant measures have been implemented such as evidence-based recommendations for consultant microbiologists and attending physicians concerning an adequate selection of antibiotic agents, guidelines for initial antibiotic therapy including antibiotic prophylaxis, restriction of certain antibiotic classes or improvement of hygiene and epidemiological measures.

The present study showed a significant relationship between aminoglycoside consumption and resistance of *Escherichia coli* and *Klebsiella pneumoniae* to gentamicin, results consistent with those in our 2014 study [43]. Moreover, there were correlations between fluoroquinolone consumption and resistance of *Klebsiella pneumoniae* to ciprofloxacin and between aminoglycoside consumption and resistance of *Pseudomonas aeruginosa* to amikacin, consistent with findings published by other authors [34,51]. Another reason for increasing bacterial resistance may be the horizontal or clonal spread of genetically identical strains of particular species among patients. In this case, the selection pressure of antibiotics may be of less importance and external environmental factors may play a role, for example, those related to healthcare staff. Examples include a study by Hricová et al. on vancomycin-resistant enterococci in patients with hematological malignancies at the University Hospital Olomouc reporting 67% clonality of isolated strains or outbreaks of epidemic MRSA clones in various parts of the world [48,52–54]. The present study, however, did not show a significant clonal spread of MRSA and meropenem-resistant strains of *Klebsiella pneumoniae* isolated from Department of Anesthesiology and Intensive Care Medicine patients, highlighting the role of horizontal resistance gene transfer in the spread of antibiotic resistance. Further, there is no doubt that the use of antibiotics contributes to the development of resistance by acquiring resistance genes and maintenance of chromosomal resistance-associated mutations [38]. However, determining the exact effect of antibiotic use on the development of resistance is problematic. Moreover, it is increasingly claimed that the emergence, maintenance and spread of resistance traits are also influenced by social, economic and genetic factors.

5. Conclusions

The presented data suggest low rates of bacterial resistance at the University Hospital Olomouc, with the only exception being an increased prevalence of meropenem-resistant strains of *Pseudomonas aeruginosa*. This confirms the importance of antibiotic stewardship and surveillance of antimicrobial resistance, including the use of molecular biology methods, for maintaining the effectiveness of antibiotics and limiting the spread of multidrug-resistant bacterial pathogens. Data on the prevalence of bacterial resistance and the results of molecular genetic analysis of multidrug-resistant strains must form the basis for practical antibiotic stewardship. These should include a definition of optimal regimens for initial antibiotic therapy and assessment of the sources and routes of spread of multidrug-resistant bacteria so that adequate hygiene and epidemiological measures may be introduced. It is apparent that besides obtaining data for the entire hospital, hospital departments need to be individually assessed and adequate antibiotic stewardship measures must be implemented based on the results.

Author Contributions: Conceptualization, M.K.; Data curation, M.H.S.; Formal analysis, J.Z.; Funding acquisition, M.K.; Investigation, M.H.S., K.U., P.M., M.R., K.H., K.M., P.K. (Pavla Kucova) and K.F.; Methodology, P.M.; Project administration, M.K.; Resources, M.H.S., K.U., P.K. (Pavla Kucova) and K.F.; Supervision, M.K.; Validation, M.R.; Visualization, M.K., M.H.S., K.U., P.M., M.R., K.H., K.M., P.K. (Pavla Kucova), K.F. and P.K. (Pavel Kurfurst); Writing—original draft, M.K., M.H.S., P.M., M.R., J.Z., and P.K. (Pavel Kurfurst); Writing—review & editing, M.K., M.H.S., K.U., P.M., M.R., K.H., K.M., P.K. (Pavla Kucova), J.Z., K.F. and P.K. (Pavel Kurfurst) All authors have read and agreed to the published version of the manuscript.

Funding: This research was funded by the Czech Health Research Council (project no. NV18-05-00340), project IGA_LF_2020_021, Junior Grant of UP in Olomouc JG_2019_005 and by MH CZ—DRO (FNOL, 00098892).

Data Availability Statement: Data sharing not applicable.

Acknowledgments: The authors thank med. Arne C. Rodloff (Facharzt für Mikrobiologie, Virologie und Infektionsepidemiologie, Krankenhaushygieniker, Germany) and Pavel Boštík (Faculty of Medicine, Charles University and University Hospital in Hradec Kralové) for critically reviewing the manuscript.

Conflicts of Interest: The authors declare no conflict of interest.

References

1. Dyar, O.J.; Huttner, B.; Schouten, J.; Pulcini, C. ESGAP (ESCMID Study Group for Antimicrobial stewardshiP). What is antimicrobial stewardship? *Clin. Microbiol. Infect.* **2017**, *23*, 793–798. [CrossRef] [PubMed]
2. Srinivasan, A. Antibiotic stewardship: Why we must, how we can. *Clevel. Clin. J. Med.* **2017**, *84*, 673–679. [CrossRef] [PubMed]
3. Luyt, C.E.; Bréchot, N.; Trouillet, J.L.; Chastre, J. Antibiotic stewardship in the intensive care unit. *Crit. Care* **2014**, *18*, 480. [CrossRef] [PubMed]
4. Barlam, T.F.; Cosgrove, S.E.; Abbo, L.M.; MacDougall, C.; Schuetz, A.N.; Septimus, E.J.; Srinivasan, A.; Dellit, T.H.; Falck-Ytter, Y.T.; Fishman, N.O.; et al. Implementing an Antibiotic Stewardship Program: Guidelines by the Infectious Diseases Society of America and the Society for Healthcare Epidemiology of America. *Clin. Infect. Dis.* **2016**, *62*, 51–77. [CrossRef] [PubMed]
5. Goff, D.A. Antibiotic Stewardship: The Health of the World Depends on It. *Hosp. Pharm.* **2018**, *53*, 214–216. [CrossRef]
6. Karam, G.; Chastre, J.; Wilcox, M.H.; Vincent, J.L. Antibiotic strategies in the era of multidrug resistance. *Crit. Care* **2016**, *20*, 136. [CrossRef]

7. Baur, D.; Gladstone, B.P.; Burkert, F.; Carrara, E.; Foschi, F.; Döbele, S.; Tacconelli, E. Effect of antibiotic stewardship on the incidence of infection and colonisation with antibiotic-resistant bacteria and *Clostridium difficile* infection: A systematic review and meta-analysis. *Lancet Infect. Dis.* **2017**, *17*, 990–1001. [CrossRef]
8. Kollef, M.H.; Bassetti, M.; Francois, B.; Burnham, J.; Dimopoulos, G.; Garnacho-Montero, J.; Lipman, J.; Luyt, C.E.; Nicolau, D.P.; Postma, M.J.; et al. The intensive care medicine research agenda on multidrug-resistant bacteria, antibiotics, and stewardship. *Intensive Care Med.* **2017**, *43*, 1187–1197. [CrossRef]
9. Laxminarayan, R.; Duse, A.; Wattal, C.; Zaidi, A.K.; Wertheim, H.F.; Sumpradit, N.; Vlieghe, E.; Hara, G.L.; Gould, I.M.; Goossens, H.; et al. Antibiotic resistance—the need for global solutions. *Lancet Infect. Dis.* **2013**, *13*, 1057–1098. [CrossRef]
10. The European Committee on Antimicrobial Susceptibility Testing. Breakpoint Tables for Interpretation of MICs and Zone Diameters, Version 1.0 December 2009–Version 10.0 January 2020. Available online: https://www.eucast.org/ (accessed on 16 December 2020).
11. WHO Collaborating Centre for Drug Statistics Methodology. ATC/DDD Index 2020. Available online: https://www.whocc.no/atc_ddd_index/ (accessed on 16 December 2020).
12. Croxatto, A.; Prod'hom, G.; Greub, G. Applications of MALDI-TOF mass spectrometry in clinical diagnostic microbiology. *FEMS Microbiol. Rev.* **2012**, *36*, 380–407. [CrossRef]
13. Htoutou Sedlakova, M.; Hanulik, V.; Chroma, M.; Hricova, K.; Kolar, M.; Latal, T.; Schaumann, R.; Rodloff, A.C. Phenotypic detection of broad-spectrum beta-lactamases in microbiological practice. *Med. Sci. Monit.* **2011**, *17*, BR147–BR152. [CrossRef] [PubMed]
14. Nordmann, P.; Poirel, L.; Dortet, L. Rapid detection of carbapenemase-producing Enterobacteriaceae. *Emerg. Infect. Dis.* **2012**, *18*, 1503–1507. [CrossRef] [PubMed]
15. Sila, J.; Sauer, P.; Kolar, M. Comparison of the prevalence of genes coding for enterotoxins, exfoliatins, Panton-Valentine leukocidin and TSST-1 between methicillin-resistant and methicillin-susceptible isolates of *Staphylococcus aureus* at the University Hospital in Olomouc. *Biomed. Pap. Med. Fac. Univ. Palacky Olomouc Czechoslov. Repub.* **2009**, *153*, 215–218. [CrossRef] [PubMed]
16. Ellington, M.J.; Kistler, J.; Livermore, D.M.; Woodford, N. Multiplex PCR for rapid detection of genes encoding acquired metallo-beta-lactamases. *J. Antimicrob. Chemother.* **2007**, *59*, 321–322. [CrossRef] [PubMed]
17. Mlynarcik, P.; Roderova, M.; Kolar, M. Primer evaluation for PCR and its application for detection of carbapenemases in Enterobacteriaceae. *Jundishapur J. Microb.* **2016**, *9*, e29314. [CrossRef] [PubMed]
18. Mlynarcik, P.; Bardon, J.; Htoutou Sedlakova, M.; Prochazkova, P.; Kolar, M. Identification of novel OXA-134-like beta-lactamases in *Acinetobacter lwoffii* and *Acinetobacter schindleri* isolated from chicken litter. *Biomed. Pap. Med. Fac. Univ. Palacky Olomouc Czech. Repub.* **2019**, *163*, 141–146. [CrossRef]
19. Husickova, V.; Cekanova, L.; Chroma, M.; Htoutou Sedlakova, M.; Hricova, K.; Kolar, M. Carriage of ESBL- and AmpC-positive Enterobacteriaceae in the gastrointestinal tract of community subjects and hospitalized patients in the Czech Republic. *Biomed. Pap. Med. Fac. Univ Palacky Olomouc Czechoslov. Repub.* **2012**, *156*, 348–353. [CrossRef]
20. Tenover, F.C.; Arbeit, R.D.; Goering, R.V.; Mickelsen, P.A.; Murray, B.E.; Persing, D.H.; Swaminathan, B. Interpreting chromosomal DNA restriction patterns produced by pulsed-field gel electrophoresis: Criteria for bacterial strain typing. *J. Clin. Microbiol.* **1995**, *33*, 2233–2239. [CrossRef]
21. Luna, C.M.; Vujacich, P.; Niederman, M.S.; Vay, C.; Gherardi, C.; Matera, J.; Jolly, E.C. Impact of BAL data on the therapy and outcome of ventilator-associated pneumonia. *Chest* **1997**, *111*, 676–685. [CrossRef]
22. Tumbarello, M.; Sanguinetti, M.; Montuori, E.; Trecarichi, E.M.; Posteraro, B.; Fiori, B.; Citton, R.; D'Inzeo, T.; Fadda, G.; Cauda, R.; et al. Predictors of mortality in patients with bloodstream infections caused by extended-spectrum-ß-lactamase-producing Enterobacteriaceae: Importance of inadequate initial antimicrobial treatment. *Antimicrob. Agents Chemother.* **2007**, *51*, 1987–1994. [CrossRef]
23. Kang, C.I.; Chung, D.R.; Ko, K.S.; Peck, K.R.; Song, J.H. Korean Network for Study of Infectious Diseases. Risk factors for infection and treatment outcome of extended-spectrum β-lactamase-producing *Escherichia coli* and *Klebsiella pneumoniae* bacteremia in patients with hematologic malignancy. *Ann. Hematol.* **2012**, *91*, 115–121. [CrossRef] [PubMed]
24. Herkel, T.; Uvizl, R.; Doubravska, L.; Adamus, M.; Gabrhelik, T.; Htoutou Sedlakova, M.; Kolar, M.; Hanulik, V.; Pudova, V.; Langova, K.; et al. Epidemiology of hospital-acquired pneumonia: Results of a Central European multicenter, prospective, observational study compared with data from the European region. *Biomed. Pap. Med. Fac. Univ. Palacky Olomouc Czechoslov. Repub.* **2016**, *160*, 448–455. [CrossRef] [PubMed]
25. De Kraker, M.E.; Wolkewitz, M.; Davey, P.G.; Koller, W.; Berger, J.; Nagler, J.; Icket, C.; Kalenic, S.; Horvatic, J.; Seifert, H.; et al. Clinical impact of antimicrobial resistance in European hospitals: Excess mortality and length of hospital stay related to methicillin-resistant *Staphylococcus aureus* bloodstream infections. *Antimicrob. Agents Chemother.* **2011**, *55*, 1598–1605. [CrossRef] [PubMed]
26. European Centre for Disease Prevention and Control. *Antimicrobial Resistance in the EU/EEA (EARS-Net)—Annual Epidemiological Report 2019*; ECDC: Stockholm, Sweden, 2020.
27. European Antimicrobial Resistance Surveillance Network (EARS-Net). Available online: https://www.ecdc.europa.eu/en/antimicrobial-resistance/surveillance-and-disease-data/data-ecdc (accessed on 16 December 2020).
28. Urbanek, K.; Kolar, M.; Strojil, J.; Koukalová, D.; Čekanová, L.; Hejnar, P. Utilization of fluoroquinolones and *Escherichia coli* resistance in urinary tract infection: Inpatients and outpatients. *Pharmacoepidemiol. Drug Saf.* **2005**, *14*, 741–745. [CrossRef]

29. Urbanek, K.; Kolar, M.; Loveckova, Y.; Strojil, J.; Santava, L. Influence of 3rd generation cephalosporin utilization on the occurrence of ESBL-positive *Klebsiella pneumoniae* strains. *J. Clin. Pharm. Ther.* **2007**, *32*, 403–408. [CrossRef]
30. Kolar, M.; Urbanek, K.; Latal, T. Antibiotic selective pressure and development of bacterial resistance. *Int. J. Antimicrob. Agents* **2001**, *17*, 357–363. [CrossRef]
31. Urbanek, K.; Kolar, M.; Cekanova, L. Utilisation of macrolides and the development of *Streptococcus pyogenes* resistance to erythromycin. *Pharm. World Sci.* **2005**, *27*, 104–107. [CrossRef]
32. Bell, B.G.; Schellevis, F.; Stobberingh, E.; Goossens, H.; Pringle, M. A systematic review and meta-analysis of the effects of antibiotic consumption on antibiotic resistance. *BMC Infectious Dis.* **2014**, *14*, 13. [CrossRef] [PubMed]
33. Kim, B.; Kim, Y.; Hwang, H.; Kim, J.; Kim, S.W.; Bae, I.G.; Choi, W.S.; Jung, S.I.; Jeong, H.W.; Pai, H. Trends and correlation between antibiotic usage and resistance pattern among hospitalized patients at university hospitals in Korea, 2004 to 2012: A nationwide multicenter study. *Medicine* **2018**, *97*, e13719. [CrossRef]
34. Mladenovic-Antic, S.; Kocic, B.; Velickovic-Radovanovic, R.; Dinic, M.; Petrovic, J.; Randjelovic, G.; Mitic, R. Correlation between antimicrobial consumption and antimicrobial resistance of *Pseudomonas aeruginosa* in a hospital setting: A 10-year study. *J. Clin. Pharm. Ther.* **2016**, *41*, 532–537. [CrossRef]
35. Zequinao, T.; Gasparetto, J.; dos Santos Oliveira, D.; Takahara Silva, G.; Telles, J.P.; Tuon, F.F. A broad-spectrum beta-lactam-sparing stewardship program in a middle-income country public hospital: Antibiotic use and expenditure outcomes and antimicrobial susceptibility profiles. *Braz. J. Infect. Dis.* **2020**, *24*, 221–230. [CrossRef] [PubMed]
36. Falagas, M.E.; Karageorgopoulos, D.E. Extended-spectrum beta-lactamase-producing organisms. *J. Hosp. Infect.* **2009**, *73*, 345–354. [CrossRef] [PubMed]
37. Che Hamzah, A.M.; Yeo, C.C.; Puah, S.M.; Chua, K.H.; Rahman, N.I.A.; Abdullah, F.H.; Othman, N.; Chew, C.H. Tigecycline and inducible clindamycin resistance in clinical isolates of methicillin-resistant *Staphylococcus aureus* from Terengganu, Malaysia. *J. Med. Microbiol.* **2019**, *68*, 1299–1305. [CrossRef] [PubMed]
38. Martinez, J.L.; Baquero, F. Mutation Frequencies and Antibiotic Resistance. *Antimicrob. Agents Chemother.* **2000**, *44*, 1771–1777. [CrossRef]
39. Zhao, X.; Drlica, K. Restricting the Selection of Antibiotic-Resistant Mutants: Measurement and Potential Uses of the Mutant Selection Window. *JID* **2002**, *185*, 561–565. [CrossRef]
40. Ho, C.M.; Ho, M.W.; Liu, Y.C.; Toh, H.S.; Lee, Y.L.; Liu, Y.M.; Huang, C.C.; Lu, P.L.; Liu, C.E.; Chen, Y.H.; et al. Correlation between carbapenem consumption and resistance to carbapenems among Enterobacteriaceae isolates collected from patients with intra-abdominal infections at five medical centers in Taiwan, 2006–2010. *Int. J. Antimicrob. Agents* **2012**, *40*, S24–S28. [CrossRef]
41. Lai, C.-C.; Wang, C.-Y.; Chu, C.-C.; Tan, C.-K.; Lu, C.-L.; Lee, Y.-C.; Huang, Y.-T.; Lee, P.-I.; Hsueh, P.-R. Correlation between antibiotic consumption and resistance of Gramnegative bacteria causing healthcare-associated infections at a university hospital in Taiwan from 2000 to 2009. *J. Antimicrob. Chemother.* **2011**, *66*, 1374–1382. [CrossRef]
42. Altunsoy, A.; Aypak, C.; Azap, A.; Ergönül, Ö.; Balik, I. The impact of a nationwide antibiotic restriction program on antibiotic usage and resistance against nosocomial pathogens in Turkey. *Int. J. Med. Sci.* **2011**, *8*, 339–344. [CrossRef]
43. Htoutou Sedlakova, M.; Urbanek, K.; Vojtova, V.; Suchankova, H.; Imwensi, P.; Kolar, M. Antibiotic consumption and its influence on the resistance in Enterobacteriaceae. *BMC Res. Notes* **2014**, *7*, 454.
44. Barbosa, T.M.; Levy, S.B. The impact of antibiotic use on resistance development and persistence. *Drug Resist. Updates* **2000**, *3*, 303–311. [CrossRef]
45. Händel, N.; Otte, S.; Jonker, M.; Brul, S.; ter Kuile, B.H. Factors that affect transfer of the IncI1 β-lactam resistance plasmid pESBL-283 between *E. coli* strains. *PLoS ONE* **2015**, *10*, e0123039. [CrossRef] [PubMed]
46. Merlin, C. Reducing the Consumption of Antibiotics: Would That Be Enough to Slow Down the Dissemination of Resistances in the Downstream Environment? *Front. Microbiol.* **2020**, *11*, 33. [CrossRef] [PubMed]
47. Kolar, M.; Cermak, P.; Hobzova, L.; Bogdanova, K.; Neradova, K.; Mlynarcik, P.; Bostik, P. Antibiotic Resistance in Nosocomial Bacteria Isolated from Infected Wounds of Hospitalized Patients in Czech Republic. *Antibiotics* **2020**, *9*, 342. [CrossRef] [PubMed]
48. Hricová, K.; Štosová, T.; Kučová, P.; Fišerová, K.; Bardoň, J.; Kolář, M. Analysis of Vancomycin-Resistant Enterococci in Hemato-Oncological Patients. *Antibiotics* **2020**, *9*, 785. [CrossRef]
49. Htoutou Sedlaková, M.; Fišerová, K.; Kolář, M. Bacteremia pathogens in the University Hospital Olomouc. *Klin. Mikrobiol. Infekc. Lek.* **2020**, *26*, 4–11.
50. Kolar, M.; Htoutou Sedláková, M.; Pudova, V.; Roderova, M.; Novosad, J.; Senkyrikova, M.; Szotkowska, R.; Indrak, K. Incidence of fecal Enterobacteriaceae producing broad-spectrum beta-lactamases in patients with hematological malignancies. *Biomed. Pap. Med. Fac. Univ. Palacky Olomouc Czechoslov. Repub.* **2014**, *159*, 100–103. [CrossRef]
51. Yang, P.; Chen, Y.; Jiang, S.; Shen, P.; Lu, X.; Xiao, Y. Association between antibiotic consumption and the rate of carbapenem-resistant Gram-negative bacteria from China based on 153 tertiary hospitals data in 2014. *Antimicrob. Resist. Infect. Control* **2018**, *7*, 137. [CrossRef]
52. Uzunović, S.; Bedenić, B.; Budimir, A.; Kamberović, F.; Ibrahimagić, A.; Delić-Bikić, S.; Sivec, S.; Meštrović, T.; Varda Brkić, D.; Rijnders, M.I.; et al. Emergency (clonal spread) of methicillin-resistant *Staphylococcus aureus* (MRSA), extended spectrum (ESBL)– and AmpC beta-lactamase-producing Gram-negative bacteria infections at Pediatric Department, Bosnia and Herzegovina. *Wien. Klin. Wochenschr.* **2014**, *126*, 747–756. [CrossRef]

53. Earls, M.R.; Coleman, D.C.; Brennan, G.I.; Fleming, T.; Monecke, S.; Slickers, P.; Ehricht, R.; Shore, A.C. Intra-Hospital, Inter-Hospital and Intercontinental Spread of ST78 MRSA From Two Neonatal Intensive Care Unit Outbreaks Established Using Whole-Genome Sequencing. *Front. Microbiol.* **2018**, *9*, 1485. [CrossRef]
54. Strauß, L.; Stegger, M.; Akpaka, P.E.; Alabi, A.; Breurec, S.; Coombs, G.; Egyir, B.; Larsen, A.R.; Laurent, F.; Monecke, S.; et al. Origin, evolution, and global transmission of community-acquired *Staphylococcus aureus* ST8. *Proc. Natl. Acad. Sci. USA* **2017**, *114*, E10596–E10604. [CrossRef]

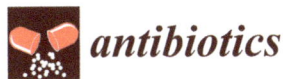

Article

In Silico Analysis of Extended-Spectrum β-Lactamases in Bacteria

Patrik Mlynarcik [1,*], Hana Chudobova [2], Veronika Zdarska [1] and Milan Kolar [1,3]

[1] Department of Microbiology, Faculty of Medicine and Dentistry, Palacky University Olomouc, Hnevotinska 3, 77515 Olomouc, Czech Republic; veronika.zdarska03@upol.cz (V.Z.); milan.kolar@fnol.cz (M.K.)
[2] Laboratory of Growth Regulators, Faculty of Science, Institute of Experimental Botany of the Czech Academy of Sciences, Palacky University, Šlechtitelů 27, 78371 Olomouc, Czech Republic; chudha01@upol.cz
[3] Institute of Molecular and Translational Medicine, Faculty of Medicine and Dentistry, Palacky University Olomouc, Hnevotinska 5, 77900 Olomouc, Czech Republic
* Correspondence: patrik.mlynarcik@upol.cz

Abstract: The growing bacterial resistance to available β-lactam antibiotics is a very serious public health problem, especially due to the production of a wide range of β-lactamases. At present, clinically important bacteria are increasingly acquiring new elements of resistance to carbapenems and polymyxins, including extended-spectrum β-lactamases (ESBLs), carbapenemases and phosphoethanolamine transferases of the MCR type. These bacterial enzymes limit therapeutic options in human and veterinary medicine. It must be emphasized that there is a real risk of losing the ability to treat serious and life-threatening infections. The present study aimed to design specific oligonucleotides for rapid PCR detection of ESBL-encoding genes and in silico analysis of selected ESBL enzymes. A total of 58 primers were designed to detect 49 types of different ESBL genes. After comparing the amino acid sequences of ESBLs (CTX-M, SHV and TEM), phylogenetic trees were created based on the presence of conserved amino acids and homologous motifs. This study indicates that the proposed primers should be able to specifically detect more than 99.8% of all described ESBL enzymes. The results suggest that the in silico tested primers could be used for PCR to detect the presence of ESBL genes in various bacteria, as well as to monitor their spread.

Keywords: ESBL; antibiotic resistance; bacteria; PCR; primer

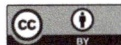

1. Introduction

The mechanisms that bacterial pathogens have developed to fight antibiotics are many, one of them being production of enzymes degrading particular antibacterial agents. In case of β-lactam antibiotics, the enzymes are β-lactamases. To date, more than 7000 β-lactamases have been described in the Beta-Lactamase DataBase (BLDB) [1], which have different characteristics in terms of their substrate specificities. A special group is made up of β-lactamases with an extended spectrum of activity (extended-spectrum β-lactamases, ESBLs), which can inactivate broad-spectrum β-lactam antibiotics (e.g., penicillins, cephalosporins and monobactams). These enzymes are classified into Ambler molecular classes A and D; within the Bush-Jacoby-Medeiros classification system, they belong to groups 2be and 2d. While a common feature of class A ESBLs is their sensitivity to the activity of inhibitors such as clavulanic acid, sulbactam and tazobactam, class D β-lactamases (oxacillinases; OXA) are resistant to them. Furthermore, class C ESBLs have also been described (e.g., ADC). Some may also hydrolyze carbapenems, like the chromosomally encoded ADC-68 enzyme described in *Acinetobacter baumannii* (*A. baumannii*), whose R2 and C-loops allow better accommodation of carbapenems [2]. Moreover, weak hydrolytic activity against carbapenems was also described for some other variants such as ACT-1, ACT-28, CMY-2 or CMY-10 (AmpC type β-lactamase) [3,4].

Regarding OXA enzymes, an OXA-23 subfamily variant (OXA-146 with an alanine duplication at position 220) possessing both ESBL and carbapenem-hydrolyzing class D β-lactamase properties has been described [5]. Recently, two novel ESBL genes probably associated with small mobilizable plasmids, named bla_{RSA1} and bla_{RSA2}, have been found in Indian river sediments, the latter also showing weak carbapenemase activity [6]. In addition, increased carbapenem resistance may be observed due to the production of ESBL enzymes if some secondary resistant mechanisms such as porin loss are present [7].

A great proportion of ESBLs are TEM (Temoneira class A extended-spectrum β-lactamase) or SHV (sulfhydryl variant of the TEM enzyme) enzyme derivatives. However, the most widespread enzymes are CTX-M (cefotaxime-hydrolyzing β-lactamase–Munich) whose production and dissemination rates have increased significantly since the mid-1990s [8]. Newly discovered and, in terms of occurrence, unusual class A ESBL enzymes include BEL, BES, GES (Guiana extended-spectrum β-lactamase), PER, VEB, SFO and TLA β-lactamases. In addition, the ESBL phenotype has been reported in other groups of β-lactamases such as CARB and L2. Additional minor ESBL types, such as FONA, BPU and YOC, have also been recently identified [9–11]. An interesting example of the minor ESBL group is SFO-1 encoded by a plasmid which includes the *ampR* regulatory gene, which allows for β-lactamase induction in a manner similar to class C β-lactamases. Minor ESBL enzymes are rare but often can associate with resistance genes against other antibiotics such as aminoglycosides or quinolones [12–14].

Many ESBL genes have been identified as a source of acquired resistance, but further studies show that ESBLs also occur naturally in clinically relevant pathogens and in environmental species. For example, many chromosomally encoded and naturally occurring ESBLs, such as CSP-1, KLUA-1, KLUC-1, OXY-1 RAHN-1 and SGM-1, have been described in various bacteria, although their role in phenotypic resistance is small [15,16]. Other enzymes with the ESBL phenotype include chromosomally encoded metallo-β-lactamases (MBLs), HMB-1, as well as KHM-1 found in multidrug-resistant bacteria [17].

GES enzymes were first classified as ESBLs due to a large number of hydrolyzable substrates including penicillins and cephalosporins with an extended spectrum. Since GES enzymes hydrolyzed, to a lesser extent, imipenem as well, they were also included among group 2f carbapenemases. Genes encoding this enzyme family can be located in integrons on plasmids. Even though they are rare, there have been reports about their presence worldwide [18].

Most SHV enzymes with an extended spectrum are derived from SHV-1 with differences in one or more amino acids; this small change is sufficient to create an extended spectrum. In particular, it is the G238S or E240K substitutions, with a serine residue being responsible for ceftazidime hydrolysis and a lysine residue for cefotaxime cleavage (both third-generation cephalosporins) [12]. Carbapenems do not belong to the hydrolytic profile of SHV enzymes, but there was a clinical isolate of *Klebsiella pneumoniae* (*K. pneumoniae*) with low sensitivity to some extended-spectrum cephalosporins as well as to imipenem. Subsequently, it has been found that a β-lactamase variant of SHV-1 with amino acid change A146V, designated SHV-38, is responsible for reduced imipenem sensitivity. Genes encoding SHV-38 are located on chromosomes, which means that it is the first SHV chromosomal enzyme with an extended spectrum of hydrolysis [19]. CTX-M enzymes do not have the ability to hydrolyze carbapenems. However, relatively recently identified CTX-M-33, a derivative of the globally widespread enzyme CTX-M-15 differing only in one amino acid substitution (N109S), exhibited the ability to hydrolyze meropenem. This property results from the substitution of N109S and strong selection of the antibiotic [20].

Enterobacteriaceae members are the main ESBL producers and they have mainly been recorded in hospital and community environments. However, the presence of ESBL producers (mainly CTX-M-15) has also been shown in foodstuffs of animal origin (e.g., cow's milk, dairy products, chicken), suggesting possible transfer through the food chain [21,22]. In addition, an increasing number of ESBL-producing enterobacteria isolated from water environments have been observed [23]. In this case, a total of 10 ESBL-positive isolates [nine *Escherichia coli* (*E. coli*) and one *K. pneumoniae*] were identified in four well waters out of 100. ESBL genotyping revealed that CTX-M-15 was present nine times and CTX-M-27 was produced once. This and many other studies suggest that, for example, ESBL-producing enterobacteria in rural waters can spread to animals and humans via drinking water.

In view of the growing clinical importance of ESBL enzymes, their detection is also necessary in routine microbiological practice. The present study was concerned with (1) in silico analysis of ESBL enzymes, and (2) designing primers serving to detect all described ESBL genes.

2. Results

2.1. In Silico Analysis of ESBL Enzymes

A search of the BLDB and BLASTn databases showed that a wide variety of class A and C β-lactamases, MBLs and class D β-lactamases such as OXA have been described for both enterobacteria and Gram-negative non-fermenting bacteria. The study of selected clinically significant ESBL enzymes (CTX-M, SHV, TEM) revealed that the most widespread group in bacterial genera were ESBL enzymes of the TEM type found in 45 genera, followed by CTX-M in 25 and SHV in 23 genera (Table 1). In addition, ESBL enzymes of the CTX-M, GES, OXA (OXA-1-like, OXA-2-like, OXA-10-like), SHV, TEM and VEB types are most commonly found in selected enterobacteria (*Enterobacter* spp., *Escherichia* spp., *Klebsiella* spp.) and Gram-negative non-fermenting rods (*Acinetobacter* spp., *Pseudomonas* spp.; data not shown).

Table 1. Distribution of (extended-spectrum β-lactamases) ESBL enzymes in bacterial genera.

Bacterial Genera	ESBL Enzymes	Bacterial Genera	ESBL Enzymes
Achromobacter	TEM	*Legionella*	TEM
Acinetobacter	CTX-M, SHV, TEM	*Lysobacter*	TEM
Aeromonas	CTX-M, SHV, TEM	*Morganella*	CTX-M, SHV, TEM
Alcaligenes	TEM	*Mycobacterium*	TEM
Atlantibacter	CTX-M, TEM	*Neisseia*	TEM
Bacillus	CTX-M, SHV, TEM	*Nocardia*	TEM
Bordetella	TEM	*Ochrobactrum*	CTX-M, SHV
Brevibacterium	CTX-M, TEM	*Pantoea*	CTX-M, TEM
Brucella	TEM	*Pasteurella*	TEM
Burkholderia	CTX-M, SHV	*Proteus*	CTX-M, SHV, TEM
Campylobacter	TEM	*Providencia*	CTX-M, TEM
Cedecea	SHV	*Pseudomonas*	CTX-M, SHV, TEM
Citrobacter	CTX-M, SHV, TEM	*Pseudochrobactrum*	CTX-M
Cronobacter	SHV, TEM	*Ralstonia*	TEM
Elizabethkingia (formerly *Chryseobacterium*)	TEM	*Raoultella*	CTX-M, SHV, TEM
Enterobacter	CTX-M, SHV, TEM	*Salmonella*	CTX-M, SHV, TEM
Enterococcus	SHV, TEM	*Serratia*	CTX-M, SHV, TEM
Erwinia	TEM	*Shewanella*	CTX-M
Escherichia	CTX-M, SHV, TEM	*Shigella*	CTX-M, SHV, TEM
Haemophilus	TEM	*Staphylococcus*	TEM
Hafnia	TEM	*Stenotrophomonas*	SHV
Kerstersia	SHV	*Streptococcus*	TEM
Klebsiella	CTX-M, SHV, TEM	*Streptomyces*	TEM
Kluyvera	CTX-M, SHV, TEM	*Superficieibacter*	SHV, TEM
Lactobacillus	TEM	*Vibrio*	CTX-M, TEM
Leclercia	CTX-M, TEM	*Yersinia*	TEM

In silico analysis of ESBL enzymes was used to detect the presence of various conserved amino acids and motifs. Several conserved amino acids such as methionine-cysteine-serine-threonine-serine-lysine at positions 71–76 (71-MCSTSK-76; numbering according to CTX-M-1; Figure 1A) were identified within studied CTX-M enzymes. In this figure, there are no remaining amino acid sections and amino acids such as methionine at position 1 (M1), glutamine at positions 34, 35 and 268 (Q34, Q35 and Q268), leucine at position

37 (L37), alanine and glutamic acid at positions 273–274 (273-AE-274), leucine and alanine at positions 280–281 (280-LA-281) and alanine at position 284 (A284).

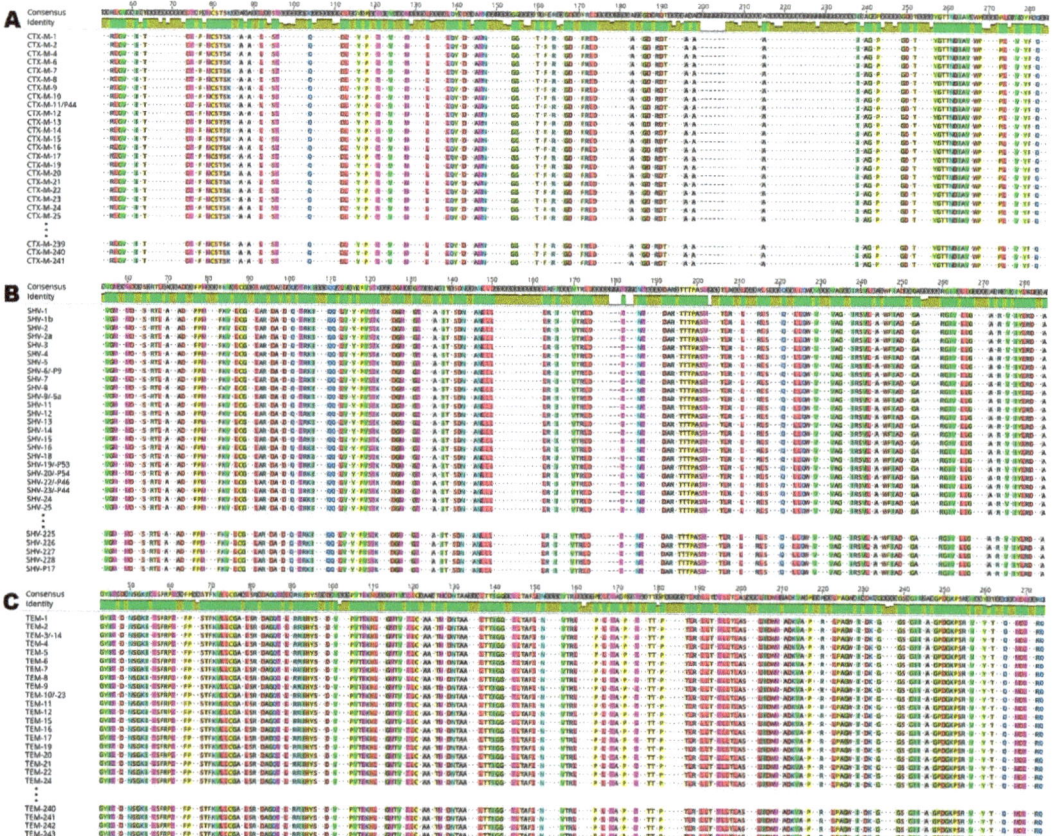

Figure 1. Comparison of 216, 199 and 199 amino acid sequences of (**A**) CTX-M (cefotaxime-hydrolyzing β-lactamase–Munich); (**B**) SHV (sulfhydryl variant of the TEM enzyme; and (**C**) TEM (Temoneira class A extended-spectrum β-lactamase enzymes), respectively. The analysis and image creation were performed in Geneious Prime. Only the same amino acid residues in all sequences are highlighted in the figure. The green panel indicates amino acids that are identical in all sequences on a given position. Different amino acids are marked with dots.

Comparison of the amino acid sequences of the selected CTX-M showed the same (55.3–99.7%) sequence identity between them. For example, CTX-M-150 and CTX-M-151 had only 55.3% amino acid identity, whereas for CTX-M-155 and CTX-M-157, it was 99.7% identity (results not shown).

Reconstruction of the phylogenetic tree allowed monitoring of the affinity of individual amino acid sequences of CTX-M enzymes. Overall, 216 types of different CTX-M were included in the analysis. CTX-M enzymes were divided into several main groups and subgroups, see Figure 2).

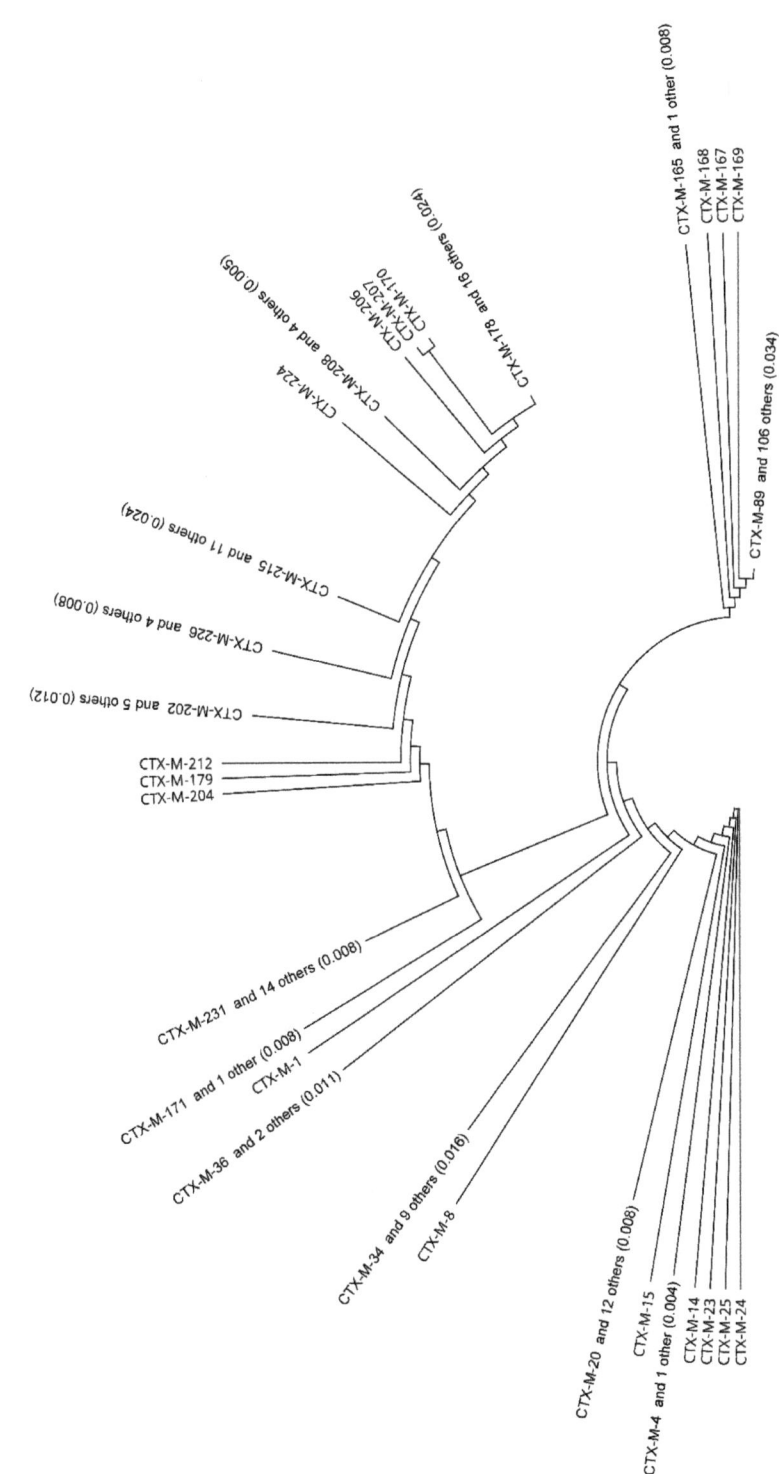

Figure 2. A phylogenetic tree obtained by comparing 216 CTX-M enzymes using Geneious PhyM and automatic subtree compression (subtree distance 0.039).

By comparing the 199 sequences of SHV enzymes, individually conserved motifs of active sites including X-X-phenylalanine-lysine were identified at positions 66–69 (66-XXFK-69; numbering according to SHV-1; Figure 1B). Other amino acid sections and amino acids which are not shown in the figure include arginine at positions 2 and 5 (R2, R5), isoleucine at positions 8 to 9 (I8, I9), leucine at positions 11 to 12, 17 and 26 (11-LL-12, L17, L26), valine at position 19 (V19), serine-proline-glutamine at positions 22–24 (22-SPQ-24), glutamine-isoleucine-lysine at positions 28–30 (28-QIK-30), serine and glutamic acid at positions 32–33 (32-SE-33), serine and glycine at positions 37–38 (37-SG-38), methionine at position 266 (M266), glutamine at position 271 (Q271), isoleucine and alanine at positions 273–274 (273-IA-274), glycine at position 277 (G277), alanine at position 279 (A279) and glutamic acid-histidine-tryptophan-glutamine at positions 282–285 (282-EHWQ-285).

In this case, the comparison of the amino acid sequences of SHV enzymes showed 93.1–99.7% sequence identity between them. For example, SHV-16 and SHV-100 had 93.1% amino acid consensus, while in the case of SHV-7 and SHV-105, the identity was 99.7% (results not shown).

The relationships of individual SHV enzymes were shown using a phylogenetic tree. A rooted phylogenetic tree enabled us to distinguish different clusters and identify several major groups and subgroups (Figure 3).

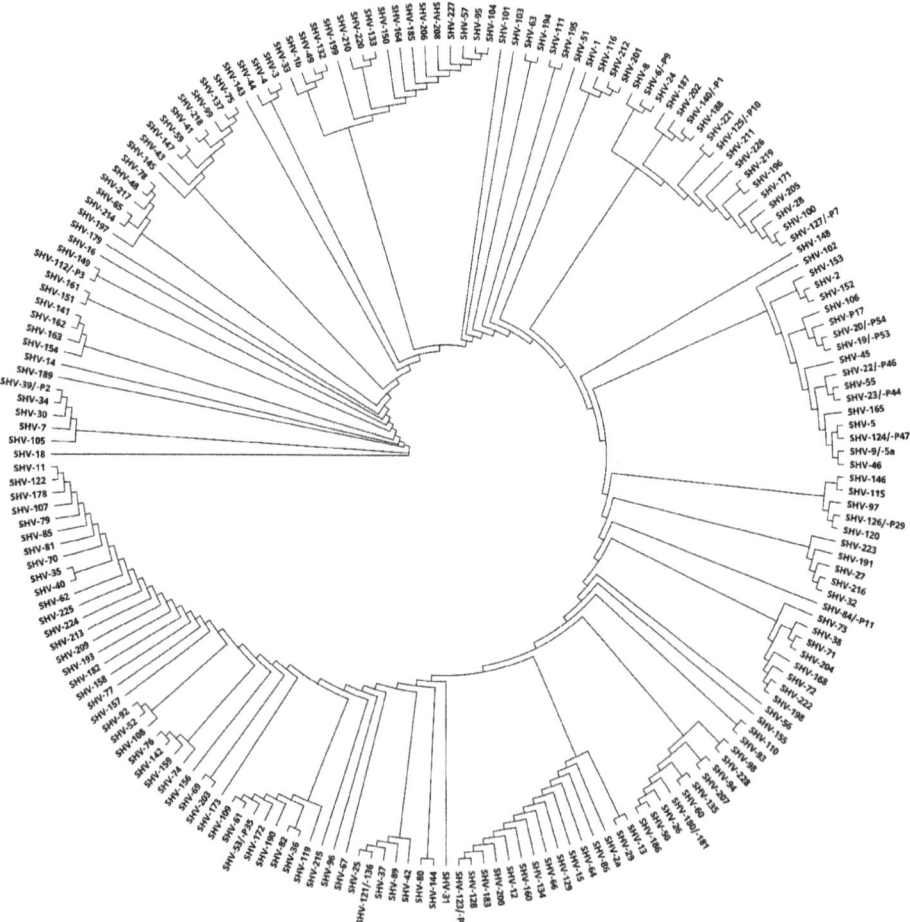

Figure 3. A phylogenetic tree obtained by comparing 199 SHV enzymes using Geneious PhyML.

Conserved amino acids and motifs including serine-threonine-phenylalanine-lysine at positions 68–71 (68-STFK-71; numbering according to TEM-1; Figure 1C) were identified by analysis of another 199 sequences of TEM enzymes. The remaining identical amino acid sections and amino acids which are not shown in the figure include methionine at position 1 (M1), histidine-phenylalanine-arginine-valine at positions 5–8 (5-HFRV-8), proline and phenylalanine at positions 12–13 (12-PF-13), alanine-alanine-phenylalanine-cysteine at positions 15–18 (15-AAFC-18), proline-valine-phenylalanine at positions 20–22 (20-PVF-22), proline at position 25 (P25), threonine at position 27 (T27), valine-lysine-valine at positions 29–31 (29-VKV-31), alanine and glutamic acid at positions 34–35 (34-AE-35), glutamic acid-isoleucine-glycine at positions 277–279 (277-EIG-279), and serine-leucine-isoleucine-lysine at positions 281–284 (281-SLIK-284).

The amino acid consensus of the studied sequences of TEM enzymes were in the range of 93.4–99.7%. The lowest 93.4% amino acid consensus was recorded, for example, at TEM-178 and TEM-194, with 99.7% consensus, for example, between TEM-189 and TEM-191 (results are not shown).

By using a phylogenetic tree, relationships among TEM enzymes were shown based on the similarity of amino acid sequences. A rooted phylogenetic tree allowed us to observe different clusters and identify several major groups and subgroups (Figure 4).

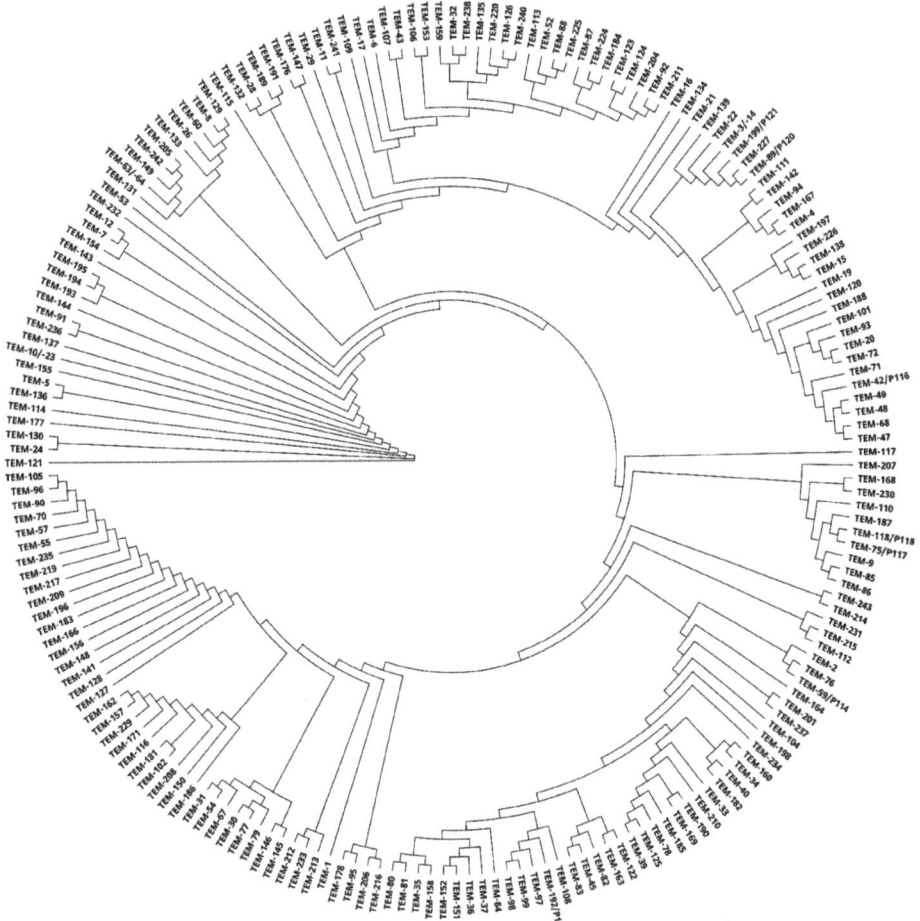

Figure 4. A phylogenetic tree obtained by comparing 199 TEM enzymes using Geneious PhyML.

Point mutation studies showed that the highest numbers of amino acid changes were observed in the CTX-M, OXY, TEM, SHV, PER and VEB types, namely 6344, 904, 534, 418, 162 and 61, respectively (Table 2). In case of CTX-M enzymes, the most common amino acid changes recorded were as follows: S → T (275 times, this amino acid change was also described in all remaining ESBL enzymes), K → Q (217 times) and Q → R (198 times). Conversely, amino acid changes recorded only once were A → I, M, Q or R, etc. The most common amino acid changes in the remaining ESBL enzymes included A → T (108 times), I → V (15 times), L → Q (73 times), E → K (82 times) and I → V (14 times) in OXY, PER, SHV, TEM and VEB, respectively.

Table 2. Point mutations in selected ESBL enzymes.

Amino Acid Change		Number of Mutations (Amino Acid Position)					
from	to	CTX-M *	OXY *	PER *	SHV *	TEM *	VEB *
A	C	7 (22)		2 (7)			
A	D	36 (32/131/157)		3 (114)	1 (264)	1 (230)	
A	E	28 (35/46/157/222/236)	21 (230)	2 (114/166)			1 (38)
A	G	158 (16/64/73/131/136/157/297)	10 (240)	1 (7)	3 (205/259)	2 (235/280)	
A	I	1 (16)					
A	K	22 (64/244)					
A	M	1 (73)					
A	N	36 (35)					
A	P	78 (59/78/272)			1 (15)	1 (183)	
A	Q	1 (157)		2 (151)			
A	R	1 (222)			1 (151)	1 (185)	
A	S	102 (35/46/151/235/244)	2 (240)	4 (109)	1 (23)	3 (9/40/266)	
A	T	110 (16/18/35/90/120/131/137/161/222/244)	108 (16/30/32/38/56/129/171/208/240/284)	1 (11)	14 (20/23/63/90/125/135/157/161/204)	12 (9/183/235/280)	4 (248)
A	V	74 (16/35/88/131/135/137/163)	32 (16/233)		20 (20/63/125/135/137/145/157/188/205/218/264/288)	18 (23/40/182/222/266/276)	
A	W				1 (299)		
C	N				1 (9)		
C	R				1 (134)		
C	S				1 (9)		
D	A	69 (36)	1 (39)	4 (155)	3 (195/231)		
D	E	160 (218/303)	1 (242)		2 (168/230)	2 (155/177)	
D	G	179 (259/270)			4 (115/195/230/231)	2 (113/161)	
D	H	23 (36/292/303)			2 (112)		
D	K	2 (303)					
D	N	40 (36/218/270/303)	28 (39/58)		1 (195)	3 (36/113/174)	
D	P	1 (292)				1 (33)	
D	Q	1 (218)					
D	S	25 (36/65/256/303)					
E	A	106 (47/177)					
E	D	35 (98/169)	22 (92/99/149/278)		2 (29/273)	1 (26)	
E	G	1 (47)		1 (33)	3 (59/75/177)	2 (164/237)	
E	K	3 (47/132/169)	1 (278)		37 (29/100/256/289)	82 (26/62/102/166/237)	
E	N	1 (169)					
E	P	1 (107)					
E	Q	85 (98/132)	4 (92)	8 (119/193/224)	1 (75)		

Table 2. Cont.

Amino Acid Change		Number of Mutations (Amino Acid Position)					
from	to	CTX-M *	OXY *	PER *	SHV *	TEM *	VEB *
E	R				1 (256)	1 (237)	
E	T	1 (98)					
E	V			3 (23)		1 (237)	
F	A	10 (12)					
F	L	1 (12)		3 (19)		3 (14/228)	
F	M	72 (12)					
F	S	21 (12)			1 (162)		
F	W			1 (22)			
F	Y						2 (64)
G	A	31 (25/217)		4 (149/190)	6 (158/191/255)		
G	C	3 (47/132/169)			1 (258)		
G	D		1 (159)		11 (98/154/167/245)	4 (39/90/194/236)	
G	E	1 (25)		1 (41)	2 (158/296)	1 (216)	
G	H	1 (304)					
G	K	1 (126)					
G	N	1 (53)				1 (236)	
G	R	4 (54/234/304)			1 (296)	2 (154/236)	
G	S	27 (25/213/234/253/304)	30 (24/75)		42 (65/155/167/255)	40 (194/236)	
G	V					2 (194/263)	
H	D			2 (134/154)			
H	F	1 (123)					
H	K	1 (152)					
H	L			2 (134)		4 (285)	
H	N					1 (156)	
H	Q	74 (152)			1 (22)		
H	R					5 (24/151)	
H	T				1 (107)		
H	Y				3 (123)		
I	A	1 (69)		2 (5/97)			
I	F	1 (119)			11 (6)	1 (11)	
I	L	1 (150)	5 (33)	3 (61/194)	2 (297/302)		
I	M			4 (111)	1 (275)	1 (259)	
I	P					4 (3)	
I	R					1 (11)	
I	S	1 (300)					
I	T	13 (69)		7 (5/40/97)	2 (275/297)	1 (275)	1 (18)
I	V	170 (69/108/266/275)	7 (111)	15 (61/162/194/245/258)	3 (6/58)	5 (125/171/256)	14 (18)
K	A	5 (109/110/299)	23 (102)	3 (102)			
K	D	1 (214)					
K	E	36 (93/122/269)	27 (180)	1 (113)		1 (32)	
K	G	1 (214)					
K	H	73 (4/214)					
K	L	1 (148)	20 (140)				
K	N	80 (3/214/286)	20 (101)		2 (209/271)		
K	P	81 (110)					
K	Q	217 (4/44/94/109/269/286)		2 (196)		1 (144)	
K	R	103 (3/44/94/109/122/229/251/299)		7 (196/246)	5 (251/271)		2 (237)
K	S	7 (110/214)					
K	T	91 (3/269)				1 (190)	

Table 2. Cont.

Amino Acid Change		Number of Mutations (Amino Acid Position)					
from	to	CTX-M *	OXY *	PER *	SHV *	TEM *	VEB *
L	A	4 (9/14/23/210)		2 (256)			
L	F	121 (14/24/30/130/305)	1 (84)		6 (124/133/189)	23 (19/55/100/136)	1 (56)
L	G	2 (30/70)					
L	I	111 (9/149/166/276)	24 (2)	1 (256)		4 (19/135/218)	
L	M	5 (9/22/102/207/242)	23 (2/11)	4 (75/260)	2 (17/237)	3 (47/219)	
L	N	1 (305)					
L	P	4 (130/149/212)	1 (262)		4 (38/62/102/301)	1 (49)	
L	Q	2 (60/180)			73 (33/62)		
L	R				5 (8/102/133/185)	1 (10)	
L	S	3 (14/23/305)					
L	V	193 (9/60/101/153/216)		3 (305)	2 (159/210)	4 (28/38/100/247)	
L	Y	15 (224/305)					
M	A	69 (14)					
M	G	1 (197)					
M	I	1 (86)	35 (12/141)	1 (160)	3 (80)	10 (66/67/153/180)	
M	K				4 (3)		
M	L	105 (228)	20 (12)	3 (160)	1 (80)	17 (67)	
M	T	21 (14)				34 (180)	
M	V				7 (80/140/228)	11 (67/184)	
N	D	89 (62/125/143)	36 (54/90/200/256)	3 (308)	2 (269/291)	12 (272)	6 (294)
N	E	1 (86)					
N	G	12 (66/100/125)					
N	H	25 (36/65/256/303)	10 (90)		2 (269)	4 (134/173)	
N	I				1 (270)	1 (173)	
N	K	2 (100/209)			1 (169)		
N	L	1 (100)					
N	Q	141 (100/209)					
N	S	27 (100/103/117/181)				3 (98/272)	
N	T	1 (66)				1 (168)	
N	W	1 (209)					
N	Y	1 (115)	1 (200)				
P	A	3 (29/178/194)		3 (123)		1 (143)	
P	G				1 (268)		
P	H	1 (178)					
P	K	105 (99)	23 (91)				
P	L	3 (178/188)	1 (269)		3 (156/268/284)		
P	N		4 (91)				
P	Q	95 (156/178/185/285)					
P	S	18 (178/283)	1 (170)		7 (18/27/190/236/243/284)	1 (143)	
P	T	29 (29/178/283)		1 (123)			
Q	A	77 (11/165/220)					
Q	D	1 (199)					
Q	E	35 (165/284)			1 (165)		
Q	H	1 (68)	23 (34/156)		2 (223/293)	1 (88)	
Q	I	1 (68)					
Q	K	2 (11/223)		2 (94/183)		38 (4/37)	
Q	L	3 (11/165/199)	4 (156/270)	1 (129)			
Q	P			1 (116)	2 (175/214)	1 (203)	
Q	R	198 (11/68/239)	27 (35/156)	1 (158)	1 (37)	3 (97/204)	
Q	S	128 (33/51/165)					
Q	T	10 (165)					

Table 2. Cont.

Amino Acid Change		Number of Mutations (Amino Acid Position)					
from	to	CTX-M *	OXY *	PER *	SHV *	TEM *	VEB *
Q	V						
R	A					4 (176/271)	
R	C				1 (72)	9 (162/241)	
R	G	2 (10/175)			2 (232)	2 (118/241)	
R	H	25 (10/271/291)	9 (43/68/194)		5 (54/72/219)	22 (162/238/241)	
R	K	131 (10/50/105/208)					
R	L	37 (10/72/195)			7 (76/175/222/232/290)	4 (241/271)	
R	M		1 (97)				
R	N		1 (43)				
R	P	73 (76/105)			1 (175)	1 (41)	
R	Q	74 (10/50/208/221/290)			4 (257/307)	6 (202/271)	
R	S	4 (10/105/175)	10 (43/225)		17 (54/109/219)	37 (63/162/241)	
R	T					1 (41)	
R	V	2 (72)					
S	A	110 (52/67/111/296)	45 (25/89/103)	1 (280)		1 (221)	
S	C	1 (245)	1 (4)			4 (2)	
S	D						
S	E			2 (280)			
S	F				1 (12)		
S	G	101 (111/134/141/158/237/245)	39 (143/231)	2 (18)	2 (36/144)	7 (128/264)	
S	H	2 (289)					
S	I	3 (134/254)	1 (192)		2 (286)		
S	K	36 (158/296)					
S	L				1 (220)		
S	N	6 (26/237/254/289)	29 (4/29/157/275)		3 (81/213)	1 (122)	
S	P					1 (104)	
S	Q	1 (97)					
S	R	83 (5/237/289)					
S	T	275 (67/97/129/141)	37 (4/44/174)	10 (12/37/121/135)	1 (117)	3 (128/233)	2 (131)
S	V	2 (219)	2 (89)				
T	A	192 (13/17/19/21/34/144/206/211/226/281/302)		11 (13/165/293)	9 (16/69/82/252)		9 (25/176/219)
T	C	81 (19)					
T	D	1 (233)					
T	G	3 (17/19)			1 (178)		
T	H	2 (226/233)					
T	I	6 (176/182/226/278)	48 (9/61)		4 (152/212)	1 (267)	
T	K	3 (34/170/211)		3 (202)		1 (186)	
T	M	134 (13/17/226)	8 (168)		1 (283)	19 (261)	10 (104)
T	N	1 (176)			2 (16/212)	1 (186)	
T	P	90 (19/21)			1 (16)	1 (112)	
T	S	130 (21/127/170/179/182/192/193/206)	34 (9/184)	3 (95/221)	4 (129/160/283)		
T	V	108 (144/206)	1 (61)	3 (24)			
V	A	98 (27/85/106/248)	20 (161)	1 (290)	2 (86/91)		2 (19)
V	E					1 (78)	7 (19)
V	F	1 (293)		3 (9)	2 (153)	1 (258)	
V	G	3 (37/247)					

Table 2. Cont.

Amino Acid Change		Number of Mutations (Amino Acid Position)					
from	to	CTX-M *	OXY *	PER *	SHV *	TEM *	VEB *
V	I	175 (2/20/37/114/159/293/301)	2 (261)	2 (235)	1 (130)	6 (82)	
V	L	22 (20/91)	11 (17/94)	3 (17)	1 (86)		
V	M	35 (2/37)			5 (86/91/95/277)		
V	P	1 (27)					
V	Q	2 (27/106)					
V	R						
V	S	2 (225/247)				1 (42)	
V	T	68 (247)					
W	C					1 (163)	
W	G					2 (163)	
W	L					1 (163)	
W	P				1 (176)		
W	R	1 (246)			1 (71)	5 (163)	
Y	C	10 (31)					
Y	F	1 (31)			8 (5)	1 (103)	
Y	G						
Y	H	22 (31)	1 (144)	4 (115)	2 (5/108)		
Y	N					1 (103)	
Y	S	1 (31)				1 (103)	
Y	W	1 (71)					

Total numbers of mutations: CTX-M: 6344, OXY: 904, PER: 162, SHV: 418, TEM: 534, VEB: 61. Numbers of amino acid insertions: CTX-M: 6, OXY: 10, PER: 0, SHV: 9, TEM: 0, VEB: 0. Numbers of amino acid deletions: CTX-M: 3, OXY: 8, PER: 0, SHV: 2, TEM: 3, VEB: 1. * Total numbers of analyzed sequences: CTX-M (216), OXY (48), PER (15), SHV (199), TEM (199), VEB (27).

2.2. Detection of ESBL-Positive Bacteria with PCR

A total of 49 different types of ESBLs were analyzed in this study, including 1438 β-lactamase genes, of which only 624 enzymes had ESBL phenotype based on BLDB database and literature search. There were 42 members of class A β-lactamases (e.g., CARB, CTX-M, GES, OXY, PER, SHV, TEM, VEB), two members of the class C β-lactamase family (ADC and YOC), two gene families of the subclass B1 (HMB and KHM), and three members of class D β-lactamases (BPU, CDD and OXA; 5 OXA subgroups, OXA-18 and OXA-45; Table 3). In case of the most numerous groups of ESBL enzymes (CTX-M, SHV, TEM), there were 216, 199 and 199 variants of these enzymes with GenBank accession numbers, respectively. The CTX-M enzymes were subclassified based on similarity of amino acid sequences into 5 groups (CTX-M-1-like, CTX-M-2-like, CTX-M-8-like, CTX-M-9-like and CTX-M-151-like). A total of 58 specific primer pairs for ESBL detection were designed (Table 3) in silico using Primer3 (Geneious, Biomatters). The primer-BLAST results showed that these primers could detect all or almost all allelic variants of these so far described types of enzymes that are commonly found in bacteria.

3. Discussion

Currently, clinically significant bacteria are increasingly resistant to carbapenems and polymyxins due to the production of ESBL, carbapenemases and phosphoethanolamine transferases of the MCR type, which can overcome the last-line antibiotics for the treatment of infections caused by multidrug-resistant Gram-negative bacterial pathogens [24–26].

For the past decade, we have observed a global rapid increase in ESBL- and carbapenemase-producing bacteria in animals intended for food production [27]. Other sources of transmission and dissemination of β-lactamases include, besides hospital or community environments, also coins and paper currency. An example is the presence of various Gram-negative bacteria producing CTX-M-type ESBLs and OXA-48 carbapenemase on the surface of Algerian currency. Especially simultaneous manipulation of money and food contributes to the spread of infectious agents and thus of bacterial resistance to antibiotics [28].

ESBLs have become a global problem in the treatment of hospitalized patients after the introduction of β-lactam antibiotics with an extended spectrum of activity into clinical practice. Most microorganisms producing these enzymes belong to the Enterobacteriaceae family, the most widespread producers being *K. pneumoniae* and *E. coli* isolated from the hospital environment. ESBL-producing bacterial strains are most commonly found in hospital patients, with the risk factors being prolonged hospital stay, disease severity, previous exposure to antibiotics, time spent in intensive care or presence of a urinary/arterial catheter [12,29].

The ever-expanding problem of ESBL resistance is largely due to frequent and unjustified prescription, especially of broad-spectrum cephalosporins. Increasing resistance to third-generation cephalosporins in *E. coli* isolates can be observed in a gradient from northern to southern countries, with the lowest and highest percentage in Northern and Southern Europe, respectively. The current resistance status can be evaluated using the EARS-NET database. For example, the percentage of *E. coli* isolates resistant to third-generation cephalosporins in 2019 was 7.8% in Sweden, compared to 30.9% in Italy. In case of *K. pneumoniae*, resistance to third-generation cephalosporins in most European countries was below 60%, but exceeded 70% in some countries such as Bulgaria (data obtained from the EARS-NET database; https://ecdc.europa.eu/en/antimicrobial-resistance/surveillance-and-disease-data/data-ecdc, accessed on 31 March 2021).

By the end of the 1990s, the majority of identified SHV- and TEM-type ESBLs originated from nosocomial isolates of *K. pneumoniae* (especially in intensive care units). In the following years, the epidemiological situation concerning ESBLs underwent dramatic changes. The main producers of ESBLs were *E. coli* strains expressing CTX-M-type β-lactamases that spread mainly through mobile genetic elements. There was also an increase in the number of isolates from the community, mostly from patients with urinary infection [30].

One of the objectives of the present study was comparison of amino acid sequences of the investigated ESBL enzymes to elucidate the conserved amino acids and motifs (sections). The presence of various conserved motifs is discussed by many authors [31]. The present study showed a large number of conserved motifs and amino acid residues in the selected ESBL enzymes (Figure 1A–C). The seemingly smaller amount of conserved amino acid residues and sections may be primarily related to the use of all variants of the studied ESBL types. Within the analyzed types of ESBL enzymes, the lowest amino acid identity was found for CTX-M enzymes, ranging from 55.3 to 99.7%, which also correlates with the highest number of point mutations (Table 2) found in this enzyme group.

Sometimes it is not easy to classify some β-lactamases into subgroups based on sequential and other properties because they are rather varied. Phylogenetic trees were created (Figures 2–4), which show similarity of the studied subtypes of ESBL enzymes. Obviously, there is a great variety between genes encoding individual types of ESBL.

In general, many proposed primers or methods described in the literature are generally useful for detecting the most common types of ESBL but do not cover all variants of these genes. Therefore, the present study aimed to design specific primers for rapid PCR detection of all known ESBL genes described in the BLDB database. Briefly, our results suggest that proposed primers (58 primer pairs; Table 3) have the ability to specifically detect 623 analyzed ESBL subtypes (99.8%) and are suitable for detection and epidemiological analysis of all described ESBL genes in various bacteria. Additional primers for detection of β-lactamase genes, including carbapenemases [e.g., bla_{KPC} (*Klebsiella pneumoniae* carbapenemase), bla_{NDM} (New Delhi MBL), bla_{VIM} (Verona integron-encoded MBL)] and OXA subgroups, are described elsewhere [27,32–34].

The CARB-F2/R2 primers were designed to detect seven CARB subtypes, including CARB-10 (ESBL) enzyme. A total of 51 subtypes of these enzymes have been described. The remaining subtypes of CARB enzymes except for CARB-42 could be verified using the specific primers described previously [34]. This could be detected with an additional primer (F-TCTCTCCTCGAGCAACAAA, R-AAGTGAGAGCTCGGTTTCT; Tm: 53, PCR product: 708 bp). The L2-F1/R1 primers can be used to detect 18 L2 subtypes, including four L2-1/-2/-3/-E-10 (ESBL) enzymes, while not being able to distinguish 4 subtypes. The remaining L2 subtypes can be detected using the L2-F2/R2 primers [34]. To confirm the presence of the bla_{KLUB}, bla_{KLUG} and bla_{KLUY} genes, the primers CTX-M-F1/R1 could be used to detect all two, five and five different subtypes listed in the BLDB database, respectively. The primers CTX-M-F/R were used to detect 215 subtypes of $bla_{CTX-M-like}$ genes but were unable to distinguish one allelic variant (CTX-M-151). Thus, a primer (F-CAGTAAAGTGATGGCGGTAG, R–ATACCACGGCAATATCGTTG; Tm: 54 °C, PCR product: 536 bp) could be used to detect it. The primers ADC-F/R (ADC-F1/R1 to ADC-F4/R4) were used to detect 31 ESBL subtypes (e.g., ADC-33, ADC-117, ADC-140) of the $bla_{ADC-like}$ genes. The remaining 12 subtypes of ADC enzymes could be detected using the specific primers described elsewhere [34]. The OXA(7)-F/R primer was aimed at detecting 38 subtypes of the $bla_{OXA-48-like}$ genes, including ESBL types OXA-163 and OXA-405. To date, a total of 41 subtypes of OXA-48-like enzymes have been described in the BLDB database. Another 3 specific OXA-48-like subtypes (OXA-436/-535/-731) could be tested using the primer (F-ACGAGAATAMACAGCAGGG, R-GATAMACAGGCACAACCGA; Tm: 56, PCR product: 228 bp).

We are currently witnessing increasing antibiotic resistance in clinically important bacteria, which is associated with the discovery of new enzymes that break down antibiotics, in our case ESBLs, which appear over time. In some cases, very numerous variants of these enzymes appear, which can significantly limit their accurate detection. Therefore, continuous analysis of all known ESBL enzymes and design of more specific primers is necessary to prevent their spread. For example, OXA enzymes represent a rapidly growing family that includes over 943 enzymes [1] that are highly diverse in terms of sequence. However, in case of OXA enzymes, another difficulty is their accurate and timely detection, since OXA-encoding genes are expressed only in the presence of functional promoters represented by insertion sequences. Another very large group is, for example, AmpC β-lactamases bla_{EC} (formerly bla_{ESC}, chromosomally encoded cephalosporinases), in which more than 2200 variants have been described and their number is growing. Although these are only chromosomally encoded β-lactamases, some exhibit the ESBL phenotype and, together with overexpression of efflux pumps and low outer membrane permeability, they are increasingly reported with regard to multidrug resistance, for example in *A. baumannii* [35]. Ultimately, this suggests that antibiotic resistance in bacteria is a complex phenomenon.

Authors often state that broad-spectrum cephalosporin-resistant isolates are ESBL-negative [36]. Therefore, we cannot rule out the possibility that these bacterial strains also contain other rare ESBL types such as CARB, KLUC or very rare OXA variants. Furthermore, we must also consider other resistance mechanisms, such as over-production of chromosomal AmpC, increased expression of an efflux pump or reduced permeability of the outer membrane, with new and non-described resistance mechanisms not being excluded. The solution seems to be transcriptome sequencing, as well as other forms of sequencing, such as whole genome sequencing, which will provide new possibilities for resistance prediction in the near future.

Table 3. Specifications of primers used in the study.

Target (Subtype)	Primer Name	Sequence (5' to 3' Direction) [a]	Natural (N) or Acquired (A)/Phenotype	Amplicon Size (bp)	Tm (°C)	Reference
ACI (1)	ACI-F/R	CCGTTGACATGGAGAATGG, GCGTGTCGGTTATGGAATT	N/ESBL	507	54	This study
ADC (178)	ADC-F1/R1	MAACCTAAAAACYCAATCGTG, YGGATAAGMAAACTCTTCCA	N/AmpC, ESBL or CARBA	417–420	58	[34]
ADC (29)	ADC-F2/R2	RGGTTCTAYCAAGTCGYA, GCGTTCTTCATTBGAATACGT		268	59	
ADC (5)	ADC-F3/R3	TGGTCTACAATCCGTTCAAGA, GCCGGGGTTAACTCGAAT		517	54	
ADC (7)	ADC-F4/R4	TATRATGTGCCGGTATGG, RTCTGTTTGTACTTCAYCTGG		318	54	This study
BEL (4)	BEL-F/R	CGTTCCTTGAAGAGTACGC, ACCCGTTACCCATGAATCA	A/ESBL	401	53	This study
BES (1)	BES-F/R	ATAAGCGGGTGCATTATGC, CTTTAAGCCAGCTCACCAG	A/ESBL	363	53	This study
BPS (11)	BPS-F/R	GCTYCAGTACAGGCACAAC, GTCKTGTTGCCGAGCATCCA	N/cephalosporinase or ESBL	270	57	This study
BPU (1)	BPU-F/R	AAGAAAAGTCCCCATGGT, CGAACTTGTTCGATGGGAG	N/ESBL	364	55	This study
CARB (8)	CARB-F2/R2	GGGAAAACGTTGGGAACAT, TAATAGCACGCGACCCATA	N or A/BSBL or ESBL	578	54	This study
CDD (2)	CDD-F/R	AACAAGTGCAAACAATGGC, TTCCTTTTACCTTTGGCCCT	N/ESBL	266	52	This study
CdiA (2)	CdiA-F/R	CGTGCTCGCTTTCTTTACT, CACCTGCTCCGTTTATC	N/penicillinase or ESBL	692	53	This study
CepA (6)	CepA-F/R	AGTGACAATAATGCCTGCG, TGCTTCGGAATCTTTCACG	N/ESBL	438	52	This study
CfxA (13)	CfxA-F/R	GAAATTGGTGTGGCGGTTA, CAGCACCAAGAGGAGATGT	N or A/BSBL or ESBL	442	53	This study
CGA (1)	CGA-F/R	AGCTACAGTCGGTGTTTCT, TTCATTTTCTGCGCCTGTT	N/ESBL	640	53	This study
CIA (4)	CIA-F/R	GATGGTTTCTGCCTTTGCT, CTTCCGAAATTTTTCCG	N/ESBL	299	53	This study
CME (3)	CME-F/R	CCAAAGTGACAACAACGA, TCCTGAATCGTTCTCAGCA	N/ESBL	376	53	This study

Table 3. Cont.

Target (Subtype)	Primer Name	Sequence (5′ to 3′ Direction) [a]	Natural (N) or Acquired (A)/Phenotype	Amplicon Size (bp)	Tm (°C)	Reference
CSP (1)	CSP-F/R	TCTGCTGAGGTTGATTGAA, TCCCACATCATTGGTAGCA	N/ESBL	346	53	This study
CTX-M (208), KLUB (2), KLUG (5), KLUY (5)	CTX-M-F1/R1	ATGTGCAGYACCAGTAARGT, TGGGTRAARTARGTSACCAGA	N or A/ESBL or CARBA	593	55	[37]
CTX-M (7)	CTX-M-F2/R2	ATGTGCAGYACCAGYAAAG, GGCCARATCACCGCRATAT		551	56	[34]
CumA (3)	CumA-F/R	ATCTCAATGCTATGGCT, TCACGAGGATCACCATGAA	N/BSBL or ESBL	483	53	This study
DES (1)	DES-F/R	GTTCCAGTTATTCCAGGCG, TGCCAGCACTTTAAAGGTG	N/ESBL	269	53	This study
ERP (1)	ERP-F/R	GTATCGGGCTGTCTCTGAT, GCTGTGCTGTCTGTAATCC	N/ESBL	477	54	This study
FAR (1)	FAR-F/R	CTGAAGAAATCTGTCGCC, AGCAGTTTCAGGATCTGT	N/ESBL	473	53	This study
FONA (8)	FONA-F/R	CCGATCTGGTCAACTACAAC, CCCTTCATCCATTCAACCAG	N/ESBL	340	55	This study
GES (45)	GES-F1/R1	ACGTTCAAGTTTCCGCTAG, GGCAACTAATTCGTCACGT	N or A/ESBL or CARBA	624	53	[25]
GES (1)	GES-F2/R2	ATGATCGTGAGTGGAGCCC, AAGAAGCCGATGTCGTTGCG		448	58	This study
HMB (1), KHM (1)	HMB, KHM-F/R	AAATCGAAGCYTTTTATCCGGG, TTTCCAGCAGCGATGCRTCG	N or A/ESBL or CARBA	237	60	This study
KLUA (12)	KLUA-F/R	CGCTCAATGTTAACGGTGA, TTCATGGCAGTATTGTGC	N/ESBL	395	52	This study
KLUC (6)	KLUC-F/R	CGATTGCGAAAAACATGT, CGCCGAGGCTAAWACATC	N or A/ESBL	521	53	This study
KPC (52)	KPC-F/R	CGCTAAACTCGAACAGGAC, CGGTCGTGTTTCCCTTTAG	N or A/ESBL or CARBA	548	54	[34]
LUT (6)	LUT-F/R	TGCTCATGAAAAGCTGGG, ACCTGTCTTATCGCCTACC	N/BSBL or ESBL	299	54	This study
L2 (18)	L2-F1/R1	TTCCCGATGTGCAGCAC, TTGCTGCCGGTCTTGTC	N/ESBL	518	53	[34]
OHIO (1)	OHIO-F/R	CTTTCCCATGATGAGCACC, CCCGCAGATAAATCACCAC	A/ESBL	599	54	This study

Table 3. Cont.

Target (Subtype)	Primer Name	Sequence (5′ to 3′ Direction) [a]	Natural (N) or Acquired (A)/Phenotype	Amplicon Size (bp)	Tm (°C)	Reference
OXA-1-like (11)	OXA(1)-F/R	TCTGTTGTTTGGGTTTCGC, TCTATGGTGTTTTCTATGGCTG	N or A/NSBL, BSBL or ESBL	245	53	[27]
OXA-2-like (22)	OXA(2)-F/R	GATAGTTGTGGCAGACGAAC, TCCATYCTGTTTGGCGTATC	N or A/ESBL	603	55	This study
OXA-10-like (38)	OXA(3)-F/R	ACAAAGAGTTCTCTGCCGAA, TCCACTTGATTAACTGCGGA	N or A/ESBL	418	53	This study
OXA-18	OXA(4)-F/R	ACCATCTGGCTGAAGGATT, CAGAAGTTTTCCGACAGGG	A/ESBL	506	54	This study
OXA-23-like (41)	OXA(5)-F/R	ACTAGGAGAAGCCATGAAGC, ATTTTCCATCTGGCTGCTC	N or A/ESBL or CARBA	369	55	[34]
OXA-45	OXA(6)-F/R	GCGGTAAACACACTGTCAT, GGGTCAATTGCTGCGAATA	A/ESBL	333	52	This study
OXA-48-like (38)	OXA(7)-F/R	ACCARGCATTTTTACCCGCA, GGCATATCCATATTCATCGC	N or A/ESBL or CARBA	538	55	This study
OXY (28)	OXY-F1/R1	TAAAGTGATGGCYGCCGC, RTTGGTGTGCCGTAATC	N/ESBL	517	54	This study
OXY (20)	OXY-F2/R2	CCCTGCCTTTATTGCTCTG, TTTATCTCCCAGACCCAG	N/ESBL	665	54	This study
PER (12)	PER-F1/R1	CTCGACGCTACTGATGGTA, TTCAATTGGTTCGGCTTGAC	N or A/ESBL	820	54	This study
PER (3)	PER-F2/R2	CTGTTAATCGTGCTGCAGT, GACAAATACCGCCACCAAT		530	53	This study
PME (1)	PME-F/R	GATCCACTTCAGCGATGAC, GACATCGTGGGTCTTGTTC	A/ESBL	478	54	This study
RAHN (2)	RAHN-F/R	ATGACGTCAGTTCAGCAAC, CATCCATTCCACCAGTTGC	N/ESBL	555	54	This study
RSA1 (1)	RSA-F1/R1	TCGACGATCCTCACTGTTT, GTTGGTGTTCAAATCGGT	N or A/ESBL or CARBA	483	53	This study
RSA2 (1)	RSA-F2/R2	TGTGGACCTTTCCGAAGAA, CGCGATCAGATTACGAGTG		475	55	This study
SGM (7)	SGM-F/R	CATGTCGTCGACCTTCAAG, ATCGGCAGCARCAGRTTGG	N/ESBL	225	58	This study
SHV (199)	SHV-F/R	TGGATGCCGNTGACNAACAGC, NTATCGGCGATAAACCAGNCC	N or A/BSBL, ESBL or CARBA	451	59	[34]

Table 3. Cont.

Target (Subtype)	Primer Name	Sequence (5′ to 3′ Direction) [a]	Natural (N) or Acquired (A)/Phenotype	Amplicon Size (bp)	Tm (°C)	Reference
SMO (1)	SMO-F/R	CTCACAGACCGTATACCGT, GAATGTCTCATCGCCGATC	N/ESBL	316	54	This study
TEM (199)	TEM-F/R	CACCAGTCACAGAAAAGCA, AGGGCTTACCATCTGC	N or A/BSBL or ESBL	450	54	[34]
SFO (1)	SFO-F/R	CTCGAGAAAACTCCGGTG, GTTAGGGTTTGCAGGCTTT	A/ESBL	473	54	This study
TLA (2)	TLA-F/R	GCTAAAGGTACGGATTCGC, CTTAACGCCAAGCTTGCTA	A/ESBL	417	54	This study
TLA2 (1)	TLA2-F/R	ATCGTGCTTGCTGTTTTGA, TCATTTGCCGCATTGTTCT	A/ESBL	623	52	This study
VEB (27)	VEB-F/R	TTTCCGATTGCTTTAGCCG, CCCAACATCATTAGTGGC	N or A/ESBL	553	54	[34]
YOC (1)	YOC-F/R	CCGGCATCAGAAGAGAAAA, GGATTCGGGTAGCTTTTGTT	N/ESBL	467	54	This study

[a] For degenerate primers: B = C or G or T; K = G or T; M = A or C; N = any base; R = A or G; S = G or C; W = A or T; Y = C or T. Abbreviations: AmpC—AmpC, ampicillin chromosomal cephalosporinase; BSBL—broad-spectrum β-lactamase; CARBA—carbapenemase; CTX-M, cefotaxime-hydrolyzing β-lactamase-Munich; ESBL—extended-spectrum β-lactamase; GES, Guiana extended-spectrum β-lactamase; KPC, Klebsiella pneumoniae carbapenemase; NDM, New Delhi metallo-β-lactamase; NSBL—narrow-spectrum β-lactamase; OXA, oxacillin carbapenemase/oxacillinase; SHV, sulfhydryl variant of the TEM enzyme; TEM, Temoneira class A extended-spectrum β-lactamase.

4. Materials and Methods

4.1. Sequence Analysis

A total of 624 sequences of genes encoding ESBLs (with definitive assignment) described in the BLDB (http://bldb.eu; last accessed in 31 May 2021) [1] were downloaded from the GenBank database. Comparison of nucleotide/amino acid sequences and mutation analysis were performed using the bioinformatics software Geneious Prime (Biomatters). Multiple sequence alignments were carried out using the default settings of the Geneious alignment algorithm (cost matrix: 51% similarity; gap open penalty: 12; and gap extension penalty: 3) to identify highly homologous regions suitable for designing primers.

4.2. Phylogenetic Tree Construction

The phylogenetic tree was made by Geneious software using PhyML based on the Le and Gascuel model. The first phylogenetic tree was obtained by comparing 216 various types of CTX-M enzymes; the second and third ones consist of 199 SHV and 199 TEM β-lactamases, respectively.

4.3. Designing Primers for PCR

Homologous regions in nucleotide sequences were used for designing primers with Primer3 (Geneious Prime) with the following requirements: an optimal melting temperature of 52–60 °C, a GC content varying from 40% to 60%, an optimal oligo length between 17 and 22 base pairs, and an amplification product size of 225 to 820 base pairs. All the oligonucleotides were tested in silico for hybridization with ESBL genes contained in the BLDB database. The primer specifications are listed in Table 3.

5. Conclusions

The present study reports 58 in silico and in vitro tested primer pairs for PCR assay that may be able to distinguish 99.8% of ESBL-producing bacteria. These may be part of diagnostic tests for the detection of observed resistance genes in bacterial pathogens. Such diagnostic tests can be used for early detection, monitoring and dissemination of ESBLs, thus contributing to reducing the spread of ESBL-positive bacteria, adequate antibiotic treatment and reducing health care costs.

Author Contributions: Conceptualization, P.M.; data curation, P.M.; formal analysis, P.M.; funding acquisition, P.M.; investigation, P.M., H.C., V.Z. and M.K.; methodology, P.M.; project administration, P.M.; resources, P.M. and M.K.; supervision, P.M.; validation, H.C. and V.Z.; visualization, P.M. and V.Z.; writing—original draft, P.M. and H.C.; writing—review & editing, P.M. and M.K. All authors have read and agreed to the published version of the manuscript.

Funding: This research was funded by Junior Grant from Palacky University Olomouc (JG_2019_005), "Increasing Internationalization of the Faculty of Medicine and Dentistry, Palacky University Olomouc" (SPP 210015017) and IGA LF 2021_022 project.

Conflicts of Interest: The authors declare no conflict of interest.

Abbreviations

A	alanine
AmpC	ampicillin chromosomal cephalosporinase
BSBL	broad-spectrum β-lactamase
C	cysteine
CARBA	carbapenemase
CTX-M	cefotaxime-hydrolyzing β-lactamase–Munich
E	glutamic acid
ESBLs	extended-spectrum β-lactamases
F	phenylalanine
G	glycine
GES	Guiana extended-spectrum β-lactamase

H	histidine
I	isoleucine
K	lysine
KPC	Klebsiella pneumoniae carbapenemase
L	leucine
M	methionine
MBLs	metallo- β-lactamases
NDM	New Delhi metallo- β-lactamase
NSBL	narrow-spectrum β-lactamase
OXA	oxacillinases
P	proline
Q	glutamine
R	arginine
S	serine
SHV	sulfhydryl variant of the TEM enzyme
T	threonine
TEM	Temoneira class A extended-spectrum β-lactamase
V	valine
W	tryptophan

References

1. Naas, T.; Oueslati, S.; Bonnin, R.A.; Dabos, M.L.; Zavala, A.; Dortet, L.; Retailleau, P.; Iorga, B.I. Beta-lactamase database (BLDB)—structure and function. *J. Enzym. Inhib. Med. Chem.* **2017**, *32*, 917–919. [CrossRef]
2. Jeon, J.H.; Hong, M.K.; Lee, J.H.; Lee, J.J.; Park, K.S.; Karim, A.M.; Jo, J.Y.; Kim, J.H.; Ko, K.S.; Kang, L.W.; et al. Structure of ADC-68, a novel carbapenem-hydrolyzing class C extended-spectrum beta-lactamase isolated from Acinetobacter baumannii. *Acta Crystallogr. D Biol. Crystallogr.* **2014**, *70*, 2924–2936. [CrossRef] [PubMed]
3. Mammeri, H.; Guillon, H.; Eb, F.; Nordmann, P. Phenotypic and biochemical comparison of the carbapenem-hydrolyzing activities of five plasmid-borne AmpC beta-lactamases. *Antimicrob. Agents Chemother.* **2010**, *54*, 4556–4560. [CrossRef] [PubMed]
4. Jousset, A.B.; Oueslati, S.; Bernabeu, S.; Takissian, J.; Creton, E.; Vogel, A.; Sauvadet, A.; Cotellon, G.; Gauthier, L.; Bonnin, R.A.; et al. False-Positive Carbapenem-Hydrolyzing Confirmatory Tests Due to ACT-28, a Chromosomally Encoded AmpC with Weak Carbapenemase Activity from Enterobacter kobei. *Antimicrob. Agents Chemother.* **2019**, *63*, e02388-18. [CrossRef]
5. Kaitany, K.C.; Klinger, N.V.; June, C.M.; Ramey, M.E.; Bonomo, R.A.; Powers, R.A.; Leonard, D.A. Structures of the class D Carbapenemases OXA-23 and OXA-146: Mechanistic basis of activity against carbapenems, extended-spectrum cephalosporins, and aztreonam. *Antimicrob. Agents Chemother.* **2013**, *57*, 4848–4855. [CrossRef] [PubMed]
6. Marathe, N.P.; Janzon, A.; Kotsakis, S.D.; Flach, C.F.; Razavi, M.; Berglund, F.; Kristiansson, E.; Larsson, D.G.J. Functional metagenomics reveals a novel carbapenem-hydrolyzing mobile beta-lactamase from Indian river sediments contaminated with antibiotic production waste. *Environ. Int.* **2018**, *112*, 279–286. [CrossRef] [PubMed]
7. Suh, B.; Bae, I.K.; Kim, J.; Jeong, S.H.; Yong, D.; Lee, K. Outbreak of meropenem-resistant Serratia marcescens comediated by chromosomal AmpC beta-lactamase overproduction and outer membrane protein loss. *Antimicrob. Agents Chemother.* **2010**, *54*, 5057–5061. [CrossRef]
8. Bonnet, R. Growing group of extended-spectrum beta-lactamases: The CTX-M enzymes. *Antimicrob. Agents Chemother.* **2004**, *48*, 1–14. [CrossRef]
9. Tanimoto, K.; Nomura, T.; Hashimoto, Y.; Hirakawa, H.; Watanabe, H.; Tomita, H. Isolation of Serratia fonticola Producing FONA, a Minor Extended-Spectrum beta-Lactamase (ESBL), from Imported Chicken Meat in Japan. *Jpn. J. Infect. Dis.* **2021**, *74*, 79–81. [CrossRef] [PubMed]
10. Zhou, D.; Sun, Z.; Lu, J.; Liu, H.; Lu, W.; Lin, H.; Zhang, X.; Li, Q.; Zhou, W.; Zhu, X.; et al. Characterization of a Novel Chromosomal Class C beta-Lactamase, YOC-1, and Comparative Genomics Analysis of a Multidrug Resistance Plasmid in Yokenella regensburgei W13. *Front. Microbiol.* **2020**, *11*, 2021. [CrossRef]
11. Toth, M.; Antunes, N.T.; Stewart, N.K.; Frase, H.; Bhattacharya, M.; Smith, C.A.; Vakulenko, S.B. Class D beta-lactamases do exist in Gram-positive bacteria. *Nat. Chem. Biol.* **2016**, *12*, 9. [CrossRef] [PubMed]
12. Bradford, P.A. Extended-spectrum beta-lactamases in the 21st century: Characterization, epidemiology, and detection of this important resistance threat. *Clin. Microbiol. Rev.* **2001**, *14*, 933–951. [CrossRef] [PubMed]
13. Paterson, D.L.; Bonomo, R.A. Extended-spectrum beta-lactamases: A clinical update. *Clin. Microbiol. Rev.* **2005**, *18*, 657–686. [CrossRef] [PubMed]
14. Naas, T.; Poirel, L.; Nordmann, P. Minor extended-spectrum beta-lactamases. *Clin. Microbiol. Infect.* **2008**, *14* (Suppl. 1), 42–52. [CrossRef]
15. Guillon, H.; Eb, F.; Mammeri, H. Characterization of CSP-1, a novel extended-spectrum beta-lactamase produced by a clinical isolate of Capnocytophaga sputigena. *Antimicrob. Agents Chemother.* **2010**, *54*, 2231–2234. [CrossRef] [PubMed]
16. Lamoureaux, T.L.; Vakulenko, V.; Toth, M.; Frase, H.; Vakulenko, S.B. A novel extended-spectrum beta-lactamase, SGM-1, from an environmental isolate of *Sphingobium* sp. *Antimicrob. Agents Chemother.* **2013**, *57*, 3783–3788. [CrossRef]
17. Pfennigwerth, N.; Lange, F.; Campos, C.B.; Hentschke, M.; Gatermann, S.G.; Kaase, M. Genetic and biochemical characterization of HMB-1, a novel subclass B1 metallo-beta-lactamase found in a Pseudomonas aeruginosa clinical isolate. *J. Antimicrob. Chemother.* **2017**, *72*, 1068–1073. [CrossRef]

18. Queenan, A.M.; Bush, K. Carbapenemases: The versatile beta-lactamases. *Clin. Microbiol. Rev.* **2007**, *20*, 440–458. [CrossRef]
19. Poirel, L.; Heritier, C.; Podglajen, I.; Sougakoff, W.; Gutmann, L.; Nordmann, P. Emergence in Klebsiella pneumoniae of a chromosome-encoded SHV beta-lactamase that compromises the efficacy of imipenem. *Antimicrob. Agents Chemother.* **2003**, *47*, 755–758. [CrossRef]
20. Poirel, L.; Ortiz de la Rosa, J.M.; Richard, A.; Aires-de-Sousa, M.; Nordmann, P. CTX-M-33, a CTX-M-15 derivative conferring reduced susceptibility to carbapenems. *Antimicrob. Agents Chemother.* **2019**, *63*, e01515-19. [CrossRef]
21. Alegria, A.; Arias-Temprano, M.; Fernandez-Natal, I.; Rodriguez-Calleja, J.M.; Garcia-Lopez, M.L.; Santos, J.A. Molecular Diversity of ESBL-Producing Escherichia coli from Foods of Animal Origin and Human Patients. *Int. J. Environ. Res. Public Health* **2020**, *17*, 1312. [CrossRef]
22. Bardon, J.; Mlynarcik, P.; Prochazkova, P.; Roderova, M.; Mezerova, K.; Kolar, M. Occurrence of bacteria with a dangerous extent of antibiotic resistance in poultry in the Central Region of Moravia. *Acta Vet. Brno* **2018**, *87*, 165–172. [CrossRef]
23. Zhang, H.; Zhou, Y.; Guo, S.; Chang, W. Prevalence and characteristics of extended-spectrum beta-lactamase (ESBL)-producing Enterobacteriaceae isolated from rural well water in Taian, China, 2014. *Environ. Sci. Pollut. Res. Int.* **2015**, *22*, 11488–11492. [CrossRef] [PubMed]
24. Abbott, I.; Cerqueira, G.M.; Bhuiyan, S.; Peleg, A.Y. Carbapenem resistance in Acinetobacter baumannii: Laboratory challenges, mechanistic insights and therapeutic strategies. *Expert Rev. Anti Infect. Ther.* **2013**, *11*, 395–409. [CrossRef] [PubMed]
25. Kolar, M.; Htoutou Sedlakova, M.; Urbanek, K.; Mlynarcik, P.; Roderova, M.; Hricova, K.; Mezerova, K.; Kucova, P.; Zapletalova, J.; Fiserova, K.; et al. Implementation of Antibiotic Stewardship in a University Hospital Setting. *Antibiotics* **2021**, *10*, 93. [CrossRef]
26. Mlynarcik, P.; Kolar, M. Molecular mechanisms of polymyxin resistance and detection of mcr genes. *Biomed. Pap. Med. Fac. Univ. Palacky Olomouc. Czech. Repub.* **2019**, *163*, 28–38. [CrossRef]
27. Mlynarcik, P.; Chalachanova, A.; Vagnerova, I.; Holy, O.; Zatloukalova, S.; Kolar, M. PCR Detection of Oxacillinases in Bacteria. *Microb Drug Resist.* **2020**. [CrossRef]
28. Bendjama, E.; Loucif, L.; Chelaghma, W.; Attal, C.; Bellakh, F.Z.; Benaldjia, R.; Kahlat, I.; Meddour, A.; Rolain, J.M. First detection of an OXA-48-producing Enterobacter cloacae isolate from currency coins in Algeria. *J. Glob. Antimicrob. Resist.* **2020**, *23*, 162–166. [CrossRef]
29. Gniadkowski, M. Evolution and epidemiology of extended-spectrum beta-lactamases (ESBLs) and ESBL-producing microorganisms. *Clin. Microbiol. Infect.* **2001**, *7*, 597–608. [CrossRef]
30. Canton, R.; Novais, A.; Valverde, A.; Machado, E.; Peixe, L.; Baquero, F.; Coque, T.M. Prevalence and spread of extended-spectrum beta-lactamase-producing Enterobacteriaceae in Europe. *Clin. Microbiol. Infect.* **2008**, *14* (Suppl. 1), 144–153. [CrossRef]
31. Bush, K. The ABCD's of beta-lactamase nomenclature. *J. Infect. Chemother.* **2013**, *19*, 549–559. [CrossRef]
32. Mlynarcik, P.; Bardon, J.; Htoutou Sedlakova, M.; Prochazkova, P.; Kolar, M. Identification of novel OXA-134-like beta-lactamases in *Acinetobacter lwoffii* and *Acinetobacter schindleri* isolated from chicken litter. *Biomed. Pap. Med. Fac. Univ. Palacky Olomouc. Czech. Repub.* **2019**, *163*, 141–146. [CrossRef]
33. Mlynarcik, P.; Roderova, M.; Kolar, M. Primer Evaluation for PCR and its Application for Detection of Carbapenemases in Enterobacteriaceae. *Jundishapur. J. Microbiol.* **2016**, *9*, e29314. [CrossRef]
34. Mlynarcik, P.; Dolejska, M.; Vagnerova, I.; Kutilová, I.; Kolar, M. Detection of clinically important β-lactamases by using PCR. *FEMS Microbiol. Lett.* **2021**, *368*, fnab068. [CrossRef] [PubMed]
35. Peleg, A.Y.; Seifert, H.; Paterson, D.L. Acinetobacter baumannii: Emergence of a successful pathogen. *Clin. Microbiol. Rev.* **2008**, *21*, 538–582. [CrossRef] [PubMed]
36. Peymani, A.; Naserpour-Farivar, T.; Zare, E.; Azarhoosh, K.H. Distribution of blaTEM, blaSHV, and blaCTX-M genes among ESBL-producing P. aeruginosa isolated from Qazvin and Tehran hospitals, Iran. *J. Prev. Med. Hyg.* **2017**, *58*, E155–E160. [PubMed]
37. Pagani, L.; Dell'Amico, E.; Migliavacca, R.; D'Andrea, M.M.; Giacobone, E.; Amicosante, G.; Romero, E.; Rossolini, G.M. Multiple CTX-M-Type extended-spectrum b-lactamases in nosocomial isolates of *Enterobacteriaceae* from a hospital in northern Italy. *J. Clin. Microbiol.* **2003**, *41*, 4264–4269. [CrossRef] [PubMed]

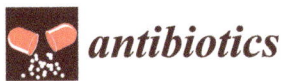

Article

Strong Antimicrobial and Healing Effects of Beta-Acids from Hops in Methicillin-Resistant *Staphylococcus aureus*-Infected External Wounds In Vivo

Radek Sleha [1], Vera Radochova [1], Jiri Malis [1,2], Alexander Mikyska [3], Milan Houska [4], Karel Krofta [5], Katerina Bogdanova [6], Sylva Janovska [1], Jaroslav Pejchal [7], Milan Kolar [6], Pavel Cermak [2] and Pavel Bostik [1,8,*]

1 Department of Epidemiology, Faculty of Military Health Sciences, University of Defence, 500 01 Hradec Kralove, Czech Republic; radek.sleha@unob.cz (R.S.); vera.radochova@unob.cz (V.R.); jiri.malis@ftn.cz (J.M.); sylva.janovska@unob.cz (S.J.)
2 Thomayer Hospital, 110 00 Prague, Czech Republic; pavel.cermak@lf3.cuni.cz
3 Research Institute of Brewing and Malting, 110 00 Prague, Czech Republic; mikyska@beerresearch.cz
4 Food Research Institute, 110 00 Prague, Czech Republic; milan.houska@vupp.cz
5 Hop Research Institute, 438 01 Zatec, Czech Republic; krofta@chizatec.cz
6 Department of Microbiology, Faculty of Medicine and Dentistry, University Hospital, Palacky University, 771 47 Olomouc, Czech Republic; katerina.bogdanova@fnol.cz (K.B.); kolar@fnol.cz (M.K.)
7 Department of Toxicology and Military Pharmacy, Faculty of Military Health Sciences, University of Defence, 500 01 Hradec Kralove, Czech Republic; jaroslav.pejchal@unob.cz
8 Institute of Clinical Microbiology, Faculty of Medicine in Hradec Kralove, Charles University and University Hospital, 500 05 Hradec Kralove, Czech Republic
* Correspondence: pavel.bostik@unob.cz

Abstract: *Staphylococcus* (S.) *aureus* is an important causative agent of wound infections with increasing incidence in the past decades. Specifically, the emergence of methicillin-resistant *S. aureus* (MRSA) causes serious problems, especially in nosocomial infections. Therefore, there is an urgent need to develop of alternative or supportive antimicrobial therapeutic modalities to meet these challenges. Purified compounds from hops have previously shown promising antimicrobial effects against MRSA isolates in vitro. In this study, purified beta-acids from hops were tested for their potential antimicrobial and healing properties using a porcine model of wounds infected by MRSA. The results show highly significant antimicrobial effects of the active substance in both the powder and Ambiderman-based application forms compared to both no-treatment control and treatment with Framycoin. Moreover, the macroscopic evaluation of the wounds during the treatment using the standardized Wound Healing Continuum indicated positive effects of the beta-acids on the overall wound healing. This is further supported by the microscopic data, which showed a clear improvement of the inflammatory parameters in the wounds treated by beta-acids. Thus, using the porcine model, we demonstrate significant therapeutic effects of hops compounds in the management of wounds infected by MRSA. Beta-acids from hops, therefore, represent a suitable candidate for the treatment of non-responsive nosocomial tissue infections by MRSA.

Keywords: hops; methicillin-resistant; *Staphylococcus aureus*; infection; porcine model

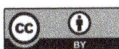

1. Introduction

Staphylococcus (S.) *aureus* is an etiologic agent of various infections in both humans and animals. These bacteria colonize the entry of the nasal cavity in up to 80% of the human population and can be found on other mucosal surfaces [1]. Its pathogenic potential is associated with a variety of diseases, ranging from minor skin infections to the life-threatening toxic shock syndrome. The skin and soft tissue infections (SSTI) caused by *S. aureus* represent one of the major current healthcare problems. SSTI are very often associated with inpatient care and *S. aureus* has become a major nosocomial pathogen worldwide [2,3].

For many years, the management of SSTI was accomplished using beta-lactam antimicrobial drugs that are effective against β-hemolytic streptococci. The emergence of antibiotic-resistant strains of *S. aureus*, commonly known as methicillin-resistant *S. aureus* (MRSA), has complicated the use of these standard treatment regimens. The increased prevalence of MRSA especially in nosocomial settings significantly increases the morbidity, mortality, length of stay, and cost burden. In addition, the utilization of standard antibiotic treatment schemes further induces bacterial resistance and can create an even higher burden for the patient [4]. To reverse this continually increasing bacterial resistance, effective non-classical antimicrobial treatment alternatives are urgently needed and have been investigated for several years. Among those, various hops extracts and individual hops compounds have shown an antimicrobial potential, and therefore, represent a useful solution for the treatment of SSTI. The biological activities of such compounds have been known for some time, including their antimicrobial and anti-inflammatory effects. The data from various laboratories, including ours, have shown potent in vitro antimicrobial activities of hops compounds (isolated from *Humulus lupulus* L.), such as xanthohumol or alfa- and beta-acids against many bacterial pathogens, such as MRSA, *Pseudomonas aeruginosa*, *Helicobacter pylori*, or *Clostridium* spp. [5–7]. With their minimal inhibitory concentrations being close to commonly used antibiotics, these compounds may represent useful treatment alternatives provided that they show these antimicrobial effects in vivo as well.

While various animal models may prove suitable for the in vivo studies of SSTI, the porcine model is commonly used in experimental wound healing and treatment experiments. The pig, therefore, is the animal of choice when developing a wound infection model due to its similarity of skin anatomy, physiology, and immune system to humans. Porcine models are well accepted as being one of the best for human dermal repair due to the similarities between porcine and human skin [8–12].

The purpose of this study was to analyze antimicrobial and therapeutic effects of natural compounds isolated from hops in the porcine model of MRSA-infected wounds.

2. Results

Our previous data showed that both xanthohumol and beta-acids from hops possess strong antimicrobial activity against MRSA in vitro under the standard testing conditions [5,13]. However, when using antimicrobial substances in vivo, especially in wounds, binding of the tested compounds to the proteins secreted during the healing process may substantially modify their efficacy. An assessment using a modified agar diffusion method in the presence of BSA was, therefore, performed to quantitate the antimicrobial effect of the hop compounds in the presence of increased concentrations of proteins (Figure 1).

The diameters of inhibition zones for individual hops compounds and a hydrophilic base—Ambiderman control—are presented in Table 1. Indeed, the presence of BSA substantially decreased the antimicrobial activities of the tested compounds. The growth inhibition of MRSA was no longer detectable in xanthohumol at any concentration used. Only beta-acids retained the antimicrobial effect, but it was achieved at higher concentrations than in standard in vitro testing conditions without the addition of BSA [13]. The tested concentrations—3%, 5%, and 10%—did not show any significant differences in the diameters of the inhibition zones. Based on these results, the further evaluation of xanthohumol in the in vivo porcine model was not performed.

The experimental porcine model was subsequently established to evaluate the antibacterial and healing effects of purified hops compounds in vivo. External wounds were created and experimentally infected with a quantified dose of bacterial suspension of MRSA. The beta-acids from hops were applied to the wounds on days 3 and 7 after infection either in a powder form or in Ambiderman base during standard surgical dressing. Framycoin was used as a positive control due to its efficacy against a wide spectrum of bacteria and general suitability in the porcine model [14]. Bacterial load in the wounds, their size and macroscopic appearance on the standardized Wound Healing Continuum [15] were assessed.

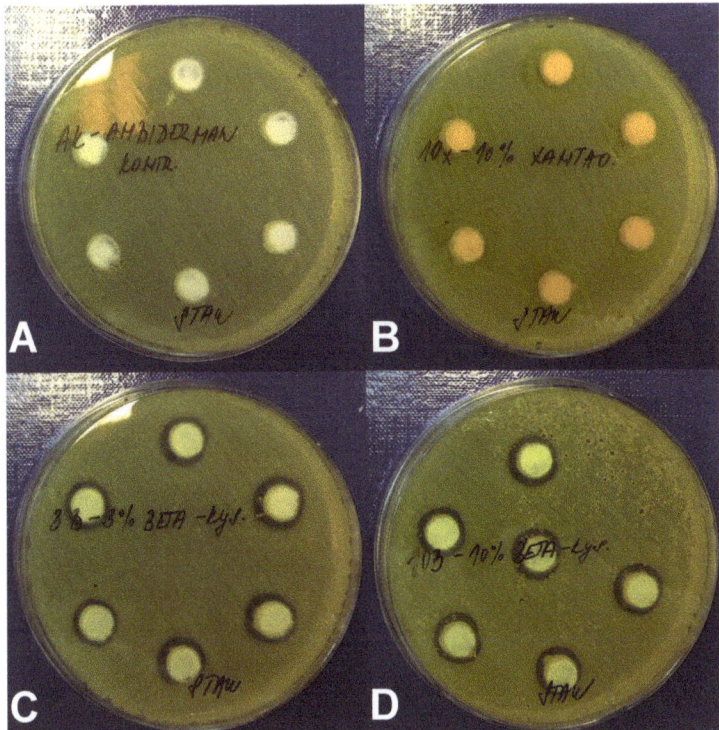

Figure 1. Antimicrobial activity of hop compounds in vitro. Agar diffusion test was performed using MRSA and compounds applied in Ambiderman base. (**A**) Ambiderman base only (negative control), (**B**) 10% xanthohumol, (**C**) 3% beta-acids and (**D**) 10% beta-acids. Inhibition zones.

Table 1. The antimicrobial activity of hops compounds against the MRSA strain obtained by the agar diffusion method.

Tested Compound	Diameter of Inhibition Zone (mm) [1]		
	3%	5%	10%
Beta-acids	11.2 ± 1.1	11.6 ± 1.3	12.8 ± 0.8
Xanthohumol	0	0	0
Ambiderman	0	0	0

[1] Data are presented as mean ± standard deviation of inhibition zone diameters ($n = 5$).

The first quantitation of MRSA in the wounds was performed on day 3 post-inoculation before the application of the first treatment to verify the infection of the wounds and then on days 7 and 10 to record the anti-microbial effect of the applied substances. The effects of beta-acids on the growth of MRSA are shown in Figure 2.

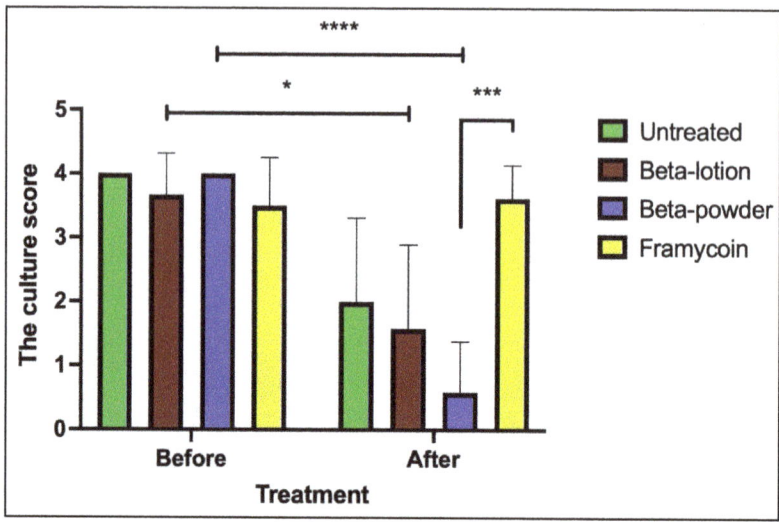

Figure 2. The effects of beta-acids on MRSA growth. Quantitation of MRSA in wounds before and on day 10 (after) of the treatment protocol is shown. Statistical significance (nonparametric Kruskal–Wallis test, multiple comparison test): * $p < 0.05$, *** $p < 0.001$, **** $p < 0.0001$.

All the wounds infected with MRSA showed a comparable bacterial growth before the treatments started. While some decrease in the culture score could be observed even in the untreated wounds, highly significant reductions of the bacterial growth were detected in the wounds treated with beta-acids in both the lotion and powder forms when compared to the pre-treatment levels ($p < 0.05$ and $p < 0.0001$, respectively). In addition, the beta-acid powder treatment exhibited a highly significant antimicrobial effect when compared to Framycoin ($p < 0.001$), which had no effect on the MRSA growth. Comparison of the bacterial growth levels in beta-acid treated wounds to the untreated ones revealed a clear positive effect of the beta-acid powder, although it was not statistically significant. These data show that the beta-acids exhibit a strong antimicrobial effect against the MRSA and this effect is pronounced the most when the substances are applied in the powder form.

To assess the effect of the compounds on wound healing, the areas of individual wounds were compared first as the general indicator of the healing process. Figure 3 shows that wound areas decreased during the experiment regardless of the infection or treatment used. Such results point to the innately high healing potential of porcine skin.

For more detailed wound assessment, the wound management framework characteristics were recorded and compared for the individual treatment modalities. In general, the signs of ongoing infection were clearly present during the first surgical dressing on day 3. The wounds with MRSA were characterized by hyperemia, redness in the surroundings, and pungent odor. On day 7, however, the wounds with beta-acids showed significant improvement compared to both the negative controls and Framycoin treatment. Wounds with beta-acids showed a decrease in redness, secretion, and odor. On day 10, the wounds treated with beta-acids were filled with fresh granulation tissue. Once again, the most pronounced effects were observed with the powder form of beta-acids. The detailed data for each wound recorded using original scales of the Wound Healing Continuum are available in Table S1 (Supplementary Material). To allow for further statistical analysis the original criteria were assigned numeric scores and the results of the color score and the total score evaluation on day 10 of the experiment are shown in Figure 4.

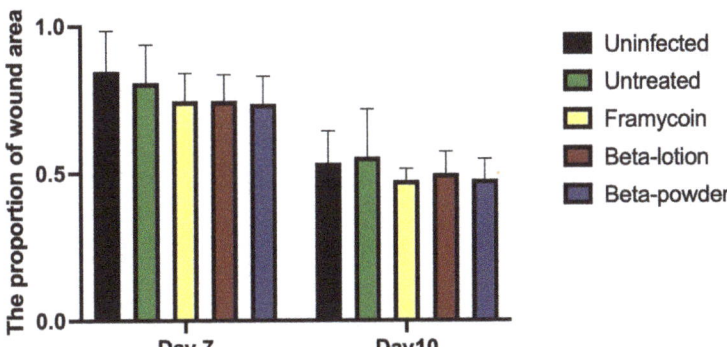

Figure 3. The effect of antibacterial treatments on the wound area. Areas of the individual wounds on days 7 and 10 were related to the respective wound area at the beginning of the experiment. The data are presented as means and standard deviations using the nonparametric Kruskal–Wallis test and multiple comparison test.

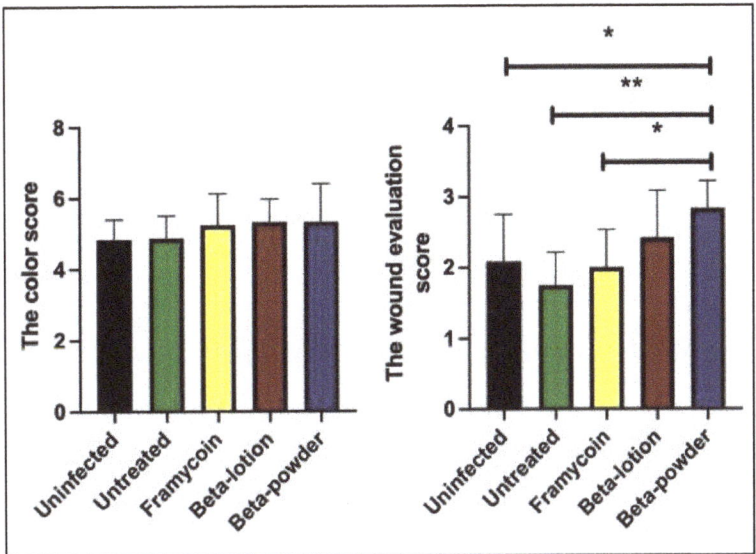

Figure 4. The wound healing evaluation. Individual wound characteristics were assigned numerical scores and the analysis for day 10 is shown. Statistical analysis was performed with the nonparametric Kruskal–Wallis test and the multiple comparison test (* $p < 0.05$ and ** $p < 0.01$).

While the color characteristics alone showed no significant differences between the individual treatments, the application of beta-acids exhibited a clear positive effect on the overall healing score. Beta-acids in powder form show marked and significant differences when compared to the untreated and Framycoin-treated wounds. Interestingly, the overall healing was improved even in comparison to the uninfected wounds, indicating a potential effect on the wound healing per se, not only in connection to its anti-microbial effects.

Finally, the effects of beta-acids on the MRSA-infected wounds were assessed on the microscopic level. Tissue samples from the wounds were processed as indicated in the Materials and Methods section, and the following categories of parameters were scored: epithelial tissue recovery, connective tissue recovery, and inflammatory parameters. The results of the effect of the treatments on the individual inflammatory parameters are shown in Figure 5.

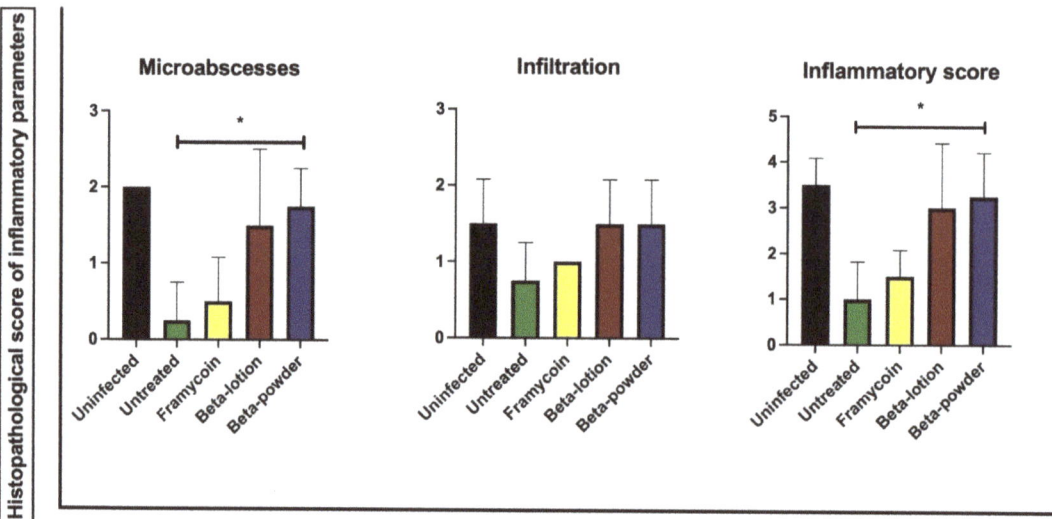

Figure 5. The histopathological score of the inflammatory response. The statistical analysis was performed with the parametric one-way ANOVA test with post hoc Dunn's comparison test (* $p < 0.05$).

The data show that beta-acids in both application forms exhibit distinct positive effects on microabscess formation and total inflammation score compared to the untreated wounds. These effects were statistically significant when beta-acids were applied in the powder form ($p < 0.05$). Representative microphotographs of the inflammatory changes in wounds after the infection and treatment with beta-acids are shown in Figure 6.

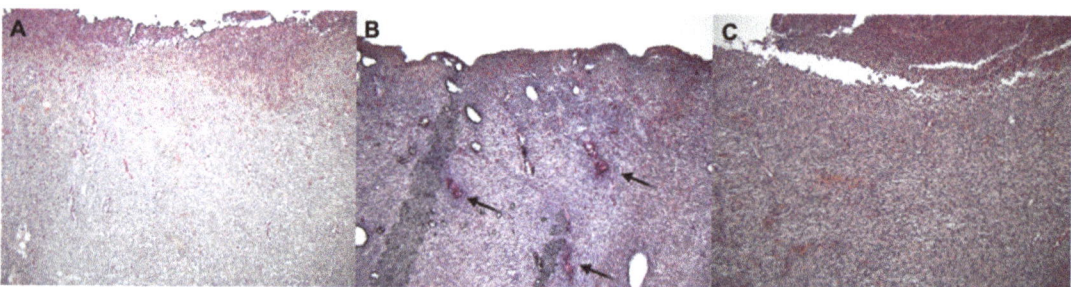

Figure 6. Histopathological changes in the wounds infected with MRSA. Naphthol AS-D chloroacetate-stained samples of porcine skin taken from the center of wounds, 100-fold the original magnification. (**A**) Non-infected samples with mild granulocyte infiltration underneath a fibrin clot. (**B**) Infected wound receiving no treatment with three microabscesses (indicated by arrows) and generally moderate granulocyte infiltration in the surrounding connective tissue. (**C**) Infected wound treated with beta-acid powder, showing mild granulocyte infiltration underneath a fibrin clot.

No effects of the infection or individual treatments were observed in the epithelial and connective tissue recovery parameters (Supplementary Figures S1–S5).

3. Discussion

Bacterial skin and soft tissue infections represented by impetigo, folliculitis, furuncle, carbuncle, erysipelas, cellulitis, fasciitis, and myonecrosis are frequently caused by *Staphylococcus aureus*. Kolar et al. proved that the most prevalent etiological agent of infected decubitus ulcers, leg ulcers, and bacterial infections of surgical wounds was *S. aureus* with an MRSA frequency of 9% [16]. At the same time, MRSA is one of the most common nosocomial pathogens with a worldwide distribution. Because of its higher resistance against regularly used antibiotics, the research of effective drugs with antimicrobial properties are still necessary. Several new antibiotics were developed in the past 20 years, which are active against certain strains of MRSA and also present a potential in the treatment of wounds (reviewed in [17]). Non-healing wounds currently represent one of the most common problems encountered in healthcare systems and hospitals. The healing process is often complicated by wound infection with nosocomial bacterial strains, which may lead to the development of chronic wounds requiring long-term treatment [18]. Given this situation, there is an urgent need for useful therapeutics providing both a healing effect and antimicrobial activity. The use of topical antibacterial treatments has clear advantages in the treatment of infected wounds [19]. However, while the antibiotic resistance of the bacteria is still on the rise, the antibiotic research and development has been stalled due to commercial and regulatory reasons [20–22].

Due to all the reasons above, there has been an increasing interest in recent years in compounds derived from plants and herbs for their medicinal properties and anti-microbial activities [17]. Thus, for example, tea tree oil and manuka honey have been shown to exert positive effects on healing of MRSA-infected wounds as adjuvant therapeutics improving the effect of antibiotics [23,24]. Numerous studies have shown that the hop cones represent an abundant source of components with apparent antimicrobial effects against selected strains of bacteria, viruses, fungi, and protozoa. One of the specific properties for the use of hop derivatives as therapeutics is their low cytotoxicity. These features lead to their safety and the absence of side effects. The antibacterial properties of some purified compounds from hops, namely xanthohumol and beta-acids, were determined for many pathogens (including MRSA) in vitro in the past [5,6,13].

The standard approach of testing individual compounds from natural sources rarely produces clinically valuable products, and potent activity against planktonic bacteria in a standard lab media rarely translates to the in vivo efficacy. Numerous studies have used porcine models to evaluate the therapeutic effects of novel compounds, treatments, or devices on wound healing processes [25–28].

In the presented study, the efficiency of the treatment with hop-isolated beta-acids was tested in the porcine model of external wounds infected with MRSA. We first successfully determined the antimicrobial activity of tested compounds against this pathogen in vitro under the conditions simulating the wound environment. The antimicrobial activity of xanthohumol on plates with 3% BSA content was no longer detectable. The antimicrobial effects of beta-acids were still detectable, but at much higher concentrations than the MICs detected using the standard conditions [13]. The effect was seen at all three concentrations used with no clear dose-dependent effects. This suggests that binding of beta-acids from hops to the proteins affects their antimicrobial properties, and therefore, the concentrations in the in vivo treatments have to be adjusted accordingly.

The in vivo activity of beta-acids was tested using a porcine model of external wounds that were previously infected with MRSA. Two modes of application of the active compounds have been used in this study—the lotion with Ambiderman base and the powder form—to investigate whether the mode of application influences the effect in the wounds. Ambiderman was selected based on our preliminary results from the in vitro tests, where it showed good release parameters for the hop compounds among the nine different bases tested (data not shown). The individual modes required differential approaches in the application and choice of dressings to ascertain that the compounds were uniformly spread in the wound and did not leak out between the individual dressings. Thus, beta-acids in lotion were applied in a standardized volume to uniformly fill each wound and covered with standard Curad dressings. The powder form was spread on each wound uniformly by a sterile loop and then covered with Polymem pads. These are non-adherent and non-absorbent polyurethane pads frequently used as dressings of skin wounds in surgery in combination with antibacterial substances [29,30]. As such, these pads prevent the leakage of the powdered substance out of the wound and its absorption into the dressing. Regardless of the application form, the amount of the active substance per wound was kept uniform to allow for direct comparisons. Both application forms of beta-acids exhibited strong antimicrobial properties against the MRSA infection in vivo. This was manifested by both the reduction of MRSA in the wounds and a decrease in inflammation when compared to the untreated controls. However, the powder form of beta-acids has shown both stronger antimicrobial effects and healing potential, which were statistically significant. This may be in part due to the mode of application, where the powder is applied to the wound and covered by a non-adherent dressing.

This study illustrates the antimicrobial and therapeutic potential of beta-bitter acids in wound healing with MRSA contamination. The obtained results show a potential of these compounds to be developed into an antimicrobial treatment scheme or to be used in combination with standardly used drugs. In fact, having all the following properties, beta-acids could represent an ideal topical antimicrobial for the use in chronic wounds: targeted antimicrobial spectrum, rapid and persistent activity allowing for infrequent dosing, low local absorption, activity in the presence of exudate, and low cost [31].

4. Materials and Methods

4.1. Hop Compounds

Pure beta-acids of hops were isolated from CO_2 extract (variety Magnum; Hopsteiner, Germany) by two purification steps according to schedule elaborated by the Hop Research Institute [32]. The first step involved partitioning of the extract solution in toluene in an alkaline medium of disodium carbonate ($c = 0.2$ mol·L^{-1}) and sodium hydroxide ($c = 1$ mol·L^{-1}). In the second step, crude extract of beta-acids containing up to 3% *w/w* of residual alpha-acids was recrystallized from the mixed solvent acetonitrile/water. The final preparation of the beta-acids was entirely free of alpha-acid residues. Residual solvent was removed by incubation at 40 °C and beta-acids of the minimal purity of 98% were then reconditioned in a refrigerator for 24 h and kept at −18 °C until further use. The lotions containing 3%, 5%, and 10% (*w/w*) of xanthohumol or beta-acids were prepared by mixing the purified compounds with hydrophilic base Ambiderman (containing 8 g of paraffinum liquidum, 12 g of paraffinum solidum, 2 g of alcohol stearilicus, 5 g of propylenglycolum, 2 g of slovasol 2430, 0.5 g of carbomera, 0.6 g of trolaminum, 0.2 g of methylparabenum, 0.05 g of propylparabenum, and 69.65 g of aqua purificata in 100 g). This formulation was previously shown to be effective in vitro [13].

4.2. Bacterial Strain and Culture Conditions

The methicillin-resistant *S. aureus* used in this study was from the collection of isolates of the Department of Microbiology of University Hospital in Olomouc (Czech Republic). The strain was cultured on blood agar, Mannitol Salt Phenol Red agar and Oxacillin Resistance Screening Agar Base (all from LabMediaServis, Jaromer, Czech Republic). Bacterial stocks for cryopreservation were prepared on porous beads (ITEST, Hradec Kralove, Czech Republic). For each experiment, fresh bacterial culture was prepared by inoculation of the porous bead with MRSA onto the blood agar plate. The subsequent culture was performed under aerobic conditions at 37 °C for 24 h.

Quantitation of bacterial growth in the wounds was performed by a semiquantitative culture analysis [33–36]. The swab samples from the wounds were inoculated onto agar plates. Then, the inocula were spread further using subsequent streaks of the loop progressing from quadrant 1 of the plate (the swab inoculum) towards quadrants 2, 3, and 4 in a step-wise fashion. The results were then reported as 1+, 2+, 3+, and 4+, indicating the number of the quadrant where the presence of bacterial growth was still detected, or as 0 for no apparent growth. The number of the quadrant with a detected growth directly correlates to the quantity of the bacteria in the inoculum.

4.3. In Vitro Antimicrobial Testing of Hops Compounds

The evaluation of antimicrobial activities of tested compounds from hops was performed using a modified protocol of agar diffusion test. Briefly, the bacterial inoculum in a physiologic solution with a turbidity of 0.5 degrees of the McFarland scale was prepared from a pure bacterial culture incubated for 24 h. Subsequently, the Mueller-Hinton agar containing culture dishes supplemented with 3% bovine albumin (BSA) were inoculated by streaking with the swab containing the inoculum. After 3–5 min of drying, the wells for the tested compounds were prepared using a sterile puncher. The distance of the center of each well from the edge of the petri dish was 24 mm and no closer than 10 to 15 mm. Afterward, each individual tested substance was applied into the wells at concentrations 3%, 5%, and 10% in a volume of 200 µL in three replicates. The agar plates were then incubated at 37 °C for 24 h and the diameter of zones of inhibition was recorded using a standardized ruler.

4.4. Animals and Housing

Six experimental adult female pigs (*Sus scrofa f. domestica*, hybrid of Czech White and Landrace breeds; weight mean 50 ± 0.3 kg) were enrolled into the study. The pigs were housed in an accredited vivarium (temperature 21 ± 1 °C, naturally light/dark cycle). All animals were fed with standard assorted A1 food (VKS Pohledecti Dvoraci, Havlickuv Brod, Czech Republic) in equal amounts twice a day and had free access to drinking water. The acclimatization period was 7 days before the experiment. The project was approved by the Institutional Review Board of the Animal Care Committee of the University of Defence (record number MO 54549/2017–684800 and MO 103191/2018–684800), Faculty of Military Health Sciences, Hradec Kralove, Czech Republic. Animals were treated in accordance with the European Convention for the Protection of Vertebrate Animals and in accordance with the ARRIVE Guidelines [37]. All workers who manipulated animals are holders of a Certificate of Professional Competence to Design Experiments and Experimental Trials under the Animal Welfare.

4.5. Experimental Model

The animals were anesthetized 30 min before start of the procedure with 30 mg/kg of ketamine (Narkamon, Bioveta, Ivanovice na Hane, Czech Republic), 40 mg·kg^{-1} azaperone (Stressnil, Janssen Pharmaceutica, Beerse, Belgium), and 0.05 mg·kg^{-1} of atropine (Atropin Biotika, Biotika Bohemia, Prague, Czech Republic), using intra-muscular injection. An intravenous application of propofol (Fresenius Kabi AG, Bad Homburg, Germany) was used for the subsequent maintenance of general anesthesia. The dorsal and lateral thorax of pigs were clipped, washed with an antimicrobial-free soap, and shaved with a razor. Each animal was intubated and prepared for surgery using isopropyl alcohol to disinfect the skin surface. The site of the wound creation was designated with a marking pen on the skin over the dorsal muscle of the pig. Ten deep surgical wounds were aseptically created by the scalpel using a sterile stainless steel template with the internal dimensions of 3.5×3.5 cm (Figure 7).

The wounds penetrated the level of the muscular fascia (approximately 0.5 cm deep). The wounds were separated by 30 mm of unwounded skin in between. Eight wounds were then inoculated with 0.1 mL of MRSA suspension at uniform concentrations of 9×10^5 CFU per mL and allowed to sit undisturbed for 2 min. Two non-infected wounds treated with 0.1 mL sterile saline solution were used in the study as a negative control. All wounds were covered with sterile compress. The wounds subsequently treated with the powder form of beta-acids were covered by non-adherent Curad dressings (Medline, Northfield, Minnesota), two layers of Omnifix Elastic (Hartmann Rico, Veverska Bityska, Czech Republic), and the entire animal loosely wrapped with elastic wrap. After each procedure, the general appearance of the animals was followed, including the willingness to eat and drink, signs of lameness or pain, and signs of systematic disease.

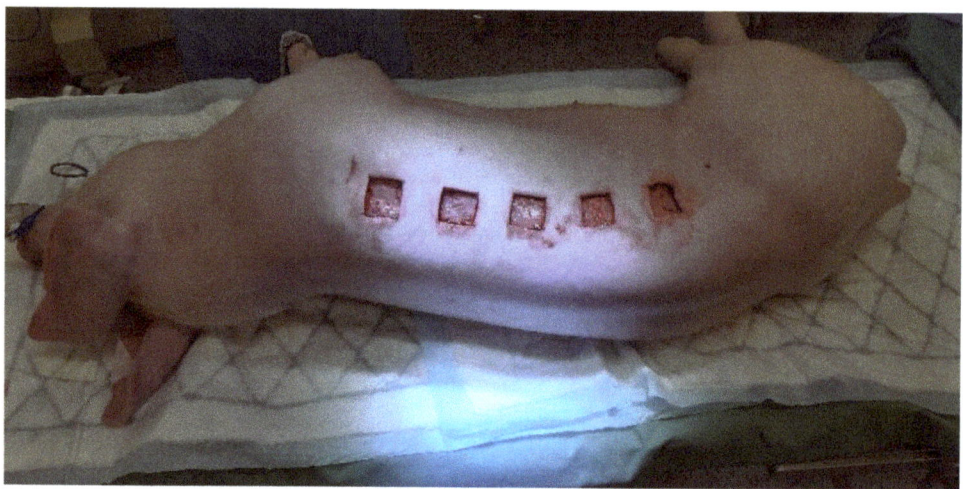

Figure 7. The creation of skin wounds.

4.6. Wound Treatments and Macroscopic Assessment

In all of the experiments, two wounds on each animal were established as negative controls (infection-free). The rest of the wounds were infected by MRSA suspension at uniform concentrations (see experimental model). The timeline of the experiment is provided in Figure 8.

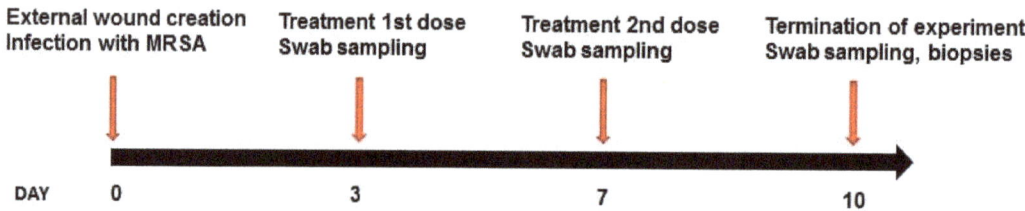

Figure 8. The timeline of the experiment.

On days 3 and 7 after the wound creation, the antibacterial compounds were applied during surgical dressings. Framycoin (active substances: zinc bacitracin 2500 IU, neomycin sulfas 52 mg in 10 g of ointment) in the amount of 1.5 g·wound^{-1} was used in two wounds on each animal as a positive control. The wounds were, thus, subsequently analyzed in the following categories—uninfected ($n = 12$), infected with no treatment ($n = 8$), Framycoin application ($n = 8$), application of beta-acids in powder form ($n = 12$), and in Ambiderman base ($n = 12$). The amount of beta-acids applied was kept uniform at 300 mg·wound^{-1}. Thus, the following procedures were used in the respective wounds: 300 mg·wound^{-1} of beta-acid powder were applied and uniformly spread on the wound surface by a sterile loop, while 3 mL of 10% beta-acid in Ambiderman base were applied to fill the wound. All dressings were performed in general anesthesia as follows. The animals were anesthetized 30 min before the procedure with 30 mg·kg^{-1} of ketamine (Narkamon, Bioveta) and 0.05 mg·kg^{-1} of atropine (AtropinBiotika, Biotika Bohemia), using intra-muscular injection. An intravenous application of propofol (Fresenius Kabi AG) was used for subsequent maintenance of general anesthesia. Before the first application of the hop substances on day 3, bacterial swab samples were taken from all wounds to evaluate the magnitude of MRSA infection. The wounds were macroscopically evaluated and pictures were taken.

After that, the active substances were applied to the wounds. The beta-acids in lotion filled the entire wound. The wounds were then covered with sterile compresses 5×5 cm and with two layers of Omnifix Elastic. The beta-acids in the powder form were dispersed over the whole wound area, after which the wound was filled with Polymem pads and covered with sterile compresses 5×5 cm and two layers of Omnifix Elastic. Wounds with Framycoin lotion were covered with compresses 5×5 cm and covered with two layers of Omnifix Elastic.

On day 7, the dressings and substance applications were performed in a similar manner, including the wound examinations. In the wounds with the lotion small irrigation with physiological saline solution was necessary to remove the dressing without wound irritation. On day 10 after the wound creation, the experiment was terminated: the last swabs were taken and, following the euthanasia, cross-sections of the wounds were sampled for histopathology.

During each surgical dressing the wound healing process was scored using The Wound Healing Continuum (color-based continuum) [15]. Briefly, this system scores selected criteria of wound appearance using colors (Black, Black-Yellow, Yellow, Yellow-Red, Red, Red-Pink, Pink) and the presence or absence of wound secretions, odor, and redness. A black wound base indicates a necrotic tissue with no healing potential. A yellow wound presents adherent fibrous material, which together with wound exudate is an ideal medium for bacterial growth and ongoing infection. The Red and Red-Pink tissue presents new vessel growth, granulation tissue matrix, and indicates wound healing.

4.7. Histopathology Examination

Collected samples were fixed in 10% neutral buffered formalin (Bamed, Ceske Budejovice, Czech Republic). Subsequently, they were histologically processed and stained with hematoxylin and eosin (both from Merck, Kenilworth, NJ, USA), according to Pejchal et al. [38]. Additionally, hydrated samples were stained with naphthol AS-D chloroacetate (specific esterase) Kit (Sigma-Aldrich, St. Louis, MO, USA) according to the manufacturer's instructions and with Masson's trichrome staining according to the procedure published previously [39].

Histopathological parameters were evaluated using an Olympus BX51 microscope (Olympus, Tokyo, Japan) by a histopathologist who was blinded to the treatment. The total histopathological score was defined as the sum of the nine parameters described in Table 2.

Table 2. Histopathological parameters of wound healing.

Score	0	1	2	3
Healing of Epithelial Layer				
Extent of the newly formed layer	Does not Reach the Cutting Edge	On the Cutting Edge	≤50% of the Wound [a]	≥50% of the Wound [a]
Differentiation	none	spinous	granular	
Healing of Connective Tissue				
Amount of Granulation Tissue	profound	moderate	scanty	absent
Collagen Fiber Orientation	vertical	mixed	horizontal	
Collagen Fiber Pattern	reticular	mixed	fascicle	
Amount of Early Collagen	profound	moderate	minimal	absent
Amount of Mature Collagen	absent	minimal	moderate	profound

Table 2. *Cont.*

Score	0	1	2	3
Inflammatory Response				
Inflammatory Infiltrate	Plenty	Moderate	Mild	A few
Presence of MicroAbscesses	≥2	1	none	

[a] does not include the cutting edge.

These parameters included healing of the epithelial layer (extent of newly formed epithelial layer and its predominant differentiation), healing of connective tissue (amount of granulation tissue, collagen fiber orientation, collagen fiber pattern, amount of early collagen, and amount of mature collagen), and the inflammatory response (inflammatory infiltrate, presence of microabscesses). Parameters 1, 2, and 3 were evaluated from hematoxylin-eosin-stained samples. Masson's trichrome-stained samples were used to measure parameters 4–7. Finally, naphthol AS-D chloroacetate-stained samples helped to score parameters 8 and 9. All these indicators were evaluated only in the area covering one microscopic field at 200-fold magnification beneath the fibrin or epithelial layer from the right to the left edge of the wound (at the surface).

4.8. Data Analysis

Data of wound monitoring were analyzed using Excel (Microsoft® 2010) software or imported into GraphPad Prism 9 (version 9.1.0, GraphPad Software Inc., San Diego, CA, USA) for further analysis. The normality was tested using the Shapiro–Wilk test. Normally distributed data were analyzed using a one-way ANOVA with post-hoc test. Non-normally distributed data were analyzed by a Kruskal–Wallis test with multiple comparison test. The differences were considered significant when $p \leq 0.05$.

5. Conclusions

Taken together, the data from our porcine model of the in vivo infection of MRSA-infected wounds show clear effects of beta-acids from hops on both the reduction of bacterial load in the wounds and improvement of macroscopic as well as microscopic parameters of wound healing. The powder application form of beta-acids shows superior results to those obtained with the active compound in the Ambiderman base. The presented study determined in the animal model that the beta-bitter from hop acids significantly improve both the wound healing process and antibacterial activity. Thus, these compounds could have potential for human application.

6. Patents

Bostik P, Sleha R, Houska M, Mikyska A, Krofta K inventors. Lecebna latka z chmele pro tezce se hojici rany jako nahrada antibiotik a zpusob jeji aplikace (Medicinal substance from hops for difficult-to-heal wounds as a substitute for antibiotics and the method of its application). Czech patent application number PV 2021–195. Industrial Property Office of the Czech Republic. Apr 19, 2021. Czech

Bostik P, Sleha R, Houska M, Mikyska A, Krofta K inventors. Lecebna latka z chmele pro tezce se hojici rany jako nahrada antibiotik a zpusob jeji aplikace (Medicinal substance from hops for difficult-to-heal wounds as a substitute for antibiotics and the method of its application). Czech utility model application number PUV 2021–38741. Industrial Property Office of the Czech Republic. 19 April 2021. Czech

Supplementary Materials: The following are available online at https://www.mdpi.com/article/10.3390/antibiotics10060708/s1, Table S1, The original wound healing evaluation scores; Figure S1, The histopathological score of epithelial tissue parameters; Figure S2, The histopathological score of connective tissue recovery; Figure S3, The total histopathological score; Figure S4, Histopathological changes in the wounds infected with MRSA; Figure S5, Histopathological changes in the wounds infected with MRSA.

Author Contributions: Conceptualization, P.B., R.S. and P.C.; methodology, R.S., J.M. and V.R.; validation, S.J., R.S. and J.P.; investigation, K.B., R.S., J.M. and V.R.; resources, A.M., K.K. and M.H.; data curation, R.S., V.R. and J.P.; writing—original draft preparation, R.S.; writing—review and editing, J.P., M.K. and P.B.; supervision, P.B. and M.K.; funding acquisition, P.B. All authors have read and agreed to the published version of the manuscript.

Funding: This research was funded by the Czech Health Research Council of Czech Republic grant NV- 17-31765A, and the Ministry of Defence of the Czech Republic—long-term organization development plan.

Institutional Review Board Statement: The study was conducted according to the guidelines of the Declaration of Helsinki and approved by the Institutional Review Board of the Animal Care Committee of the University of Defence (record number MO 54549/2017–684800 and MO 103191/2018–684800), Faculty of Military Health Sciences, Hradec Kralove, Czech Republic.

Informed Consent Statement: Not applicable.

Data Availability Statement: Data are available on request due to ethical restrictions.

Conflicts of Interest: The authors declare no conflict of interest. The funders had no role in the design of the study, in the collection, analyses, or interpretation of data, in the writing of the manuscript, or in the decision to publish the results.

References

1. Sakr, A.; Bregeon, F.; Mege, J.L.; Rolain, J.M.; Blin, O. *Staphylococcus aureus* Nasal Colonization: An Update on Mechanisms, Epidemiology, Risk Factors, and Subsequent Infections. *Front. Microbiol.* **2018**, *9*, 2419. [CrossRef] [PubMed]
2. Lone, A.G.; Atci, E.; Renslow, R.; Beyenal, H.; Noh, S.; Fransson, B.; Abu-Lail, N.; Park, J.J.; Gang, D.R.; Call, D.R. *Staphylococcus aureus* induces hypoxia and cellular damage in porcine dermal explants. *Infect. Immun.* **2015**, *83*, 2531–2541. [CrossRef] [PubMed]
3. McCaig, L.F.; McDonald, L.C.; Mandal, S.; Jernigan, D.B. *Staphylococcus aureus*-associated skin and soft tissue infections in ambulatory care. *Emerg. Infect. Dis.* **2006**, *12*, 1715–1723. [CrossRef] [PubMed]
4. Turner, N.A.; Sharma-Kuinkel, B.K.; Maskarinec, S.A.; Eichenberger, E.M.; Shah, P.P.; Carugati, M.; Holland, T.L.; Fowler, V.G., Jr. Methicillin-resistant *Staphylococcus aureus*: An overview of basic and clinical research. *Nat. Rev. Microbiol.* **2019**, *17*, 203–218. [CrossRef]
5. Bogdanova, K.; Roderova, M.; Kolar, M.; Langova, K.; Dusek, M.; Jost, P.; Kubelkova, K.; Bostik, P.; Olsovska, J. Antibiofilm activity of bioactive hop compounds humulone, lupulone and xanthohumol toward susceptible and resistant staphylococci. *Res. Microbiol.* **2018**, *169*, 127–134. [CrossRef] [PubMed]
6. Cermak, P.; Olsovska, J.; Mikyska, A.; Dusek, M.; Kadleckova, Z.; Vanicek, J.; Nyc, O.; Sigler, K.; Bostikova, V.; Bostik, P. Strong antimicrobial activity of xanthohumol and other derivatives from hops (*Humulus lupulus* L.) on gut anaerobic bacteria. *APMIS* **2017**, *125*, 1033–1038. [CrossRef]
7. Roehrer, S.; Behr, J.; Stork, V.; Ramires, M.; Medard, G.; Frank, O.; Kleigrewe, K.; Hofmann, T.; Minceva, M. Xanthohumol C. A minor bioactive hop compound: Production, purification strategies and antimicrobial test. *J. Chromatogr. B Analyt. Technol. Biomed. Life Sci.* **2018**, *1095*, 39–49. [CrossRef]
8. Barington, K.; Dich-Jorgensen, K.; Jensen, H.E. A porcine model for pathomorphological age assessment of surgically excised skin wounds. *Acta Vet. Scand.* **2018**, *60*, 33. [CrossRef]
9. Dai, T.; Kharkwal, G.B.; Tanaka, M.; Huang, Y.Y.; Bil de Arce, V.J.; Hamblin, M.R. Animal models of external traumatic wound infections. *Virulence* **2011**, *2*, 296–315. [CrossRef]
10. Jensen, L.K.; Johansen, A.S.B.; Jensen, H.E. Porcine Models of Biofilm Infections with Focus on Pathomorphology. *Front. Microbiol.* **2017**, *8*, 1961. [CrossRef]
11. Meyer, W.; Schwarz, R.; Neurand, K. The skin of domestic mammals as a model for the human skin, with special reference to the domestic pig. *Curr. Probl. Dermatol.* **1978**, *7*, 39–52. [CrossRef]
12. Zurawski, D.V.; Black, C.C.; Alamneh, Y.A.; Biggemann, L.; Banerjee, J.; Thompson, M.G.; Wise, M.C.; Honnold, C.L.; Kim, R.K.; Paranavitana, C.; et al. A Porcine Wound Model of Acinetobacter baumannii Infection. *Adv. Wound Care (New Rochelle)* **2019**, *8*, 14–27. [CrossRef] [PubMed]
13. Bogdanova, K.; Kolar, M.; Langova, K.; Dusek, M.; Mikyska, A.; Bostikova, V.; Bostik, P.; Olsovska, J. Inhibitory effect of hop fractions against Gram-positive multi-resistant bacteria. A pilot study. *Biomed. Pap. Med. Fac. Univ. Palacky. Olomouc Czech Repub* **2018**. [CrossRef] [PubMed]
14. Bacitracin—Natural Peptide with Minimal Resistance Issues. Available online: https://www.thepigsite.com/articles/bacitracin-natural-peptide-with-minimal-resistance-issues (accessed on 15 May 2018).

15. Gray, D.; White, R.; Cooper, P.; Kingsley, A. Applied Wound Management and Using the Wound Healing Continuum in Practice. *Wound Essent.* **2010**, *5*, 131–139.
16. Kolar, M.; Cermak, P.; Hobzova, L.; Bogdanova, K.; Neradova, K.; Mlynarcik, P.; Bostik, P. Antibiotic Resistance in Nosocomial Bacteria Isolated from Infected Wounds of Hospitalized Patients in Czech Republic. *Antibiotics (Basel)* **2020**, *9*, 342. [CrossRef]
17. Dou, J.L.; Jiang, Y.W.; Xie, J.Q.; Zhang, X.G. New is old, and old is new: Recent advances in antibiotic-based, antibiotic-free and ethnomedical treatments against methicillin-resistant *Staphylococcus aureus* wound infections. *Int. J. Mol. Sci* **2016**, *17*, 617. [CrossRef]
18. Nusbaum, A.G.; Gil, J.; Rippy, M.K.; Warne, B.; Valdes, J.; Claro, A.; Davis, S.C. Effective method to remove wound bacteria: Comparison of various debridement modalities in an in vivo porcine model. *J. Surg. Res.* **2012**, *176*, 701–707. [CrossRef]
19. Lio, P.A.; Kaye, E.T. Topical antibacterial agents. *Infect. Dis. Clin. N. Am.* **2009**, *23*, 945–963. [CrossRef]
20. Arias, C.A.; Murray, B.E. Antibiotic-resistant bugs in the 21st century—A clinical super-challenge. *N. Engl. J. Med.* **2009**, *360*, 439–443. [CrossRef]
21. Boucher, H.W.; Talbot, G.H.; Bradley, J.S.; Edwards, J.E.; Gilbert, D.; Rice, L.B.; Scheld, M.; Spellberg, B.; Bartlett, J. Bad bugs, no drugs: No ESKAPE! An update from the Infectious Diseases Society of America. *Clin. Infect. Dis.* **2009**, *48*, 1–12. [CrossRef] [PubMed]
22. Spellberg, B.; Powers, J.H.; Brass, E.P.; Miller, L.G.; Edwards, J.E., Jr. Trends in antimicrobial drug development: Implications for the future. *Clin. Infect. Dis.* **2004**, *38*, 1279–1286. [CrossRef]
23. Edmondson, M.; Newall, N.; Carville, K.; Smith, J.; Riley, T.V.; Carson, C.F. Uncontrolled, open-label, pilot study of tea tree (Melaleuca alternifolia) oil solution in the decolonisation of methicillin-resistant *Staphylococcus aureus* positive wounds and its influence on wound healing. *Int. Wound J.* **2011**, *8*, 375–384. [CrossRef]
24. Jenkins, R.; Cooper, R. Improving antibiotic activity against wound pathogens with manuka honey in vitro. *PLoS ONE* **2012**, *7*, e45600. [CrossRef]
25. Davis, S.C.; Li, J.; Gil, J.; Head, C.; Valdes, J.; Glinos, G.D.; Solis, M.; Higa, A.; Pastar, I. Preclinical evaluation of a novel silver gelling fiber dressing on *Pseudomonas aeruginosa* in a porcine wound infection model. *Wound Repair Regen.* **2019**, *27*, 360–365. [CrossRef] [PubMed]
26. Hadad, I.; Johnstone, B.H.; Brabham, J.G.; Blanton, M.W.; Rogers, P.I.; Fellers, C.; Solomon, J.L.; Merfeld-Clauss, S.; DesRosiers, C.M.; Dynlacht, J.R.; et al. Development of a porcine delayed wound-healing model and its use in testing a novel cell-based therapy. *Int J. Radiat. Oncol. Biol. Phys.* **2010**, *78*, 888–896. [CrossRef]
27. Malmsjo, M.; Ingemansson, R.; Martin, R.; Huddleston, E. Negative-pressure wound therapy using gauze or open-cell polyurethane foam: Similar early effects on pressure transduction and tissue contraction in an experimental porcine wound model. *Wound Repair Regen.* **2009**, *17*, 200–205. [CrossRef]
28. Mokhtari, A.; Gustafsson, R.; Sjogren, J.; Nilsson, J.; Lindstedt, S.; Malmsjo, M.; Ingemansson, R. Haemodynamic effects of -75 mmHg negative pressure therapy in a porcine sternotomy wound model. *Int. Wound J.* **2009**, *6*, 48–54. [CrossRef] [PubMed]
29. Dos Santos, M.R.; Alcaraz-Espinoza, J.J.; da Costa, M.M.; de Oliveira, H.P. Usnic acid-loaded polyaniline/polyurethane foam wound dressing: Preparation and bactericidal activity. *Mater. Sci. Eng. C Mater. Biol. Appl.* **2018**, *89*, 33–40. [CrossRef]
30. Lee, J.W.; Song, K.Y. Evaluation of a polyurethane foam dressing impregnated with 3% povidone-iodine (Betafoam) in a rat wound model. *Ann. Surg. Treat. Res.* **2018**, *94*, 1–7. [CrossRef]
31. Lipsky, B.A.; Hoey, C. Topical antimicrobial therapy for treating chronic wounds. *Clin. Infect. Dis.* **2009**, *49*, 1541–1549. [CrossRef] [PubMed]
32. Krofta, K.; Liskova, H.; Vrabcova, S. Process for Preparing Pure Beta Acids of Hop. CZ303017B6, 29 February 2012.
33. Elmarsafi, T.; Garwood, C.S.; Steinberg, J.S.; Evans, K.K.; Attinger, C.E.; Kim, P.J. Effect of semiquantitative culture results from complex host surgical wounds on dehiscence rates. *Wound Repair Regen.* **2017**, *25*, 210–216. [CrossRef]
34. Hashimoto, S.; Shime, N. Evaluation of semi-quantitative scoring of Gram staining or semi-quantitative culture for the diagnosis of ventilator-associated pneumonia: A retrospective comparison with quantitative culture. *J. Intensive Care* **2013**, *1*, 2. [CrossRef] [PubMed]
35. Jault, P.; Leclerc, T.; Jennes, S.; Pirnay, J.P.; Que, Y.A.; Resch, G.; Rousseau, A.F.; Ravat, F.; Carsin, H.; Le Floch, R.; et al. Efficacy and tolerability of a cocktail of bacteriophages to treat burn wounds infected by Pseudomonas aeruginosa (PhagoBurn): A randomised, controlled, double-blind phase 1/2 trial. *Lancet Infect. Dis.* **2019**, *19*, 35–45. [CrossRef]
36. Kallstrom, G. Are quantitative bacterial wound cultures useful? *J. Clin. Microbiol.* **2014**, *52*, 2753–2756. [CrossRef] [PubMed]
37. Kilkenny, C.; Browne, W.J.; Cuthi, I.; Emerson, M.; Altman, D.G. Improving bioscience research reporting: The ARRIVE guidelines for reporting animal research. *Vet. Clin. Pathol.* **2012**, *41*, 27–31. [CrossRef] [PubMed]
38. Pejchal, J.; Novotny, J.; Marak, V.; Osterreicher, J.; Tichy, A.; Vavrova, J.; Sinkorova, Z.; Zarybnicka, L.; Novotna, E.; Chladek, J.; et al. Activation of p38 MAPK and expression of TGF-beta1 in rat colon enterocytes after whole body gamma-irradiation. *Int. J. Radiat. Biol.* **2012**, *88*, 348–358. [CrossRef]
39. Pavlik, V.; Sobotka, L.; Pejchal, J.; Cepa, M.; Nesporova, K.; Arenbergerova, M.; Mrozkova, A.; Velebny, V. Silver distribution in chronic wounds and the healing dynamics of chronic wounds treated with dressings containing silver and octenidine. *FASEB J.* **2021**, *35*, e21580. [CrossRef]

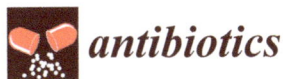

Article

Strong Antimicrobial Effects of Xanthohumol and Beta-Acids from Hops against *Clostridioides difficile* Infection In Vivo

Radek Sleha [1], Vera Radochova [1], Alexander Mikyska [2], Milan Houska [3], Radka Bolehovska [4], Sylva Janovska [1], Jaroslav Pejchal [5], Lubica Muckova [5], Pavel Cermak [6] and Pavel Bostik [1,4,7,*]

1. Department of Epidemiology, Faculty of Military Health Sciences, University of Defence, 500 03 Hradec Kralove, Czech Republic; radek.sleha@unob.cz (R.S.); vera.radochova@unob.cz (V.R.); sylva.janovska@unob.cz (S.J.)
2. Research Institute of Brewing and Malting, 110 00 Prague, Czech Republic; mikyska@beerresearch.cz
3. Food Research Institute, 110 00 Prague, Czech Republic; milan.houska@vupp.cz
4. Institute of Clinical Microbiology, University Hospital, 500 03 Hradec Kralove, Czech Republic; radka.bolehovska@fnhk.cz
5. Department of Toxicology and Military Pharmacy, Faculty of Military Health Sciences, University of Defence, 500 03 Hradec Kralove, Czech Republic; jaroslav.pejchal@unob.cz (J.P.); Lubica.Muckova@unob.cz (L.M.)
6. Thomayer Hospital, 110 00 Prague, Czech Republic; pavel.cermak@ftn.cz
7. Department of Clinical Microbiology, Faculty of Medicine in Hradec Kralove, Charles University, 500 03 Hradec Kralove, Czech Republic
* Correspondence: pavel.bostik@unob.cz

Citation: Sleha, R.; Radochova, V.; Mikyska, A.; Houska, M.; Bolehovska, R.; Janovska, S.; Pejchal, J.; Muckova, L.; Cermak, P.; Bostik, P. Strong Antimicrobial Effects of Xanthohumol and Beta-Acids from Hops against *Clostridioides difficile* Infection In Vivo. *Antibiotics* **2021**, *10*, 392. https://doi.org/10.3390/antibiotics10040392

Academic Editor: Ashish Pathak

Received: 25 February 2021
Accepted: 3 April 2021
Published: 6 April 2021

Publisher's Note: MDPI stays neutral with regard to jurisdictional claims in published maps and institutional affiliations.

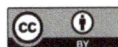

Copyright: © 2021 by the authors. Licensee MDPI, Basel, Switzerland. This article is an open access article distributed under the terms and conditions of the Creative Commons Attribution (CC BY) license (https://creativecommons.org/licenses/by/4.0/).

Abstract: *Clostridioides* (C.) *difficile* is an important causative pathogen of nosocomial gastrointestinal infections in humans with an increasing incidence, morbidity, and mortality. The available treatment options against this pathogen are limited. The standard antibiotics are expensive, can promote emerging resistance, and the recurrence rate of the infection is high. Therefore, there is an urgent need for new approaches to meet these challenges. One of the possible treatment alternatives is to use compounds available in commonly used plants. In this study, purified extracts isolated from hops—alpha and beta acids and xanthohumol—were tested in vivo for their inhibitory effect against *C. difficile*. A rat model of the peroral intestinal infection by *C. difficile* has been developed. The results show that both xanthohumol and beta acids from hops exert a notable antimicrobial effect in the *C. difficile* infection. The xanthohumol application showed the most pronounced antimicrobial effect together with an improvement of local inflammatory signs in the large intestine. Thus, the hops compounds represent promising antimicrobial agents for the treatment of intestinal infections caused by *C. difficile*.

Keywords: hops; *C. difficile*; infection; rat model

1. Introduction

C. difficile (formerly *Clostridium difficile*) is an anaerobic, spore-forming Gram-positive bacterium, which is widely found in the mammalian gastrointestinal tract (GIT), including in humans. Its growth is under physiological circumstances suppressed by the intestinal microbiome. One of the main virulence factors of *C. difficile* is the ability to form aerotolerant spores allowing bacteria to persist within the host and to disseminate by patient-to-patient contact or environmental contamination. Clostridial toxins A and B represent other important pathogenetic factors. These exotoxins have enterotoxic and cytotoxic activity that cause primary symptoms of the disease [1–3].

C. difficile is opportunistic bacteria, a pathological role which usually manifests in hospital settings in patients with antibiotic treatment that alter the colonic microbiome. The extensive antibiotic resistance of *C. difficile* leads to its proliferation in the colon and toxin production. The other patient-related risk factors affecting this process are advanced age, increased severity of underlying illness, prior hospitalization, use of feeding tubes, gastrointestinal surgery, and therapy using proton-pump inhibitors. Clinical symptoms of *C. difficile* infection manifest by signs ranging from mild diarrhea to pseudomembranous colitis, toxic megacolon, bowel perforation, and sepsis [4,5].

The treatment strategy of the *C. difficile*-induced infection depends on the health status of the patient and comorbidities. The first step in treating *C. difficile* is to discontinue the antibiotic therapy that triggered the *C. difficile* overgrowth leading to symptoms or, if necessary, to replace the antibiotic with another one. In intermediate and severe cases, antibiotics remain the recommended treatment. Vancomycin and metronidazole are the antibiotics of choice. They are the most efficient ones in clinical practice. The other drugs utilized in such cases include fidaxomicin, tigecycline, or teicoplanin. Recurrent *C. difficile* infections occur in up to 35% of cases due to the relapse of infection or reinfection with another strain [6–9]. Preserving physiological microbiome and microbial diversity in the gastrointestinal tract may prevent or even treat the disease. Other potential therapeutical modalities represent non-antibiotic therapies, such as the application of probiotics, intravenous immunoglobulins, and fecal transplants [2,5,10].

However, the commonly used antibiotic therapy could induce bacterial resistance and create a burden for the patient. Therefore, effective non-antibiotic alternatives are urgently needed and have been a focus of research for several years, including plant derivatives. Among those, various hops extracts and individual hops compounds have been known for some time for their antimicrobial activity. Strong antimicrobial activity of hops compounds (isolated from *Humulus lupulus* L.), including xanthohumol or alfa- and beta-bitter acids, has been reported against *C. difficile* in vitro. With minimal inhibitory concentrations being close to commonly used antibiotics, these compounds may represent a potential alternative for treating *C. difficile* infections [11–16].

Various animals pretreated with antibiotic regimens followed by oral challenge with *C. difficile* have been used as suitable models for *C. difficile*-induced disease [1,5,17–20].

The aim of this study was to determine the antibacterial properties of pure hops extracts of alpha- and beta-bitter acids and xanthohumol in *C. difficile* infection in vivo. For this purpose, a rat model of infection was developed.

2. Results

To evaluate the in vivo antibacterial effect of purified hops compounds, the experimental animals were first conditioned using an antibiotic regimen to clear their intestines from microflora and the endogenous *C. difficile* infection. The animals were then experimentally infected with a quantified dose of ribotyped hypervirulent *C. difficile* strain. Several different bacterial isolates were first tested for their pathogenicity in rats leading to the selection of the most pathogenic one (data not shown). A total of 35 animals divided into five experimental groups were then monitored for both the general signs of *C. difficile*-induced disease and for the presence of the bacteria in feces. Prior to the infection of animals with the experimental strain, only two animals tested positive for the endogenous colonization with *C. difficile*. Both of them belonged to the group subsequently treated with beta-bitter acids. One of these rats died during the experiment. Within three days post-infection, all animals were culture positive for the presence of vegetative form or spores of *C. difficile*. The general clinical symptoms of *C. difficile* infection were also observed in all animals (apathy, bristle coat). At this time point, the administration of antibacterial substances started (xanthohumol, beta-acids, xanthohumol + beta-acids, or vancomycin), except for the control group which received no treatment. Alpha bitter acids were not included in this study as they showed only a limited effectivity in vitro [13] and no effect in a preliminary experiment in vivo (data not shown).

The body weight of each animal was monitored during the entire experiment. Until day 3 post-infection, all infected animals suffered weight loss, and several rats also exhibited symptoms of diarrhea. After the onset of antimicrobial treatment, the body weight of each treated animal started to improve rapidly. As illustrated in Figure 1, all tested hops compounds and vancomycin effectively stopped further weight loss of animals and led to the normalization of their body weight compared to the untreated control group. All treated groups showed significant differences in body weight on days 7, 8, and 9 ($p < 0.05$) compared to the untreated control. The most profound and rapid positive effect of the hops compound was observed especially in the beta-bitter acid group. This was despite the fact that the animals in all three hops compound-treated groups exhibited the most pronounced weight loss after the infection but before the treatment. The other clinical symptoms in animals in the treated groups improved as well.

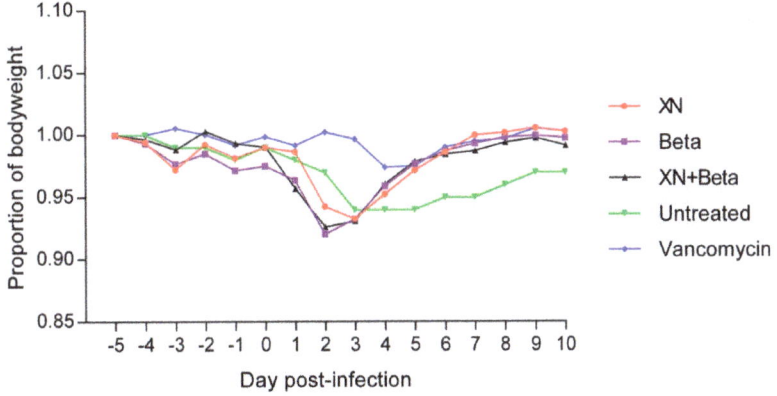

Figure 1. The proportion of body weight of infected rats during the *C. difficile* infection. Data are presented as means of the animal body weights at the individual time points relative to their body weight at the onset of the experiment (day-5). The animals were infected on day 0, and treatments started on day 3. XN—xanthohumol, Beta—beta-acids.

The quantitative determination of *C. difficile* in fecal samples showed the ability of tested compounds to reduce the bacterial load (Figure 2). During the treatment period (samples collected on days 3, 5, 7, and 9 post-infection), all three hops-compound treatment modalities showed similar inhibitory effects when compared to the untreated control. The reduction of the bacterial load was observed from day 3 post-infection. In all three treatment groups the differences in bacterial load of *C. difficile* were significant ($p < 0.05$) when compared to the untreated controls. Treatment by vancomycin in the positive control group showed a rapid decline of the bacterial load from day 5 (Figure 2).

We further evaluated the effect of treatments on the infection in intestines in experimental animals both at the macroscopical and microscopical levels after the termination of the experiment. The macroscopical evaluation showed marked hyperemia and swelling of the bowel in the animals from the untreated group. All the administered treatments led to a physiological bowel appearance after the termination of the experiment. Representative examples are shown in Figure 3.

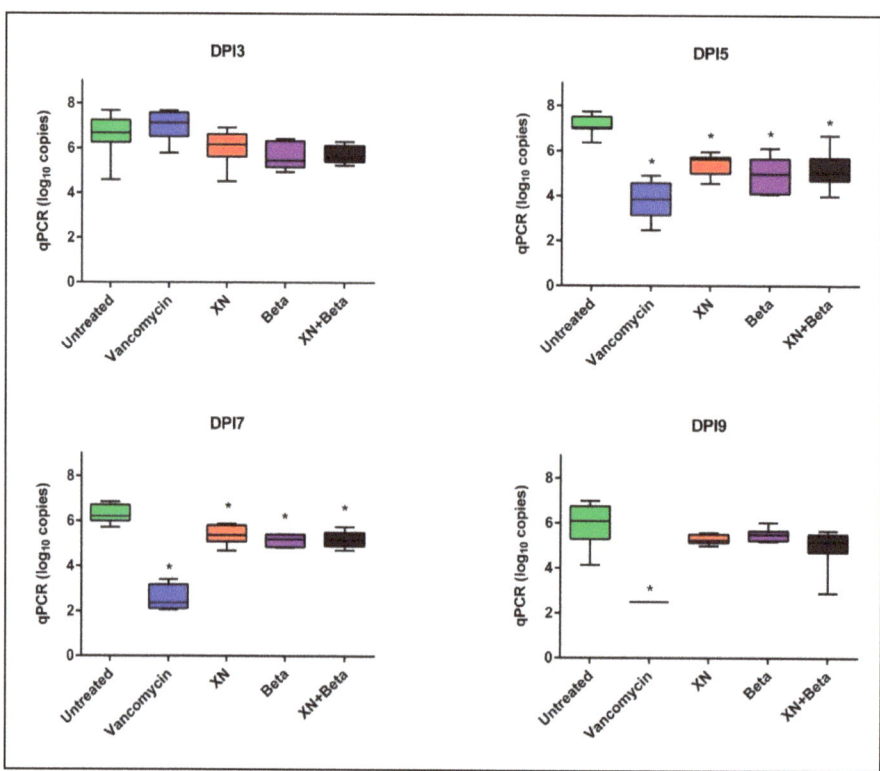

Figure 2. Bacterial load ($\log_{10}$ copies per reaction) of *C. difficile* per g of stool from rats. * Significant differences compared to untreated controls ($p < 0.05$). DPI—day post-infection, XN—xanthohumol, Beta—beta-acids.

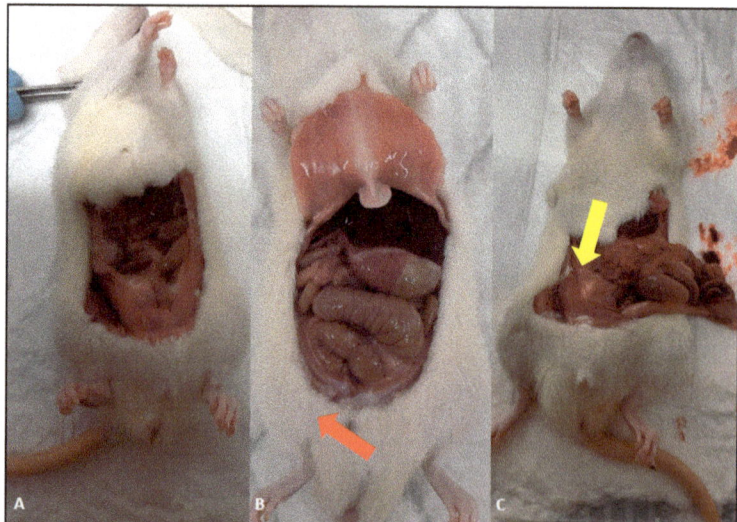

Figure 3. Macroscopical evaluation of *C. difficile* infection in the large and small intestines. (**A**) Normal macroscopical finding in the Xanthohumol treated rat; (**B**) edema in the large intestine (red arrow) and (**C**) hyperemia in the small intestine in infected untreated rats (yellow arrow).

The histopathological samples were collected at the end of the experiment (day 10). Microscopical examination showed *C. difficile* infection-induced edema and leukocyte infiltration in the large intestine of untreated animals. These findings were significantly reduced by all treatments (examples shown in Figure 4).

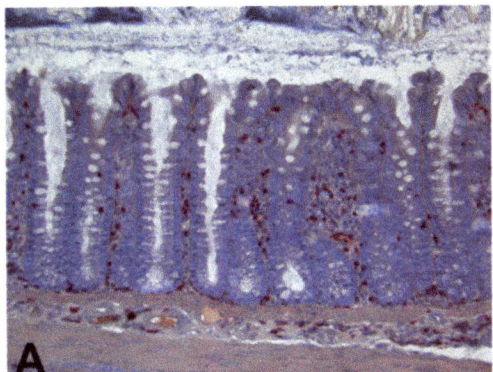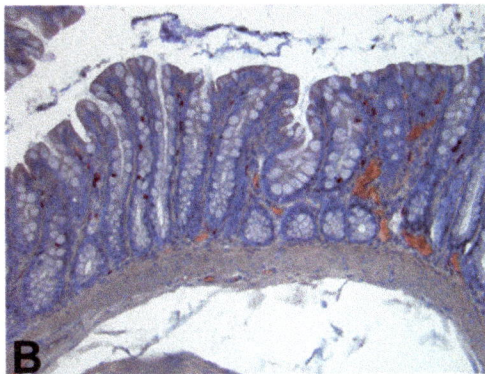

Figure 4. Histopathological changes in the colon from rats infected with *C. difficile* 10 days post-infection (**A**) with no treatment and (**B**) treated with xanthohumol. Tissue samples are stained with a naphthol AS-D chloroacetate kit and counterstained with hematoxylin (200-fold original magnification). *C. difficile* infection leads to high neutrophil infiltration (red color) and edema (**A**), which is substantially reduced by the xanthohumol treatment (**B**).

Further analysis showed (Figure 5) that treatments with xanthohumol or beta-bitter acids reduced the edema in the large intestine. Additionally, the individual compounds significantly reduced the histopathological score of inflammation. Quantitation of neutrophils in the mucosal and submucosal tissues showed that all treatment modalities led to significant decreases in the numbers of neutrophils per microscopic field.

The extent of histopathological changes in the small intestine of infected rats was generally low, even in untreated controls (data not shown).

Taken together, xanthohumol and beta-bitter acids show a clear antimicrobial effect against *C. difficile* infection in vivo, leading to both notable decreases in bacterial load (significant especially at days 5 and 7 post-infection) and normalization of inflammatory markers in the mucosal and submucosal tissues of the large intestine. The best antimicrobial effects in this model in vivo are obtained with the administration of either xanthohumol alone or a mixture of xanthohumol and beta-bitter acids from hops. In addition, the developed and presented animal model in rats provides a useful tool in studies of the pathogenesis and therapy of colitis induced by *C. difficile* infection.

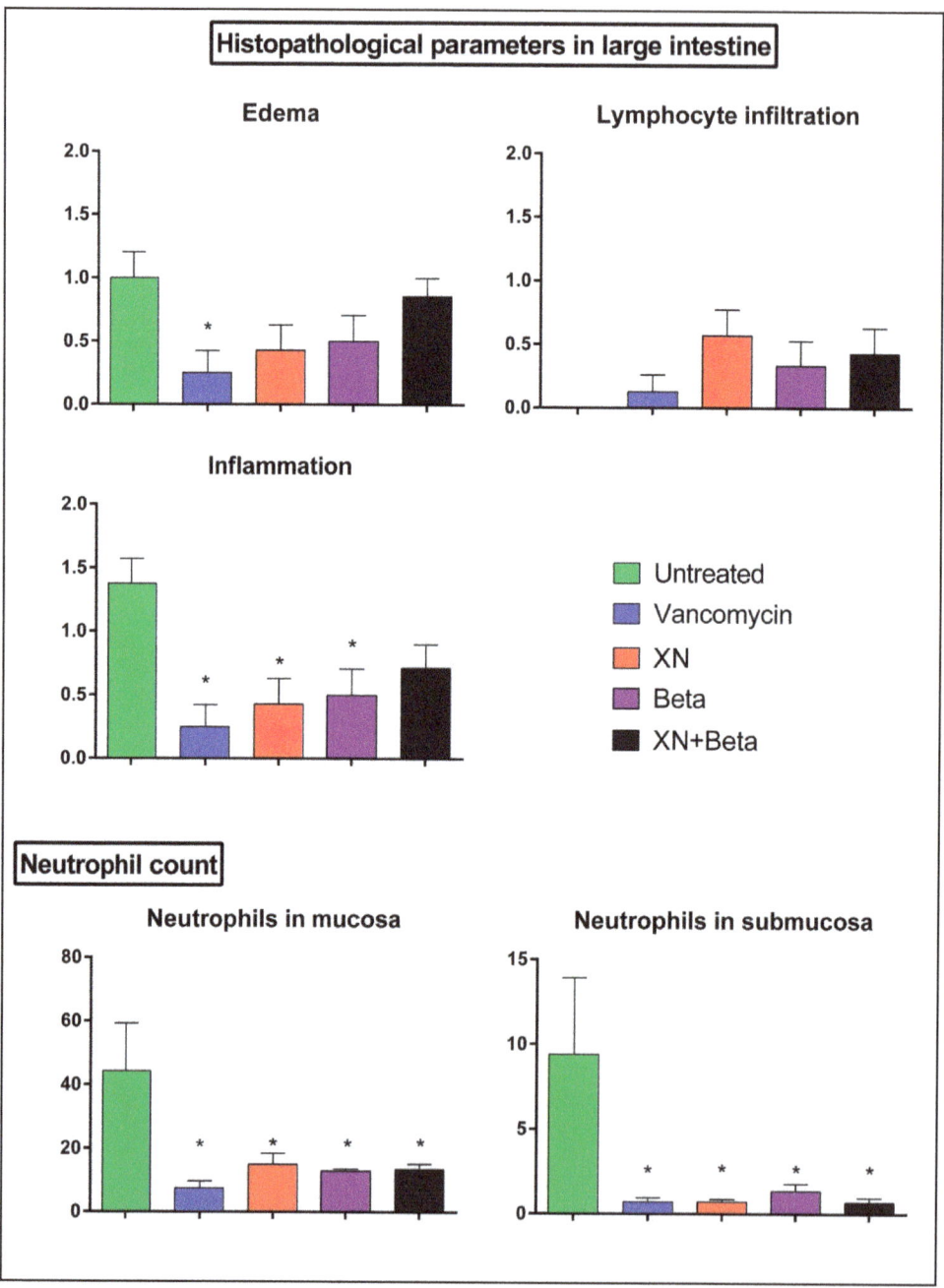

Figure 5. Histopathological analysis of the effect of treatments in large intestines of rats in the individual cohorts. Data are presented as mean ± standard deviation. * indicates significant differences compared to untreated controls ($p < 0.05$).

3. Discussion

C. difficile is one of the most common nosocomial pathogens with a worldwide distribution. It has been associated with pseudomembranous colitis, often leading to life-threatening diarrhea with increased morbidity and mortality rates. The currently used therapeutic management of *C. difficile* infection is achieved by the termination of "unnecessary" antibiotics that may lead to the development of the condition and administration of antimicrobials effective against *C. difficile*. The currently used ones are represented by vancomycin and metronidazole. However, the infection has a relatively high recurrence rate. The recurrent disease and fulminant courses require an intra-intestinal or parenteral administration of antibiotics. Some drugs, such as metronidazole, are characterized by a high resorption rate and present with serious side effects. Thus, there is an ongoing search for alternative therapies for this disease. One of those is, for example, the fecal microbial transplantation [9,21,22].

Another possible approach explored is the use of compounds with antimicrobial effects available in commonly used plants. Numerous studies have shown that the hops cones represent an abundant source of components with apparent antimicrobial effects against certain bacteria, viruses, fungi, and protozoa. Some of the specific properties for using these hops derivatives as therapeutics is their low cytotoxicity, specifically for the use in the GIT, and their very low adsorption. These features lead to their safety and the absence of side effects. The antibacterial properties of some purified compounds from hops, namely xanthohumol and beta-bitter acids, were determined in vitro for many pathogens, including *C. difficile*, in the past [13].

In the present study, the efficiency of the treatment with two compounds isolated from hops and their mixture was tested in an animal model of the *C. difficile*-induced gastrointestinal infection. We first successfully established the rat model for the *C. difficile* bowel infection. In this model, the bacteria from the hypervirulent human strain were atraumatically introduced into the GIT of animals pre-conditioned with a regimen of antibiotics. In contrast to the hamster model historically used for *C. difficile* infection, the course of the infection in rats is not fulminant and lethal, which allows for an extended antimicrobial efficacy testing. Thus, the rat model is more similar to the disease course of *C. difficile* bowel infection in humans, which will allow not only for in vivo testing of novel antimicrobials but potentially for studies of disease pathogenesis as well.

The results of this study show that all the hops derivatives tested possess antimicrobial properties against the *C. difficile* infection in vivo. However, the pure xanthohumol exhibited higher antimicrobial potential in our model than the other hops compounds tested. It significantly decreased the bacterial load of *C. difficile* in fecal samples after two days of application. These results further corroborate our previously published data of the high in vitro activity of xanthohumol against *C. difficile* determined by the broth dilution method. Similar antimicrobial effects were observed for the combination of xanthohumol and beta-bitter acids. Treatments by these substances also had positive effects on body weight and other general signs of the disease in experimental animals compared to the untreated control.

Finally, this work illustrates the antimicrobial potential of the tested compounds against *C. difficile* in in vivo testing. These results show that namely xanthohumol has the potential of being developed into an antimicrobial treatment regimen or to be used in combination with standardly used drugs. The advantage of xanthohumol for such use is its minimal resorption in the intestine, thus allowing for the administration of large doses with no or minimal side effects.

Mechanisms underlying antimicrobial activity of hops-derived compounds have not been extensively studied. Several reports suggest that these compounds affect bacterial cell membrane integrity, interfere with fatty acid metabolism, and lead to an accumulation of protons intracellularly and subsequent cell starvation [23–25]. A combination of these mechanisms may underlie effects of these compounds against *C. difficile* observed in the presented study. However, the elucidation of the exact mechanism will need further investigation. Taken together, the results show the purified substances from hops are promising candidates for further development and use in difficult-to-treat infections in humans, such as colitis caused by *C. difficile*.

4. Materials and Methods

4.1. Hops Compounds

A pure isolate of beta-acids was prepared at the Hop Research Institute in Zatec and further purified at the Research Institute of Brewing and Malting according to the procedure described by Krofta et al. [26]. The first step involved partitioning the CO_2 hops extract solution in an alkaline medium of sodium carbonate and sodium hydroxide to separate the alpha-acids and beta-acids fractions. In the next step, the crude beta-fraction has been used for the isolation of pure beta-acids (99.7% w/w) through crystallization from the solvent mixture. The isolate of xanthohumol (84.3% w/w) was prepared following the procedure described by Biendl [27]. The process consists of the selective sorption of prenylflavonoids from ethanolic hops extract on polyvinylpyrrolidone. The isolate contains, in addition to xanthohumol, the whole spectrum of different hops prenylflavonoids. A stock solution with a concentration of xanthohumol or beta-acids of 100 mg/1 mL was prepared by dissolving the isolates in dimethyl sulfoxide.

4.2. Bacterial Strain and Culture Conditions

The bacterial strain of *C. difficile* used in this study was from the collection of isolates of the Department of Medical Microbiology of Thomayer Hospital in Prague (Czech Republic). The hypervirulent strain 176 was isolated and ribotyped at the Institute of Microbiology, University Hospital and Second Medical Faculty, Charles University in Prague. The ribotype analysis was performed using PCR ribotyping and detection of the presence of toxin production governing genes (tcdA (A), tcdB (B), cdtA, and cdtB (binary)) was performed by a multiplex PCR. The strain was cultured on selective *C. difficile* blood agar (LabMediaServis, Jaromer, Czech Republic) supplemented with norfloxacin (12 µg/mL) and moxalactam (32 µg/mL). Bacterial stocks for cryopreservation were prepared on porous beads (ITEST, Hradec Kralove, Czech Republic). For each experiment, fresh bacterial culture was prepared as follows. The porous bead with *C. difficile* was inoculated onto the agar plate. The culture was performed under anaerobic conditions using an anaerobic gas chamber and an AnaeroGen sachet (Oxoid, Basingstoke, UK) at 37 °C for 48 h.

4.3. Animals and Housing

Male Wistar rats (weight 330–460 g) were purchased from VELAZ (Prague, Czech Republic). The animals were housed under veterinary control and standard conditions (light cycle 12 h/12 h, standard laboratory diet, and water ad libitum). All the experiments were performed with permission and under the supervision of the Ethics Committee of the Faculty of Military Health Sciences (Hradec Kralove, Czech Republic).

4.4. Experimental Model

The experimental animals were subjected to the following protocol to establish a suitable animal model for testing the compound's in vivo antibacterial activity. On day 5, water containing antibiotic mixture, consisting of amikacin (9.66 mg/kg, Braun Medical, Prague, Czech Republic), colistin (4.2 mg/kg, Teva Pharmaceuticals, Prague, Czech Republic), gentamicin (3.5 mg/kg, LONZA, Basel, Switzerland), metronidazole (21.5 mg/kg, Braun Medical, Prague, Czech Republic), and vancomycin (4.5 mg/kg, Mylan SAS, Saint Priest, France), was given to each animal by intragastric gavage in a total volume of 1 mL. This was followed with identical doses of amikacin, gentamicin, and colistin at day 2. A single dose of clindamycin (10 mg/kg; Fresenius Cabi, Germany) was given intraperitoneally at day 1. On day 0, the stool samples were sampled before the experimental bacterial infection to screen for any endogenous colonization with *C. difficile*. Then each rat was administered with a single dose of *C. difficile* suspension (3×10^8 cells in 1 mL) by intragastric gavage. Rats were then monitored every day for general signs of infection (diarrhea, weight loss, and infection symptoms), and stool samples were collected for *C. difficile* identification until day 10 post-infection by culture and quantification at day 3, 5, 7, 9 post-infection by qPCR (Figure 6). For the evaluation of antibacterial effects of hops compounds, the animals were divided into 5 experimental groups of 7 animals each. There were two control groups: animals in the negative control group I received no antibacterial treatment, while those in the positive control group II received vancomycin (150 mg/L, Mylan SAS, St. Priest, France) as the "standard" antibiotic used in the treatment of pseudomembranous colitis. Animals in groups III, IV, and V were treated with xanthohumol, beta-bitter acids, or a mixture of both substances at the concentration 5 mg/kg, respectively. All antibacterial agents were administered every day by intragastric gavage from day 3 post-infection. On day 10 post-infection, the animals were euthanized, and samples from the small and large intestine were collected for further histological examination.

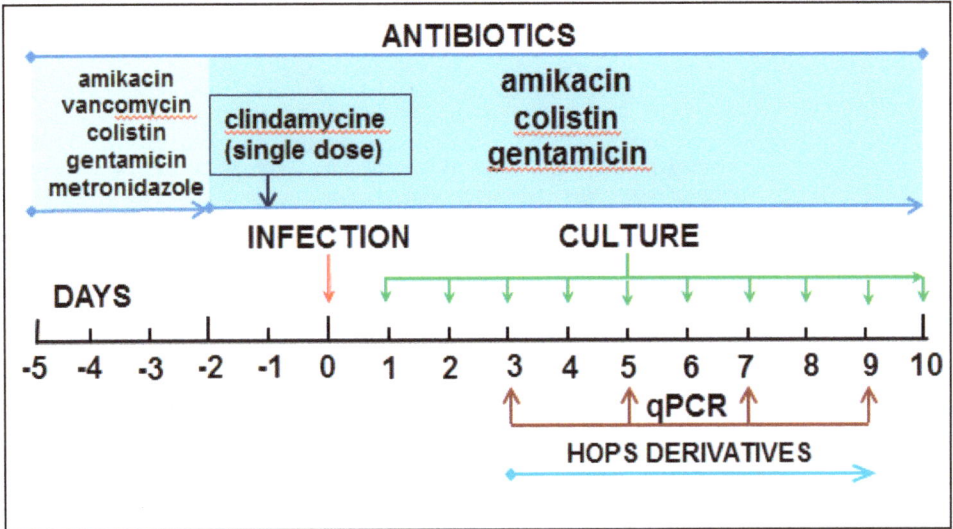

Figure 6. Time course of the experiment.

4.5. DNA Isolation and Real-Time PCR

The DNA from stool samples of rats was isolated by HigherPurity Stool DNA Isolation kit (Canvax Biotech S.L., Córdoba, Spain) according to the manufacturer's instructions. DNA samples were then stored at $-20\,°C$ until qPCR analysis.

The qPCR assay was performed using *C. difficile* Genesig Advanced Kit (PrimerDesign, Camberley, UK). The amplification reactions were carried out in a final volume of 20 µL, which consisted of 5 µL of the template and 15 µL of the master mix, containing Oasig 2X qPCR Master Mix, 300 nM of each primer and 150 nM fluorescence-labeled probe and distilled water. The assay was performed with the CFX Touch Real-Time PCR Detection System (Biorad, Hercules, CA, USA). The amplification conditions consisted of an initial enzyme activation at $95\,°C$ for 2 min, followed by 50 cycles of denaturation at $95\,°C$ for 10 s, primer annealing at $54\,°C$ for 30 s, and data collection at $60\,°C$ for 1 min. Fluorogenic data was collected through the FAM and VIC channels.

4.6. Histopathology Examination

Collected samples were fixed in 10% neutral buffered formalin (Bamed, Ceske Budejovice, Czech Republic). Subsequently, they were histologically processed and stained with hematoxylin and eosin (both from Merck, Kenilworth, NJ, USA), according to Pejchal et al. [28]. The histopathological analysis was performed using a BX-51 microscope (Olympus, Tokyo, Japan) and a semiquantitative scale developer by Shelby et al. [20].

Neutrophil granulocytes were detected using Naphthol AS-D Chloroacetate (specific esterase) Kit (Sigma-Aldrich, St. Louis, MO, USA) according to the manufacturer's instructions. Naphthol AS-D Chloroacetate positive cells were measured in 6 randomly selected microscopic fields in the mucosal and submucosal compartments at 400fold original magnification on a BX-51 microscope.

4.7. Data Analysis

Data obtained by the qPCR assay and weight monitoring were analyzed using Excel (Microsoft® 2010) software or imported into GraphPad Prism 6 (version 6.05, GraphPad Software Inc., San Diego, CA USA) for further analysis. The normality was tested using the Shapiro–Wilk test. Normally distributed data were analyzed using one-way ANOVA with post hoc Student's *t*-test. Non-normally distributed data were analyzed by Kruskal–Wallis test with post hoc Mann–Whitney test. The differences were considered significant when $p \leq 0.05$.

Author Contributions: Conceptualization, P.B., R.S. and P.C.; methodology, R.S., J.P. and V.R.; software, L.M.; validation, S.J., R.S. and J.P.; investigation, R.B., R.S. and V.R.; resources, A.M. and M.H.; data curation, R.S., V.R. and L.M.; writing—original draft preparation, R.S.; writing—review and editing, J.P. and P.B.; supervision, P.B.; funding acquisition, P.B. All authors have read and agreed to the published version of the manuscript.

Funding: This research was funded by the Czech Health Research Council of Czech Republic, grant NV-17-31765A and the Ministry of Defence of the Czech Republic—long-term organization development plan.

Institutional Review Board Statement: The study was conducted according to the guidelines of the Declaration of Helsinki and approved by the Ethics Committee of the Faculty of Military Health Sciences, Hradec Kralove, Czech Republic (protocol code MO 103191/2018-6848, date of approval 12 April 2018).

Informed Consent Statement: Not applicable.

Data Availability Statement: Data available on request due to ethical restrictions.

Conflicts of Interest: The authors declare no conflict of interest. The funders had no role in the design of the study, in the collection, analyses, or interpretation of data, in the writing of the manuscript, or in the decision to publish the results.

References

1. Oka, K.; Osaki, T.; Hanawa, T.; Kurata, S.; Sugiyama, E.; Takahashi, M.; Tanaka, M.; Taguchi, H.; Kamiya, S. Establishment of an Endogenous Clostridium difficile Rat Infection Model and Evaluation of the Effects of Clostridium butyricum MIYAIRI 588 Probiotic Strain. *Front. Microbiol.* **2018**, *9*, 1264. [CrossRef] [PubMed]
2. Shah, D.; Dang, M.D.; Hasbun, R.; Koo, H.L.; Jiang, Z.D.; DuPont, H.L.; Garey, K.W. Clostridium difficile infection: Update on emerging antibiotic treatment options and antibiotic resistance. *Expert Rev. Anti-Infect. Ther.* **2010**, *8*, 555–564. [CrossRef]
3. Zhu, D.; Sorg, J.A.; Sun, X. Clostridioides difficile Biology: Sporulation, Germination, and Corresponding Therapies for C. difficile Infection. *Front. Cell. Infect. Microbiol.* **2018**, *8*, 29. [CrossRef] [PubMed]
4. Janoir, C. Virulence factors of Clostridium difficile and their role during infection. *Anaerobe* **2016**, *37*, 13–24. [CrossRef] [PubMed]
5. Koenigsknecht, M.J.; Theriot, C.M.; Bergin, I.L.; Schumacher, C.A.; Schloss, P.D.; Young, V.B. Dynamics and establishment of Clostridium difficile infection in the murine gastrointestinal tract. *Infect. Immun.* **2015**, *83*, 934–941. [CrossRef] [PubMed]
6. Dharbhamulla, N.; Abdelhady, A.; Domadia, M.; Patel, S.; Gaughan, J.; Roy, S. Risk Factors Associated With Recurrent Clostridium difficile Infection. *J. Clin. Med. Res.* **2019**, *11*, 1–6. [CrossRef]
7. Dieterle, M.G.; Rao, K.; Young, V.B. Novel therapies and preventative strategies for primary and recurrent Clostridium difficile infections. *Ann. N. Y. Acad. Sci.* **2019**, *1435*, 110–138. [CrossRef] [PubMed]
8. Ooijevaar, R.E.; van Beurden, Y.H.; Terveer, E.M.; Goorhuis, A.; Bauer, M.P.; Keller, J.J.; Mulder, C.J.J.; Kuijper, E.J. Update of treatment algorithms for Clostridium difficile infection. *Clin. Microbiol. Infect.* **2018**, *24*, 452–462. [CrossRef]
9. Singh, T.; Bedi, P.; Bumrah, K.; Singh, J.; Rai, M.; Seelam, S. Updates in Treatment of Recurrent Clostridium difficile Infection. *J. Clin. Med. Res.* **2019**, *11*, 465–471. [CrossRef]

10. Wilcox, M.H.; Gerding, D.N.; Poxton, I.R.; Kelly, C.; Nathan, R.; Birch, T.; Cornely, O.A.; Rahav, G.; Bouza, E.; Lee, C.; et al. Bezlotoxumab for Prevention of Recurrent Clostridium difficile Infection. *N. Engl. J. Med.* **2017**, *376*, 305–317. [CrossRef]
11. Bartmanska, A.; Walecka-Zacharska, E.; Tronina, T.; Poplonski, J.; Sordon, S.; Brzezowska, E.; Bania, J.; Huszcza, E. Antimicrobial Properties of Spent Hops Extracts, Flavonoids Isolated Therefrom, and Their Derivatives. *Molecules* **2018**, *23*, 2059. [CrossRef]
12. Bogdanova, K.; Roderova, M.; Kolar, M.; Langova, K.; Dusek, M.; Jost, P.; Kubelkova, K.; Bostik, P.; Olsovska, J. Antibiofilm activity of bioactive hop compounds humulone, lupulone and xanthohumol toward susceptible and resistant staphylococci. *Res. Microbiol.* **2018**, *169*, 127–134. [CrossRef] [PubMed]
13. Cermak, P.; Olsovska, J.; Mikyska, A.; Dusek, M.; Kadleckova, Z.; Vanicek, J.; Nyc, O.; Sigler, K.; Bostikova, V.; Bostik, P. Strong antimicrobial activity of xanthohumol and other derivatives from hops (Humulus lupulus L.) on gut anaerobic bacteria. *APMIS* **2017**, *125*, 1033–1038. [CrossRef] [PubMed]
14. Jeliazkova, E.; Zheljazkov, V.D.; Kacaniova, M.; Astatkie, T.; Tekwani, B.L. Sequential Elution of Essential Oil Constituents during Steam Distillation of Hops (Humulus lupulus L.) and Influence on Oil Yield and Antimicrobial Activity. *J. Oleo Sci.* **2018**, *67*, 871–883. [CrossRef] [PubMed]
15. Mody, D.; Athamneh, A.I.M.; Seleem, M.N. Curcumin: A natural derivative with antibacterial activity against Clostridium difficile. *J. Glob. Antimicrob. Resist.* **2020**, *21*, 154–161. [CrossRef] [PubMed]
16. Roehrer, S.; Behr, J.; Stork, V.; Ramires, M.; Medard, G.; Frank, O.; Kleigrewe, K.; Hofmann, T.; Minceva, M. Xanthohumol C, a minor bioactive hop compound: Production, purification strategies and antimicrobial test. *J. Chromatogr. B Analyt. Technol. Biomed. Life Sci.* **2018**, *1095*, 39–49. [CrossRef] [PubMed]
17. Best, E.L.; Freeman, J.; Wilcox, M.H. Models for the study of Clostridium difficile infection. *Gut Microbes* **2012**, *3*, 145–167. [CrossRef]
18. De Wolfe, T.J.; Kates, A.E.; Barko, L.; Darien, B.J.; Safdar, N. Modified Mouse Model of Clostridioides difficile Infection as a Platform for Probiotic Efficacy Studies. *Antimicrob. Agents Chemother.* **2019**, *63*, e00111-19. [CrossRef] [PubMed]
19. Deng, H.; Yang, S.; Zhang, Y.; Qian, K.; Zhang, Z.; Liu, Y.; Wang, Y.; Bai, Y.; Fan, H.; Zhao, X.; et al. Bacteroides fragilis Prevents Clostridium difficile Infection in a Mouse Model by Restoring Gut Barrier and Microbiome Regulation. *Front. Microbiol.* **2018**, *9*, 2976. [CrossRef]
20. Shelby, R.D.; Tengberg, N.; Conces, M.; Olson, J.K.; Navarro, J.B.; Bailey, M.T.; Goodman, S.D.; Besner, G.E. Development of a Standardized Scoring System to Assess a Murine Model of Clostridium difficile Colitis. *J. Investig. Surg.* **2020**, *33*, 887–895. [CrossRef] [PubMed]
21. Gupta, S.; Allen-Vercoe, E.; Petrof, E.O. Fecal microbiota transplantation: In perspective. *Ther. Adv. Gastroenterol.* **2016**, *9*, 229–239. [CrossRef] [PubMed]
22. Hui, W.; Li, T.; Liu, W.; Zhou, C.; Gao, F. Fecal microbiota transplantation for treatment of recurrent C. difficile infection: An updated randomized controlled trial meta-analysis. *PLoS ONE* **2019**, *14*, e0210016. [CrossRef] [PubMed]
23. Bocquet, L.; Sahpaz, S.; Bonneau, N.; Beaufay, C.; Mahieux, S.; Samaillie, J.; Roumy, V.; Jacquin, J.; Bordage, S.; Hennebelle, T.; et al. Phenolic Compounds from Humulus lupulus as Natural Antimicrobial Products: New Weapons in the Fight against Methicillin Resistant Staphylococcus aureus, Leishmania mexicana and Trypanosoma brucei Strains. *Molecules* **2019**, *24*, 1024. [CrossRef]
24. Karabin, M.; Hudcova, T.; Jelinek, L.; Dostalek, P. Biologically Active Compounds from Hops and Prospects for Their Use. *Compr. Rev. Food Sci. Food Saf.* **2016**, *15*, 542–567. [CrossRef]
25. Cheon, D.; Kim, J.; Jeon, D.; Shin, H.C.; Kim, Y. Target Proteins of Phloretin for Its Anti-Inflammatory and Antibacterial Activities Against Propionibacterium acnes-Induced Skin Infection. *Molecules* **2019**, *24*, 1319. [CrossRef]
26. Krofta, K.; Liskova, H.; Vrabcova, S. Process for Preparing Pure Beta Acids of Hop. Patent Number CZ303017B6, 29 February 2012.
27. Biendl, M. Isolation of Prenylflavovnoids from Hops. International Society for Horticultural Science. Available online: http://www.actahort.org/books/1010/1010_15.htm (accessed on 15 January 2021).
28. Pejchal, J.; Novotny, J.; Marak, V.; Osterreicher, J.; Tichy, A.; Vavrova, J.; Sinkorova, Z.; Zarybnicka, L.; Novotna, E.; Chladek, J.; et al. Activation of p38 MAPK and expression of TGF-beta1 in rat colon enterocytes after whole body gamma-irradiation. *Int. J. Radiat. Biol.* **2012**, *88*, 348–358. [CrossRef] [PubMed]

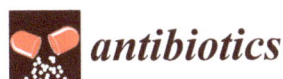

Article

Analysis of Vancomycin-Resistant Enterococci in Hemato-Oncological Patients

Kristýna Hricová, Taťána Štosová, Pavla Kučová, Kateřina Fišerová *, Jan Bardoň and Milan Kolář

Department of Microbiology, University Hospital Olomouc and Faculty of Medicine and Dentistry, Palacký University Olomouc, 77900 Olomouc, Czech Republic; hricova.k@email.cz (K.H.); tatana.stosova@fnol.cz (T.Š.); pavla.kucova@fnol.cz (P.K.); jbardon@svuol.cz (J.B.); milan.kolar@fnol.cz (M.K.)
* Correspondence: katerina.fiserova@fnol.cz; Tel.: +420-585-639-511

Received: 28 September 2020; Accepted: 6 November 2020; Published: 7 November 2020

Abstract: Enterococci are important bacterial pathogens, and their significance is even greater in the case of vancomycin-resistant enterococci (VRE). The study analyzed the presence of VRE in the gastrointestinal tract (GIT) of hemato-oncological patients. Active screening using selective agars yielded VRE for phenotypic and genotypic analyses. Isolated strains were identified with MALDI-TOF MS, (Matrix-Assisted Laser Desorption/Ionization Time-of-Flight Mass Spectrometry) their susceptibility to antibiotics was tested, and resistance genes (*vanA*, *vanB*, *vanC-1*, *vanC2-C3*) and genes encoding virulence factors (*asa1*, *gelE*, *cylA*, *esp*, *hyl*) were detected. Pulsed-field gel electrophoresis was used to assess the relationship of the isolated strains. Over a period of three years, 103 VanA-type VRE were identified in 1405 hemato-oncological patients. The most frequently detected virulence factor was extracellular surface protein (84%), followed by hyaluronidase (40%). Unique restriction profiles were observed in 33% of strains; clonality was detected in 67% of isolates. The study found that 7% of hemato-oncological patients carried VRE in their GIT. In all cases, the species identified was *Enterococcus faecium*. No clone persisted for the entire 3-year study period. However, genetically different clusters were observed for shorter periods of time, no longer than eight months, with identical VRE spreading among patients.

Keywords: VRE; GIT; hemato-oncological patients; clonality

1. Introduction

In today's medicine, important bacterial pathogens are enterococci. As etiological agents, they are responsible for community as well as healthcare-associated infections (HAIs), particularly in patients with prolonged hospital stays, severe underlying disease, or previous broad-spectrum antibiotic therapy [1]. Sievert et al. reported that enterococci belong to the most common bacterial pathogens causing HAIs in the USA [2]. According to a 2017 U.S. study, enterococci were implicated in 14% of HAIs in the country [3]. Using results from a large multicenter study involving 15 centers in the Czech Republic, Kolář et al. documented that 9% of bloodstream infections were due to enterococci [4]. Herkel et al. found that enterococci accounted for 5% of all bacterial pathogens causing healthcare-associated pneumonia [5]. In these cases, they originated in the upper gastrointestinal tract (GIT), with pneumonia developing as a result of gastric content regurgitation and subsequent microaspiration [6]. Since approximately the 1970s, a vast majority of enterococcal HAIs have been caused by *Enterococcus faecium* and *Enterococcus faecalis* [7].

Treatment of enterococcal infections is considerably influenced not only by their natural resistance to many antibacterial agents, but also by acquired resistance, representing a factor limiting antibiotic therapy. A therapeutic challenge and real threat to patients are vancomycin-resistant enterococci (VRE). The most widespread VRE type is the VanA phenotype, determined by the D-alanyl-D-lactate structure encoded by the *vanA* gene that is very often located on transposon Tn1546 [8–11]. The first description of VRE comes from the UK and was published in 1988 [12]. In the Czech Republic, VRE were first detected in hemato-oncological patients at the University Hospital Olomouc in 1997 [13].

At present, a serious public issue is the presence of multidrug-resistant bacteria including VRE in the GIT as components of the normal microflora. The clinical significance of multidrug-resistant bacteria in the GIT was documented by Kolář et al. In their study, an ESBL-positive strain of *Klebsiella pneumoniae* and an AmpC-positive strain of *Enterobacter cloacae*, isolated from rectal swabs and thus being part of gastrointestinal bacterial flora, were found to be identical with strains causing bacterial infections, namely urinary tract infection and bloodstream infection [14]. Arias and Murray reported translocation of enterococci across the GIT wall into the bloodstream with subsequent endocarditis [7]. This fact is of utmost importance in VRE that may be part of GIT microflora, with the length of hospital stay or interventions such as hemodialysis, transplantation, and application of artificial materials playing an important role [15–17]. Heisel et al. showed that the proportion of patients with VRE colonization of the GIT changed from 3% before hospital admission to 59% during their hospital stay [18]. Another important factor promoting the presence of VRE in the GIT is the selection pressure of antibiotics. Kolář et al. documented the positive selection pressure of third-generation cephalosporins and glycopeptides with regard to the presence of VRE [19]. Paterson et al. found that after treatment with piperacillin-tazobactam or cefepime, 26% and 31%, respectively, of patients primarily tested negative for VRE were colonized with these bacteria [20].

Data from the EARS-Net provide information on the current prevalence of VRE in the Czech Republic [21]. The percentage of vancomycin-resistant strains of *E. faecium* ranges from 4% to 13% [22–24]. However, this prominent European database only considers blood isolates and cannot provide more accurate comprehensive data on the prevalence of VRE in both the community and hospital human populations including GIT carriage. In the Czech Republic, such data were last published by Kolář et al. in 2006 [19,25]. In their study on the prevalence of VRE in hemato-oncological patients in a Czech university hospital, these strains accounted for 5% of all isolated enterococci. The most frequent strains were VanA-type *E. faecium* (78%) and VanB-type *E. faecalis* (10%). The fact that VRE were most frequently isolated from rectal swabs (55%) illustrates the significance of their carriage in the GIT [19].

A key role in the etiopathogenesis of infections caused by enterococci may be played by selected virulence factors. These are essential for biofilm formation and subsequent colonization [26]. The presence of selected virulence factors in VRE was studied by Yang et al. For *E. faecium*, the most frequent gene was *esp*, encoding extracellular surface protein, detected in 90% of strains. Additionally present (28%) was the *hyl* (hyaluronidase) gene. The combination of these two genes (*esp* + *hyl*) was noted in 26% of isolates. Genes encoding aggregation substance (*asa1*), cytolysin (*cylA*), or gelatinase (*gelE*) were not detected in *E. faecium*, but only in *E. faecalis* strains, which were considerably less frequently detected in the study [27].

The present study aimed to determine the presence of VRE in the GIT of hemato-oncological patients in the University Hospital Olomouc and to carry out their genetic analysis including the assessment of selected virulence factors.

2. Results

Over a 3-year study period, stool samples and perianal swabs obtained from 1405 subjects were analyzed and a total of 103 VRE were isolated, suggesting that 7.3% of hemato-oncological patients carried VRE in their GIT. In all cases, the species identified was *E. faecium*.

The results of VRE susceptibility testing showed very high susceptibility to linezolid (100%) and tigecycline (96%) and, conversely, 100% resistance to ampicillin and teicoplanin (Table 1).

Table 1. Susceptibility of vancomycin-resistant enterococci (VRE) to selected antibiotics (percentages).

Year/Antibiotic	AMP	TIG	TET	TEI	FUR	LNZ
2016	0	100	71	0	100	100
2017	0	88	43	0	84	100
2018	0	100	35	0	48	100
2016–2018	0	96	48	0	76	100

Legend: AMP—ampicillin, TIG—tigecycline, TET—tetracycline, TEI—teicoplanin, FUR—nitrofurantoin, LNZ—linezolid.

In all isolated VRE, the *vanA* gene was present. Strains with VanB, VanC-1, and VanC2-C3 phenotypes were not detected.

Analysis of the selected virulence factors showed that extracellular surface protein (*esp*) was most frequent. It was present in 84% of isolates, either alone (53%) or in combination with hyaluronidase (*esp* + *hyl*) in 31% of isolates. Hyaluronidase (*hyl*) was found in 40% of isolates (alone in 9%). No virulence factor was present in 7% of isolates.

Based on the pulsed-field gel electrophoresis (PFGE) results, a dendrogram was produced, as shown in Figure 1. Among the 103 VRE, a total of 69 strains were identified and distributed into 18 groups (A–R) based on their similarity (tolerance 1.5; cut-off, 95%). Thus, the overall clonality was 67%. The remaining 34 strains (33%) had unique restriction profiles. Within individual clonal groups, isolates showed 98% similarity. Clone G was the largest cluster, containing 12 strains. Genotypes A, E, F, H, I, J, O, P, and Q were relatively small, all containing two strains. Clones D, N, and R contained three strains each. Five strains in Clone M were isolated from patients staying in the same ward over a period of one month. Analysis of the time–spatial relationships of these patients confirmed transmission of a single VRE clone, but failed to identify the index patient or other source of the outbreak. Clone G consisted of 12 strains isolated from patients over a period of eight months. Clone K consisted of eight strains, all of which were isolated over a period of three months, namely September–November 2017. Similarly, Clone C consisted of eight strains, isolated over four months (September–December 2018). Clone B contained five strains isolated over three months (January–March 2017) and clone L consisted of fours strains obtained over six months in 2018. The timeline of the prevalence of VRE clones throughout the study duration is shown in Figure 2.

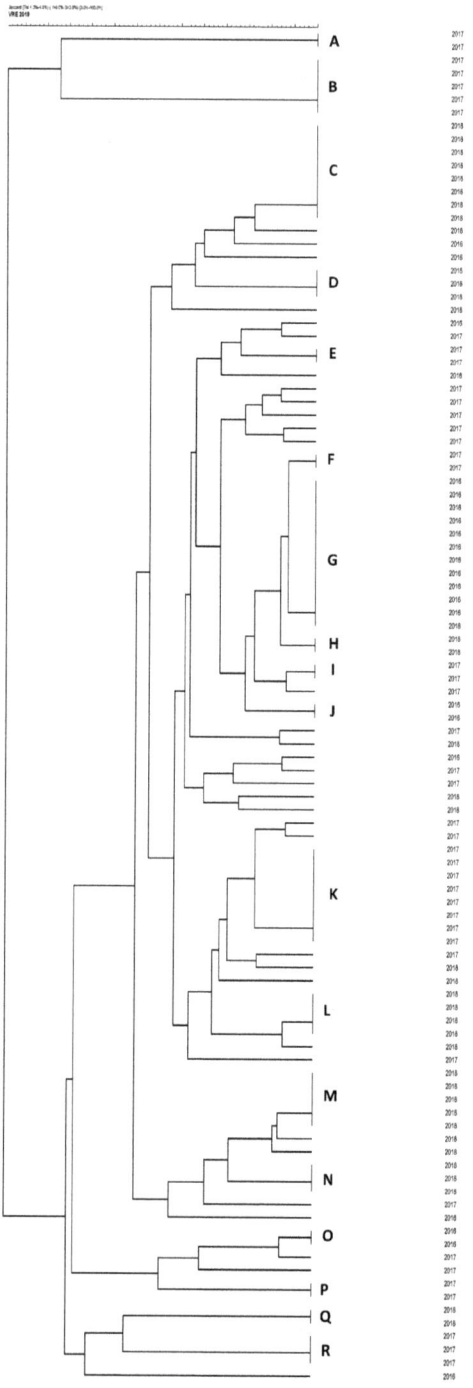

Figure 1. Pulsed-field gel electrophoresis (PFGE) dendrogram of 103 vancomycin-resistant *E. faecium* isolates. The letters represent 18 clonal groups of VRE (A–R) based on their similarity.

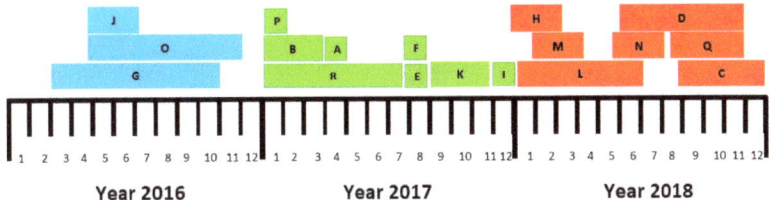

Figure 2. Timeline of the prevalence of VRE clones throughout the study duration. The letters represent 18 clonal groups of VRE (A–R) based on their similarity.

3. Discussion

Infections caused by VRE are often preceded by gastrointestinal colonization with these significant bacterial pathogens. A meta-analysis of 45 studies comprising over 8000 patients with malignancies showed approximately 20% colonization of the GIT with VRE [28]. In a 2019 study on GIT colonization with resistant bacteria in patients with acute myeloid leukemia, Ballo et al. even detected a much higher rate of 74% VRE colonization [29]. In the same year, another study found that VRE-colonized patients were as much as 24 times more likely to develop bloodstream infections caused by these strains [30]. Of importance is also the increase in the prevalence of VRE in the GIT of nursing facility patients from 10% to 29%, with MRSA detection rates declining from 37% to 13% over the 2003–2016 period [31]. In the present study, VRE were detected in the GIT of only 7% of hemato-oncological patients. This may be explained by very low prevalence of VRE (below 1%, unpublished data) in the GIT of people living in the community in the region from which the monitored patients come. Another important reason is the implementation of bacteriological surveillance in hemato-oncological patients including active search for bacterial strains with dangerous resistance phenotypes (e.g., VRE, ESBL-, AmpC- and KPC-positive enterobacteria) in the microflora of the upper respiratory tract and GIT. In the case of positive detection, barrier measures were strictly observed in these patients.

A study by Pudová et al. showed that the GIT is an important source of enterococci causing healthcare-associated pneumonia [6]. If VRE were implicated, the situation would be much more serious due to potential failure of initial antibiotic therapy. Therefore, these dangerous bacteria need to be detected in the GIT of patients, especially immunocompromised ones. All VRE isolated in our study belong to the VanA phenotype of *E. faecium* strains. In a 2006 study conducted in the same department, genetic analysis of VRE revealed that in hemato-oncological patients, the most frequent source was the GIT (55%) and the strains were mostly VanA-positive *E. faecium* (78%) and VanB-positive *E. faecalis* (10%) [19].

In Europe, the most frequent VRE phenotype is VanA [32]. This was confirmed by the results of genetic analysis of VRE in the present study showing that the *vanA* gene was present in 100% of the tested isolates while the *vanB*, *vanC-1*, and *vanC2/C3* genes were completely absent. This is consistent with results from a 2018 Serbian study by Jovanović et al. investigating VRE isolated from the oropharynx and stools of hemato-oncological patients. They also showed 100% presence of the *vanA* gene and 0% presence of the *vanB* gene [33].

Virulence factors are likely to play an important role in the etiopathogenesis of enterococcal infections [34,35]. These factors contribute to colonization, biofilm formation, and the production of enzymes potentially increasing the severity of developing infections [7]. In the present study, selected virulence factors were identified in 93% of isolated VRE. The presence of the most frequent virulence factor (*esp*) was lower than that in a similar 2018 study [36]. While Marchi et al. reported 97% prevalence of the *esp* gene in VRE, there were 84% of *esp*-positive VRE in hemato-oncological patients in the present study. Molecular analysis of virulence factors in VRE isolated from oncological patients is available in a 2013 Mexican study. Compared to our study, the *esp* gene was less frequent, being present in 50% of VRE isolates. The *hyl* gene was detected in 17% of cases compared with 40% in the present study. The *esp* + *hyl* gene combination was equally present in both studies, namely in

31% in the present study and in 33% in the study by Ochoa et al. [37]. Comparison of the presence of virulence factors between individual VRE clones did not show significant differences.

Even though VRE are widespread globally, their epidemiology varies by region. The spread of VRE between various hospitals was illustrated by a study from Ireland that had long faced high VRE prevalence rates, reaching approximately 45% [24,38]. Recurring VRE outbreaks remained an unresolved problem in the healthcare system. Only adequately selected molecular typing methods may confirm or rule out epidemiologically related cases. If a new outbreak or merely increased rate of VRE is reasonably suspected, the clonal relationship of strains needs to be analyzed to reveal the source or route of transmission of the infection. In the present study, the clonal relationship of strains was assessed with PFGE. Despite certain limitations, PFGE continues to be considered a gold-standard method as its results may be quantified with high discriminatory ability and reproducibility [39,40]. In the present study, molecular typing results confirmed clonal spread of identical strains in 67% of tested VRE isolates. This confirms the possibility of colonization in staff members and subsequent transmission to hospitalized patients via various environmental vectors. Apparently, the hands of the staff members are the most important one. The literature also mentions wastewater in a commode as an appropriate vehicle for VRE survival, enabling spread in the form of aerosol or by contact with hands or clothes [41]. With regard to the finding of unique profiles in 33% of analyzed VRE, their endogenous origin from the GIT is to be admitted, with the following selection caused by broad-spectrum antibiotic therapy.

Analysis of the restriction profiles of individual clones yielded clonal groups containing two to 12 strains obtained from various patients. The study results suggest that no single epidemic clone was spreading at the hemato-oncology department for a longer period of time and that individual epidemic clones were present for limited time intervals of one to eight months. It can be assumed that the time of occurrence of individual VRE clones was mainly conditioned by the length of hospital stay. There were no changes in the environmental parameters during the study (e.g., remodeling of the rooms or new ventilation).

4. Materials and Methods

Between 1 January 2016 and 31 December 2018, stool samples and perianal swabs were collected from patients staying at the Department of Hemato-Oncology, University Hospital Olomouc to isolate enterococci using standard procedures. All samples were inoculated onto both blood agar plates and Brilliance VRE Agar chromogenic screening plates (Oxoid, Brno, Czech Republic). Species identification of isolates was carried out with MALDI-TOF MS (Biotyper Microflex, Bruker Daltonics, Billerica, MA, USA). From each patient, only one isolate identified as the first one was included. Strains were stored in cryotubes at −80 °C (Cryobank B, ITEST, Hradec Králové, Czech Republic). Stool samples and perianal swabs were collected only as part of standard clinical care.

Susceptibility to antibiotics (ampicillin, tigecycline, tetracycline, teicoplanin, nitrofurantoin, and linezolid) was tested using the microdilution method as recommended by the EUCAST [42]. *Staphylococcus aureus* ATCC 29213 and *Enterococcus faecalis* ATCC 29212 reference strains were used for quality control.

DNA for genetic analysis was isolated with a Qiagen Kit (DNeasy Blood and Tissue Kit, Qiagen, Hilden, Germany). A PCR (polymerase chain reaction) method was used to detect glycopeptide resistance genes (*vanA*, *vanB*, *vanC-1*, *vanC2-C3*) with primers as specified in Table 2 [43]. The amplification conditions were as follows: initial denaturation at 95 °C for 7 min, followed by 35 denaturation cycles at 95 °C/30 s, annealing at 62 °C/30 s, extension at 72 °C/60 s, and final extension at 72 °C for 7 min. Selected virulence factors were identified with multiplex PCR [44]. The presence of genes encoding gelatinase (*gelE*), aggregation substance (*asa1*), hyaluronidase (*hyl*), cytolysin (*cylA*), and extracellular surface protein (*esp*) was investigated using the primers listed in Table 2. The reaction was run under the following conditions: initial denaturation at 95 °C for 15 min, followed by 30 denaturation cycles at 95 °C/60 s, annealing at 62 °C/60 s, extension at 72 °C/60 s, and final extension at 72 °C for 10 min. The final products were separated in 1.5% agarose gel at 110 V for 60 min using SYBR Safe DNA Gel Stain (Thermo Fisher Scientific, Waltham, MA, USA). Visualization was carried out under UV light with a UV transilluminator (Transluminator Discovery™, UltraLum, Claremont, CA, USA).

Table 2. PCR primers and products for detecting *van* genes and virulence factor genes.

Gene	Sequence (5'→3')	Size (bp)	Reference
van Genes			
vanA	GGGAAAACGACAATTGC GTACAATGCGGCCGTTA	732	[42]
vanB	ATGGGAAGCCGATAGTC GATTTCGTTCCTCGACC	635	
vanC-1	GGTATCAAGGAAACCTC CTTCCGCCATCATAGCT	822	
vanC2-C3	CTCCTACGATTCTCTTG CGAGCAAGACCTTTAAG	439	
Virulence Factor Genes			
asa1	GCACGCTATTACGAACTATGA TAAGAAAGAACATCACCACGA	375	[43]
gelE	TATGACAATGCTTTTTGGGAT AGATGCACCCGAAATAATATA	213	
cylA	ACTCGGGGATTGATAGGC GCTGCTAAAGCTGCGCTT	688	
esp	AGATTTCATCTTTGATTCTTGG AATTGATTCTTTAGCATCTGG	510	
hyl	ACAGAAGAGCTGCAGGAAATG GACTGACGTCCAAGTTTCCAA	276	

Molecular typing of all isolated VRE was performed using PFGE. Intact DNA was obtained according to a previously described protocol [45]. Restriction cleavage of blocks with DNA was carried out in a *SmaI* restriction enzyme solution (Takara Biotechnology, Kyoto, Japan) containing 5 µL of *SmaI* restriction buffer, 5 µL of 0.1% BSA, 50 µL of deionized water, and 10U of *SmaI*. The blocks were incubated at 30 °C overnight. Restriction fragments were separated in 1.2% (w/v) agarose gel in the CHEF-DRII system (Bio-Rad, Hercules, CA, USA). The parameters selected for analysis were as follows: 24 h, voltage 6 V·cm^{-1}, and pulse times 2–35 s. The restriction fragments were assessed with GelCompare, version 2.0 (Applied Maths, Kortrijk, Belgium). The similarity coefficient was calculated using the Dice algorithm (based on the Dice coefficient of similarity of macrorestriction profiles set at 2%). Individual clusters were analyzed with the UPGMA (unweighted pair group method with arithmetic mean) algorithm and the results were interpreted using criteria defined by Tenover et al. [46].

5. Conclusions

The results of PFGE showed no significant outbreak of clonal spread of VRE, but confirmed repeated smaller outbreaks. As seen from the constructed timeline, there was no single hospital strain with an unchanged genetic profile to repeatedly occur over the three-year study period. During that time, a total of 18 clonal groups were identified. In 2016, an identical VRE clone detected in 12 patients persisted for as long as eight months. The year 2017 seems to be most diverse, with only 1-month persistence of a clone replaced by a genetically different clone being noted in four cases. The number of clone groups in the last year was comparable to that in 2017 as it only decreased by one group. However, identical strains persisted for a longer time in various patients and no clone persisted for less than three months. Moreover, the study revealed the presence of genetically unique isolates accounting for 33% of all VRE. One of the risk factors for colonization is the long-term hospital stay of patients sharing the same room combined with the ability of enterococci to persist in the hospital environment [19].

It is those small groups of clones identified in two or three patients in the present study that suggest their spread among patients hospitalized at the same time. The potential routes of transmission are the hands of both patients and healthcare professionals or even family members visiting patients. Considering the selection pressure of antibiotics used, the immune status of hemato-oncological patients and chemotherapy, if administered, the likely source of VRE is their GIT.

Author Contributions: Conceptualization, M.K., K.H., and J.B.; Methodology, M.K., K.H., and T.Š.; Validation, T.Š. and P.K.; Investigation, K.H., T.Š., and P.K.; Resources, M.K., K.H., and J.B.; Data curation, K.H.; Writing—original draft preparation, K.H. and M.K.; Writing—review and editing, M.K., K.H., J.B. and K.F.; Visualization, K.H. and K.F.; Supervision, M.K.; Project administration, M.K.; Funding acquisition, J.B. All authors have read and agreed to the published version of the manuscript.

Funding: This research was funded by the Czech Health Research Council (project no. NV18-05-00340).

Conflicts of Interest: The authors declare no conflict of interest.

References

1. Kolář, M. Vancomycin-resistant enterococci. *Klin. Mikrobiol. Infekc. Lek.* **2018**, *24*, 50–56.
2. Sievert, D.M.; Ricks, P.; Edwards, J.R.; Schneider, A.; Patel, J.; Srinivasan, A.; Kallen, A.; Limbago, B.; Fridkin, S.; National Healthcare Safety Network (NHSN) Team and Participating NHSN Facilities. Antimicrobial-resistant pathogens associated with healthcare-associated infections: Summary of data reported to the National Healthcare Safety Network at the Centers for Disease Control and Prevention, 2009–2010. *Infect. Control Hosp. Epidemiol.* **2013**, *34*, 1–14. [CrossRef]
3. Michael, K.E.; No, D.; Roberts, M.C. VanA-positive multi-drug-resistant Enterococcus spp. isolated from surfaces of a US hospital laundry facility. *J. Hosp. Infect.* **2017**, *95*, 218–223. [CrossRef]
4. Kolář, M.; Heinigeová, B.; Bartoníková, N.; Čermák, P.; Burgetová, D.; Dorníková, G.; Dovalová, M.; Frýbortová, V.; Horová, E.; Chmelařová, E.; et al. Gram-positive pathogens in bloodstream infections—A multicenter study. *Klin. Mikrobiol. Inf. Lek.* **2003**, *9*, 244–252.
5. Herkel, T.; Uvizl, R.; Doubravska, L.; Adamus, M.; Gabrhelik, T.; Htoutou Sedlakova, M.; Kolar, M.; Hanulik, V.; Pudova, V.; Langova, K.; et al. Epidemiology of hospital-acquired pneumonia: Results of a Central European multicenter, prospective, observational study compared with data from the European region. *Biomed. Pap. Med. Fac. Univ. Palacky Olomouc Czech Repub.* **2016**, *160*, 448–455. [CrossRef]
6. Pudová, V.; Htoutou Sedláková, M.; Kolář, M.; Working Group. Clonality of bacterial pathogens causing hospital-acquired pneumonia. *Curr. Microbiol.* **2016**, *73*, 312–316. [CrossRef]
7. Arias, C.A.; Murray, B.E. The rise of the *Enterococcus*: Beyond vancomycin resistance. *Nat. Rev. Microbiol* **2012**, *10*, 266–278. [CrossRef]
8. Arthur, M.; Reynolds, P.E.; Depardieu, F.; Evers, S.; Dutka-Malen, S.; Quintiliani, R., Jr.; Courvalin, P. Mechanisms of glycopeptide resistance in enterococci. *J. Infect.* **1996**, *32*, 11–16. [CrossRef]
9. Murray, B.E. Vancomycin-resistant enterococci. *Am. J. Med.* **1997**, *102*, 284–293. [CrossRef]
10. Reynolds, P.E.; Courvalin, P. Vancomycin resistance in enterococci due to synthesis of precursors terminating in D-alanyl-D-serine. *Antimicrob. Agents Chemother.* **2005**, *49*, 21–25. [CrossRef]
11. Courvalin, P. Vancomycin resistance in gram-positive cocci. *Clin. Infect. Dis.* **2006**, *42* (Suppl. S1), S25–S34. [CrossRef]
12. Uttley, A.H.; Collins, C.H.; Naidoo, J.; George, R.C. Vancomycin-resistant enterococci. *Lancet* **1988**, *1*, 57–58. [CrossRef]
13. Kolář, M.; Vágnerová, I.; Kohnová, I. Detection of vancomycin-resistant enterococci in Teaching Hospital, Olomouc. *Klin. Mikrobiol. Inf. Lek.* **1997**, *3*, 189–191.
14. Kolar, M.; Htoutou Sedlakova, M.; Pudova, V.; Roderova, M.; Novosad, J.; Senkyrikova, M.; Szotkowska, R.; Indrak, K. Incidence of fecal Enterobacteriaceae producing broad-spectrum beta-lactamases in patients with hematological malignancies. *Biomed. Pap. Med. Fac. Univ. Palacky Olomouc Czech Repub.* **2015**, *159*, 100–103. [CrossRef] [PubMed]
15. Heath, C.H.; Blackmore, T.K.; Gordon, D.L. Emerging resistance in *Enterococcus* spp. *Med. J. Aust.* **1996**, *164*, 116–120. [CrossRef]

16. Weber, D.J.; Rutala, W.A. Role of environmental contamination in the transmission of vancomycin-resistant enterococci. *Infect. Control Hosp. Epidemiol.* **1997**, *18*, 306–309. [CrossRef] [PubMed]
17. Jordens, J.Z.; Bates, J.; Griffiths, D.T. Faecal carriage and nosocomial spread of vancomycin-resistant *Enterococcus faecium*. *J. Antimicrob. Chemother.* **1994**, *34*, 515–528. [CrossRef]
18. Heisel, R.W.; Sutton, R.R.; Mascara, G.P.; Winger, D.G.; Weber, D.R.; Lim, S.H.; Oleksiuk, L.M. Vancomycin-resistant enterococci in acute myeloid leukemia and myelodysplastic syndrome patients undergoing induction chemotherapy with idarubicin and cytarabine. *Leuk. Lymphoma* **2017**, *58*, 2565–2572. [CrossRef]
19. Kolar, M.; Pantucek, R.; Vagnerova, I.; Kesselova, M.; Sauer, P.; Matouskova, I.; Doskar, J.; Koukalova, D.; Hejnar, P. Genotypic characterisation of vancomycin-resistant *Enterococcus faecium* isolates from haemato-oncological patients at Olomouc University Hospital, Czech Republic. *Clin. Microbiol. Infect.* **2006**, *12*, 353–360. [CrossRef] [PubMed]
20. Paterson, D.L.; Muto, C.A.; Ndirangu, M.; Linden, P.K.; Potoski, B.A.; Capitano, B.; Bonomo, R.A.; Aron, D.C.; Donskey, C.J. Acquisition of rectal colonization by vancomycin-resistant *Enterococcus* among intensive care unit patients treated with piperacillin-tazobactam versus those receiving cefepime-containing antibiotic regimens. *Antimicrob. Agents Chemother.* **2008**, *52*, 465–469. [CrossRef]
21. European Antimicrobial Resistance Surveillance Network (EARS-Net). Available online: https://ecdc.europa.eu/en/about-us/partnerships-and-networks/disease-and-laboratory-networks/ears-net (accessed on 6 August 2019).
22. European Centre for Disease Prevention and Control (ECDC) Antimicrobial Resistance Surveillance in Europe 2015. Available online: https://ecdc.europa.eu/en/publications-data/antimicrobial-resistance-surveillance-europe-2015 (accessed on 6 August 2019).
23. European Centre for Disease Prevention and Control. Antimicrobial Resistance Surveillance in Europe 2016. Available online: https://ecdc.europa.eu/en/publications-data/antimicrobial-resistance-surveillance-europe-2016 (accessed on 6 August 2019).
24. European Centre for Disease Prevention and Control. Antimicrobial Resistance Surveillance in Europe 2017. Available online: https://ecdc.europa.eu/sites/portal/files/documents/EARS-Net-report-2017-update-jan-2019.pdf (accessed on 6 August 2019).
25. Kolar, M.; Pantucek, R.; Vagnerova, I.; Sauer, P.; Kesselova, M.; Cekanova, L.; Koukalova, D.; Doskar, J.; Ruzickova, V. Prevalence of vancomycin-resistant enterococci in hospitalized patients and those living in the community in the Czech Republic. *New Microbiol.* **2006**, *29*, 121–125.
26. AbdelKhalek, A.; Abutaleb, N.S.; Mohammad, H.; Seleem, M.N. Repurposing ebselen for decolonization of vancomycin-resistant enterococci (VRE). *PLoS ONE* **2018**, *13*, e0199710. [CrossRef]
27. Yang, J.X.; Li, T.; Ning, Y.Z.; Shao, D.H.; Liu, J.; Wang, S.Q.; Liang, G.W. Molecular characterization of resistance, virulence and clonality in vancomycin-resistant *Enterococcus faecium* and *Enterococcus faecalis*: A hospital-based study in Beijing, China. *Infect. Genet. Evol.* **2015**, *33*, 253–260. [CrossRef] [PubMed]
28. Alevizakos, M.; Gaitanidis, A.; Nasioudis, D.; Tori, K.; Flokas, M.E.; Mylonakis, E. Colonization with vancomycin-resistant enterococci and risk for bloodstream infection among patients with malignancy: A systematic review and meta-analysis. *Open Forum Infect. Dis.* **2016**, *4*, ofw246. [CrossRef]
29. Ballo, O.; Tarazzit, I.; Stratmann, J.; Reinheimer, C.; Hogardt, M.; Wichelhaus, T.A.; Kempf, V.; Serve, H.; Finkelmeier, F.; Brandts, C. Colonization with multidrug resistant organisms determines the clinical course of patients with acute myeloid leukemia undergoing intensive induction chemotherapy. *PLoS ONE* **2019**, *14*, e0210991. [CrossRef]
30. Weber, S.; Hogardt, M.; Reinheimer, C.; Wichelhaus, T.A.; Kempf, V.; Kessel, J.; Wolf, S.; Serve, H.; Steffen, B.; Scheich, S. Bloodstream infections with vancomycin-resistant enterococci are associated with a decreased survival in patients with hematological diseases. *Ann. Hematol* **2019**, *98*, 763–773. [CrossRef] [PubMed]
31. Mantey, J.; Min, L.; Cassone, M.; Gibson, K.E.; Mody, L. Changing dynamics of colonization in nursing facility patients over time: Reduction in methicillin-resistant *Staphylococcus aureus* (MRSA) offset by increase in vancomycin-resistant *Enterococcus* (VRE) prevalence. *Infect. Control Hosp. Epidemiol.* **2019**, *40*, 1069–1070. [CrossRef] [PubMed]
32. Talaga, K.; Odrowąż-Konduracka, D.; Paradowska, B.; Jagiencarz-Starzec, B.; Wolak, Z.; Bulanda, M.; Szcypta, A. Typing of *Enterococcus* spp. strains in 4 hospitals in the Małopolska region in Poland. *Adv. Clin. Exp. Med.* **2018**, *27*, 111–117. [CrossRef]

33. Jovanović, M.; Tošić, T.; Jovanović, S.; Stošović, R.; Stevanović, G.; Velebit, B.; Zervos, M.J. Presence of the esp gene in *Enterococcus faecium* derived from oropharyngeal microbiota of haematology patients. *Arch. Oral Biol.* **2018**, *88*, 54–59. [CrossRef]
34. Vu, J.; Carvalho, J. *Enterococcus*: Review of its physiology, pathogenesis, diseases and the challenges it poses for clinical microbiology. *Front. Biol.* **2011**, *6*, 357–366. [CrossRef]
35. Farahani, A. State of globe: Enterococci: Virulence factors and biofilm formation. *J. Glob. Infect. Dis.* **2016**, *8*, 1–2. [CrossRef]
36. Marchi, A.P.; Perdigão Neto, L.V.; Martins, R.C.R.; Rizek, C.F.; Camargo, C.H.; Moreno, L.Z.; Moreno, A.M.; Batista, M.V.; Basqueira, M.S.; Rossi, F.; et al. Vancomycin-resistant enterococci isolates colonizing and infecting haematology patients: Clonality, and virulence and resistance profile. *J. Hosp. Infect.* **2018**, *99*, 346–355. [CrossRef] [PubMed]
37. Ochoa, S.A.; Escalona, G.; Cruz-Córdova, A.; Dávila, L.B.; Saldaña, Z.; Cázares-Domímguez, V.; Eslava, C.A.; López-Martínez, B.; Hernández-Castro, R.; Aquino-Jarquin, G.; et al. Molecular analysis and distribution of multidrug-resistant *Enterococcus faecium* isolates belonging to clonal complex 17 in a tertiary care center in Mexico City. *BMC Microbiol.* **2013**, *13*, 291. [CrossRef] [PubMed]
38. Ryan, L.; O'Mahony, E.; Wrenn, C.; FitzGerald, S.; Fox, U.; Boyle, B.; Schaffer, K.; Werner, G.; Klare, I. Epidemiology and molecular typing of VRE bloodstream isolates in an Irish tertiary care hospital. *J. Antimicrob. Chemother.* **2015**, *70*, 2718–2724. [CrossRef] [PubMed]
39. Gozalan, A.; Coskun-Ari, F.F.; Ozdem, B.; Unaldi, O.; Celikbilek, N.; Kirca, F.; Aydogan, S.; Muderris, T.; Guven, T.; Acikgoz, Z.C.; et al. Molecular characterization of vancomycin-resistant *Enterococcus faecium* strains isolated from carriage and clinical samples in a tertiary hospital, Turkey. *J. Med. Microbiol.* **2015**, *64*, 759–766. [CrossRef]
40. Bressan, R.; Knezevich, A.; Monticelli, J.; Campanile, F.; Busetti, M.; Santagati, M.; Dolzani, L.; Milan, A.; Bongiorno, D.; Di Santolo, M.; et al. Spread of vancomycin-resistant *Enterococcus faecium* isolates despite validated infection control measures in an Italian hospital: Antibiotic resistance and genotypic characterization of the endemic strain. *Microb. Drug Resist.* **2018**, *24*, 1148–1155. [CrossRef]
41. Noble, M.A.; Isaac-Renton, J.L.; Bryce, E.A.; Roscoe, D.L.; Roberts, F.J.; Walker, M.; Scharf, S.; Walsh, A.; Altamirano-Dimas, M.; Gribble, M. The toilet as a transmission vector of vancomycin-resistant enterococci. *J. Hosp. Infect.* **1998**, *40*, 237–241. [CrossRef]
42. The European Committee on Antimicrobial Susceptibility Testing—EUCAST 2018. Available online: http://www.eucast.org/ (accessed on 6 August 2019).
43. Dutka-Malen, S.; Evers, S.; Courvalin, P. Detection of glycopeptide resistance genotypes and identification to the species level of clinically relevant enterococci by PCR [published correction appears in J Clin Microbiol. 1995 May;33:1434]. *J. Clin. Microbiol.* **1995**, *33*, 24–27. [CrossRef]
44. Vankerckhoven, V.; Van Autgaerden, T.; Vael, C.; Lammens, C.; Chapelle, S.; Rossi, R.; Jabes, D.; Goossens, H. Development of a multiplex PCR for the detection of asa1, gelE, cylA, esp, and hyl genes in enterococci and survey for virulence determinants among European hospital isolates of *Enterococcus faecium*. *J. Clin. Microbiol.* **2004**, *42*, 4473–4479. [CrossRef]
45. Pantůček, R.; Götz, F.; Doskar, J.; Rosypal, S. Genomic variability of *Staphylococcus aureus* and the other coagulase-positive *Staphylococcus* species estimated by macrorestriction analysis using pulsed-field gel electrophoresis. *Int. J. Syst. Bacteriol.* **1996**, *46*, 216–222. [CrossRef]
46. Tenover, F.C.; Arbeit, R.D.; Goering, R.V.; Mickelsen, P.A.; Murray, B.E.; Persing, D.H.; Swaminathan, B. Interpreting chromosomal DNA restriction patterns produced by pulsed-field gel electrophoresis: Criteria for bacterial strain typing. *J. Clin. Microbiol.* **1995**, *33*, 2233–2239. [CrossRef]

Publisher's Note: MDPI stays neutral with regard to jurisdictional claims in published maps and institutional affiliations.

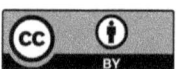

© 2020 by the authors. Licensee MDPI, Basel, Switzerland. This article is an open access article distributed under the terms and conditions of the Creative Commons Attribution (CC BY) license (http://creativecommons.org/licenses/by/4.0/).

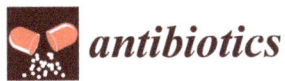

Article

Antibiotic Resistance, *spa* Typing and Clonal Analysis of Methicillin-Resistant *Staphylococcus aureus* (MRSA) Isolates from Blood of Patients Hospitalized in the Czech Republic

Katarina Pomorska [1], Vladislav Jakubu [1,2,3], Lucia Malisova [1,3], Marta Fridrichova [3], Martin Musilek [4] and Helena Zemlickova [1,2,3,*]

[1] Centre for Epidemiology and Microbiology, National Reference Laboratory for Antibiotics, National Institute of Public Health, 10000 Prague, Czech Republic; katarina.pomorska@szu.cz (K.P.); vladislav.jakubu@szu.cz (V.J.); lucia.malisova@szu.cz (L.M.)
[2] Department of Clinical Microbiology, Faculty of Medicine and University Hospital, Charles University, 53002 Hradec Kralove, Czech Republic
[3] Department of Microbiology, 3rd Faculty of Medicine Charles University, University Hospital Kralovske Vinohrady, National Institute of Public Health, 10000 Prague, Czech Republic; marta.fridrichova@fnkv.cz
[4] Centre for Epidemiology and Microbiology, National Reference Laboratory for Meningococcal Infections, National Institute of Public Health, 10000 Prague, Czech Republic; martin.musilek@szu.cz
* Correspondence: hzemlickova@szu.cz

Abstract: *Staphylococcus aureus* is one of the major causes of bloodstream infections. The aim of our study was to characterize methicillin-resistant *Staphylococcus aureus* (MRSA) isolates from blood of patients hospitalized in the Czech Republic between 2016 and 2018. All MRSA strains were tested for antibiotic susceptibility, analyzed by *spa* typing and clustered using a Based Upon Repeat Pattern (BURP) algorithm. The representative isolates of the four most common *spa* types and representative isolates of all *spa* clonal complexes were further typed by multilocus sequence typing (MLST) and staphylococcal cassette chromosome *mec* (SCC*mec*) typing. The majority of MRSA strains were resistant to ciprofloxacin (94%), erythromycin (95.5%) and clindamycin (95.6%). Among the 618 strains analyzed, 52 different *spa* types were detected. BURP analysis divided them into six different clusters. The most common *spa* types were t003, t586, t014 and t002, all belonging to the CC5 (clonal complex). CC5 was the most abundant MLST CC of our study, comprising of 91.7% (n = 565) of *spa*-typeable isolates. Other CCs present in our study were CC398, CC22, CC8, CC45 and CC97. To our knowledge, this is the biggest nationwide study aimed at typing MRSA blood isolates from the Czech Republic.

Keywords: *Staphylococcus aureus*; MRSA; *spa* typing; MLST; SCC*mec* typing; clonal analysis; epidemiology

1. Introduction

Staphylococcus aureus is an important opportunistic pathogen both in communities and in hospitals. It can cause broad spectrum of diseases, e.g., skin, soft tissue infections, heart, pleuropulmonary and osteoarticular infections [1]. It is considered to be one of the major causes of bloodstream infections (BSI) in Europe [2]. It was reported that a patient with bacteremia caused by methicillin-resistant *Staphylococcus aureus* (MRSA) is at a higher risk of all-cause mortality than a patient infected by methicillin-susceptible *Staphylococcus aureus* (MSSA) [3]. According to the European Antimicrobial Resistance Surveillance Network (EARS-Net) data, the proportion of MRSA isolates from blood from 2005 (until 2018) in the Czech Republic was around 14% (in the preceding years it was lower, from 4.3% to 8.5%) [4]. It is important to type MRSA isolates to get an insight into epidemiology, limit its possible spread or imply the infection control measures. Studies conducted over time engaged with typing Czech MRSA strains using different molecular methods such as multilocus sequence typing (MLST), staphylococcal cassette chromosome *mec* (SCC*mec*) typing, pulsed-field gel electrophoresis (PFGE) and ribotyping revealed clonal replacements. In 1996–1997 the most common MRSA clone was Brazilian clone (ST239, SCC*mec*IIIA, PFGE type B, ribotype H1) and Iberian clone (ST247, SCC*mec*IA, PFGE type A, ribotype H2) [5]. Around the year 2000, Brazilian clone was replaced by a unique "Czech clone". They differed only in PFGE type and ribotype (F and H6 for the Czech clone, respectively) [6]. After 2001, epidemic clone EMRSA-15 (ST22, SCC*mec*IV) was detected increasingly [7]. Another clonal replacement was detected using staphylococcal protein A typing method (*spa* typing). Grundmann et al. [8] in his multicentric European study showed that the majority of Czech MRSA blood isolates from 2006–2007 period were typed as t003 (t003/ST225/SCC*mec*II). The retrospective typing of staphylococcal protein A gene of Czech MRSA blood isolates revealed that the clonal replacement took place in 2004, when the most common *spa* type t030 isolates were replaced by t003 isolates [9]. It was accompanied by the shift of antibiotic susceptibility of rifampicin and gentamicin [9]. Type t003 was the second most common MRSA *spa* type from bloodstream infections in 2011 in Europe [3]. As the previous studies have shown, the dominance of MRSA clones undergoes dynamic changes. The aim of our study was to type Czech MRSA blood isolates phenotypically (antibiotic susceptibility), genotypically (*spa* typing, MLST, SCC*mec* typing) and to infer their clonal relatedness by clustering them using Based Upon Repeat Pattern (BURP) algorithm.

2. Results

2.1. Antimicrobial Susceptibility of MRSA Strains

In total, in the 2016–2018 period, 618 single-patient MRSA blood isolates from the participating Czech EARS-Net laboratories were sent and analyzed in the National Reference Laboratory for Antibiotics (NRL for ATB), National Institute of Public Health (Prague, the Czech Republic). Resistance to methicillin (screened by cefoxitine disc [30 μg]) was confirmed by PCR for *mec* genes. All MRSA strains possessed an *mecA* gene (and were *mecC* negative). The majority of strains were resistant to erythromycin (n = 590; 95.5%), clindamycin (n = 591 (including 76 strains with inducible resistance); 95.6%), and ciprofloxacin (n = 581; 94.0%). Only 77 strains (12.5%) were resistant to gentamicin, 53 (8.6%) to chloramphenicol and 48 (7.8%) to tetracycline. The resistance to other antibiotics was rare: 15 strains (2.4%) were resistant to fusidic acid, 13 (2.1%) to rifampicin, 9 (1.5%) to trimethoprim/sulfamethoxazole and 6 (1.0%) to ceftaroline. All the confirmed MRSA isolates were susceptible to tigecycline, vancomycin and linezolid. The frequency of antibiotic resistance (%) over the study period is shown in Figure 1. The majority of strains (n = 600; 97.1%) were multidrug-resistant (MDR; i.e., non-susceptibility to at least one agent in three or more antimicrobial categories [10]). The most common MDR antibiotic resistance profile (resistance to cefoxitine, erythromycin, clindamycin and ciprofloxacin) was present in 429 (69.4%) strains. The more detailed characteristics of all the isolates from our study are shown in the Supplementary Table S1.

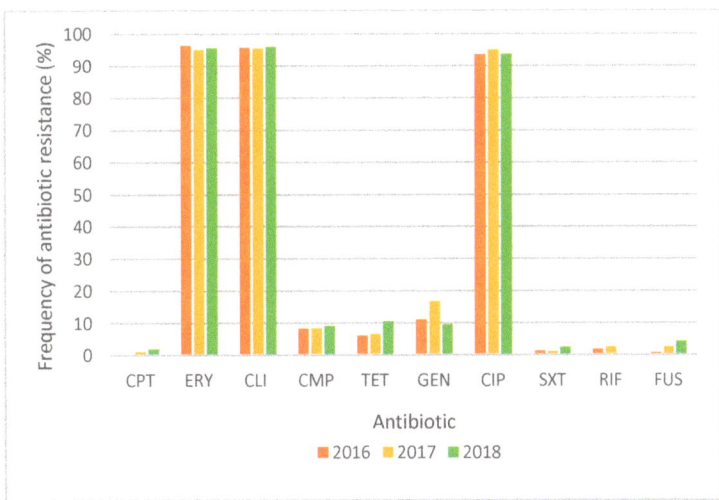

Figure 1. Frequency of antibiotic resistance (%) of the 618 single-patient MRSA blood isolates over the study period (2016–2018). CPT: ceftaroline, ERY: erythromycin, CLI: clindamycin, CMP: chloramphenicol, TET: tetracycline, GEN: gentamicin, CIP: ciprofloxacin, SXT: trimethoprim/sulfamethoxazole, RIF: rifampicin, FUS: fusidic acid. All the isolates were resistant to cefoxitine and susceptible to tigecycline, vancomycin and linezolid.

2.2. spa Typing, Cluster Analysis and Antibiotic Susceptibility within spa CCs

Altogether, 52 different *spa* types were detected in this study (Figure 2). Four *spa* types were dominant: t003 (n = 239; 38.8%), t586 (n = 129; 20.9%), t014 (n = 121; 19.6%) and t002 (n = 27; 4.4%). They were followed by t034 (n = 8; 1.3%), t045 (n = 8; 1.3%) and t127 (n = 7; 1.1%). Several *spa* types (n = 28; 53.8%) were detected only once. Two strains out of 618 (0.3%) were not typeable by *spa* typing.

The proportion of t003 and t002 did not differ much over the studied period (34.7–41.6% and 3.3–5.1%, respectively). The proportion of t586 isolates increased from 11.6% in 2016 to around 25% in the subsequent years. The proportion of t014 isolates decreased to 14.2% in 2018 (from more than 20% in the preceding years).

The majority of the *spa*-typeable isolates (n = 465; 75.5%) were grouped into 6 different clusters (4 *spa* CCs) (Figure 2). Cluster 5 and 6 did not have any founder and were not assigned into any *spa* CC (n = 5 strains; 0.8%). Several strains (n = 17; 2.8%) belonging to 6 different *spa* types were singletons. BURP algorithm excluded 134 (21.8%) strains from the analysis because of an inadequate number of repeats (Figure 2).

spa CC003 (cluster number 1) comprised of the greatest number of strains and the three most common *spa* types (t003, t002 and t014) (Figure 2). The majority of these strains were resistant to erythromycin, clindamycin and ciprofloxacin (Table 1). The second cluster, *spa* CC011, was the only cluster with a high proportion of tetracycline resistance (n = 13; 92.9%). The majority of isolates (>50%) within the two remaining *spa* CCs (2436 and 024) were resistant to erythromycin and ciprofloxacin. Five isolates (71.4%) from *spa* CC2436 were also clindamycin resistant; the resistance was inducible in 4 out of 5 aforementioned isolates. Gentamicin resistance (66.7%) was higher among isolates belonging to the cluster number 6 (no founder); however, this cluster did not consist of the representative number of isolates. The percentage of MDR strains and the number of resistances to different antibiotics for each *spa* CC is shown in Table 1.

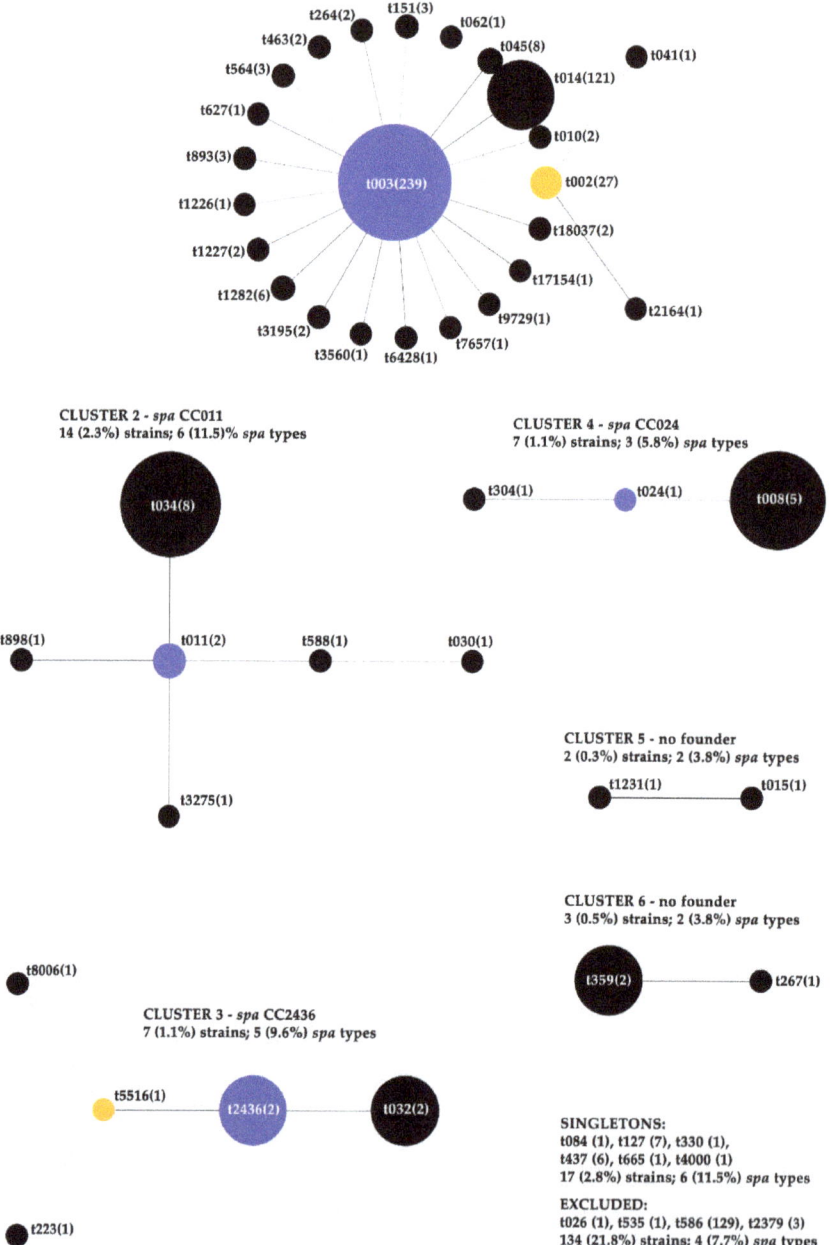

Figure 2. Based Upon Repeat Pattern (BURP) clustering of the *spa*-typed isolates. Isolates were clustered by Ridom Staph Type software using the following parameters: *spa* types were clustered if the cost was less or equal 6 and *spa* types that were shorter than 4 repeats were excluded from the analysis. The number in brackets represents number of isolates. The majority of the *spa* typeable isolates (75.5%) were grouped into 6 different clusters; 21.8% of the isolates were excluded from analysis and 2.8% of isolates were evaluated as singletons.

Table 1. Antibiotic resistance profiles of different *spa* clusters (clonal complexes) and multidrug-resistance within *spa* clusters.

Cluster	*spa* CC	No. (%) of Strains [1]	No. (%) of Strains Resistant to Antibiotics [2]										No. (%) of MDR Strains	No. of Resistant ATB (Mean Value) [3]
			CPT	ERY	CLI	CMP	TET	GEN	CIP	SXT	RIF	FUS		
1	003	432 (70.1)	5 (1.2)	426 (98.6)	426 (98.6)	36 (8.3)	10 (2.3)	35 (8.1)	428 (99.1)	6 (1.4)	8 (1.9)	10 (2.3)	427 (98.8)	4.2
2	011	14 (2.3)	0	7 (50.0)	12 (85.7)	0	13 (92.9)	2 (14.3)	6 (42.9)	1 (7.1)	1 (7.1)	0	14 (100)	4.0
3	2436	7 (1.1)	0	5 (71.4)	5 (71.4)	0	0	0	6 (85.7)	0	0	0	5 (71.4)	3.3
4	024	7 (1.1)	0	5 (71.4)	2 (28.6)	0	0	2 (28.6)	4 (57.1)	0	0	1 (14.3)	4 (57.1)	3
5	no founder	2 (0.3)	0	0	0	0	0	0	0	0	0	0	0	1
6	no founder	3 (0.5)	0	0	0	0	0	2 (66.7)	0	0	0	1 (33.3)	1 (33.3)	2

CC: clonal complex, MDR: multidrug-resistance, ATB: antibiotics, CPT: ceftaroline, ERY: erythromycin, CLI: clindamycin, CMP: chloramphenicol, TET: tetracycline, GEN: gentamicin, CIP: ciprofloxacin, SXT: trimethoprim/sulfamethoxazole, RIF: rifampicin, FUS: fusidic acid; [1] (%) are calculated from the total number of *spa*-typeable strains; [2] all the isolates were resistant to cefoxitine and susceptible to tigecycline, vancomycin and linezolid; [3] number of resistances to the different antibiotics including cefoxitine.

2.3. spa Types and Resistance to Tetracycline

The high proportion of tetracycline resistance within *spa* CC011 prompted us to investigate its prevalence among the different *spa* types further. A high prevalence was detected in strains belonging to *spa* type t011 (n = 2; 100%), t034 (n = 7; 87.5%), t127 (n = 6; 85.7%) and t437 (n = 4; 66.7%). These *spa* types either belonged to *spa* CC011 (t011 and t034) or were classified as singletons (t127, t437). The four most common *spa* types, t586, t003, t014 and t002, had a low proportion of resistance to tetracycline: n = 13 (10.1%), n = 6 (2.5%), n = 3 (2.5%) and n = 0 (0%), respectively.

2.4. MLST, SCCmec Typing and MLST CCs in Relation to the Different spa CCs (BURP Clustering)

Representative isolates differing in antibiotic susceptibility profile of each *spa* CC (or cluster), together with singletons and strains excluded from BURP analysis, were further analyzed by MLST and SCC*mec* typing. Altogether, 40 isolates were typed: nine isolates belonging to *spa* cluster 1 (*spa* CC003), five isolates from cluster 2 (*spa* CC011), four isolates from cluster 3 (*spa* CC2436), three isolates from cluster 4 (*spa* CC024), two isolates belonging to cluster 5, three isolates from cluster 6, six isolates classified as singletons and eight strains excluded from BURP analysis because of inadequate number of repeats (Table 2).

In total, thirteen different MLST sequence types (STs) were typed among the 40 aforementioned isolates: ST1 (n = 1), ST5 (n = 2), ST8 (n = 3), ST22 (n = 4), ST45 (n = 4), ST59 (n = 1), ST72 (n = 1), ST97 (n = 3), ST225 (n = 13), ST398 (n = 5), ST1472 (n = 1), ST1535 (n = 1) and ST5688 (n = 1, new ST). They belonged to MLST CC1 (ST1), CC5 (ST225, ST5, ST5688), CC8 (ST8, ST72), CC15 (ST1535), CC22 (ST22), CC30 (ST1472), CC45 (ST45), CC59 (ST59), CC97 (ST97) and CC398 (ST398).

Strains were clustered in the same way either by BURP analysis or by Bionumerics software (MLST CC) with the exception of the two *spa* types. t4000 and t330 (classified as singletons by BURP analysis) belonged to MLST CC8 and CC45, respectively. For the more detailed relationship between different *spa* types and MLST CCs, see Table 2.

Four different SCC*mec* types were detected in our study. Isolates belonging to MLST CC5 were mainly typed as SCC*mec*II (15/16 isolates). Isolates belonging to other MLST CCs possessed either SCC*mec*IV, V or V_T type (Table 2).

Table 2. Results of the more detailed genotyping of the representative isolates differing in antibiotic susceptibility profiles belonging to the different *spa* clusters, singletons or strains excluded from BURP analysis.

Strain	spa Type	spa Cluster	spa CC	MLST ST	MLST CC	SCCmec Type	Resistance to Antibiotics [1]
B0040949	t003	1	003	225	CC5	II	CIP, GEN, ERY, CLI
B0041781	t003	1	003	225	CC5	II	CMP, CIP, RIF, ERY, CLI
B0047063	t003	1	003	225	CC5	II	CIP, ERY, CLI
B0034821	t586	excluded	excluded	225	CC5	II	CMP, CIP, GEN, ERY, CLI,
B0038966	t586	excluded	excluded	225	CC5	II	CIP, ERY, CLI
B0043165	t586	excluded	excluded	225	CC5	II	CIP, GEN, ERY, CLI, TET
B0037533	t014	1	003	225	CC5	II	CIP, GEN
B0040744	t014	1	003	225	CC5	II	CIP, GEN, ERY, CLI
B0047366	t014	1	003	225	CC5	II	CIP, ERY, CLI
B0037993	t002	1	003	5	CC5	II	CMP, CIP, GEN, ERY, CLI
B0040837	t002	1	003	5688	CC5	IV	-
B0042384	t002	1	003	5	CC5	II	CIP, ERY, CLI
B0033841	t535	excluded	excluded	225	CC5	II	CIP, ERY, CLI
B0039941	t2379	excluded	excluded	225	CC5	II	CIP, ERY, CLI
B0040619	t2379	excluded	excluded	225	CC5	II	CIP, ERY, CLI
B0047250	t2379	excluded	excluded	225	CC5	II	CIP, ERY, CLI
B0038416	t011	2	011	398	CC398	V	CIP, TET
B0046007	t011	2	011	398	CC398	IV	CIP, GEN, SXT, TET
B0037087	t034	2	011	398	CC398	V	CLI, TET
B0043212	t034	2	011	398	CC398	V	CIP, CLI, TET
B0044843	t034	2	011	398	CC398	V	ERY, CLI, TET

Table 2. Cont.

Strain	spa Type	spa Cluster	spa CC	MLST ST	MLST CC	SCCmec Type	Resistance to Antibiotics [1]
B0034866	t032	3	2436	22	CC22	IV	CIP
B0039472	t032	3	2436	22	CC22	IV	CIP, ERY, CLI
B0036602	t2436	3	2436	22	CC22	IV	CIP, ERY, CLI
B0040230	t2436	3	2436	22	CC22	IV	CIP, ERY, CLI
B0034699	t008	4	024	8	CC8	nt	ERY
B0043674	t008	4	024	8	CC8	IV	CIP, ERY
B0043848	t008	4	024	8	CC8	IV	CIP, ERY, CLI
B0045550	t4000	singleton	singleton	72	CC8	nt	GEN, FUS
B0043746	t015	5	no founder	45	CC45	IV	-
B0044462	t1231	5	no founder	45	CC45	IV	-
B0032812	t026	excluded	excluded	45	CC45	IV	-
B0033429	t330	singleton	singleton	45	CC45	IV	ERY, CLI
B0040776	t267	6	no founder	97	CC97	V	GEN
B0037227	t359	6	no founder	97	CC97	V	GEN, FUS
B0048151	t359	6	no founder	97	CC97	IV	-
B0048051	t084	singleton	singleton	1535	CC15	V	GEN, FUS, TET
B0042118	t127	singleton	singleton	1	CC1	IV	ERY, CLI, TET
B0040853	t437	singleton	singleton	59	CC59	V_T	CMP, ERY, CLI, TET
B0033532	t665	singleton	singleton	1472	CC30	IV	CIP, ERY, TET

CC: clonal complex, ST: sequence type, ERY: erythromycin, CLI: clindamycin, CMP: chloramphenicol, TET: tetracycline, GEN: gentamicin, CIP: ciprofloxacin, SXT: trimethoprim/sulfamethoxazole, RIF: rifampicin, FUS: fusidic acid; [1] cefoxitine is not listed in the antibiotic resistance profiles, since all the isolates were resistant.

2.5. Distribution of the Major spa Types and MLST CCs among the Czech Regions

Figure 3 and Table 3 show the distribution of the four major *spa* types and MLST CCs among the Czech regions. t003 strains were sent to NRL for ATB from all the Czech regions (n = 13; except the Moravian-Silesian, from which we did not obtain any MRSA strains). t003 was ubiquitous. It was dominant in the eastern part of the country: in the Olomouc region it was the only *spa* type detected and in Zlin region it represented more than 90% of the isolates. t586 strains (≥25% of the strains) were mainly isolated from the northwestern, southwestern and middle western part of the country. t014 strains were not detected in three regions (eastern/southeastern part of the country) and t002 strains in five regions.

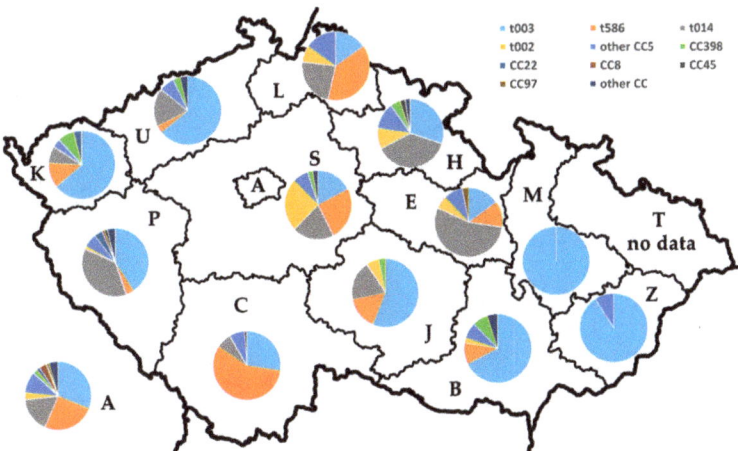

Figure 3. The distribution of the major *spa* types and MLST CCs among the Czech regions. A: Prague Region; S: Central Bohemian Region; C: South Bohemian Region; P: Pilsen Region; K: Karlovy Vary Region; U: Usti nad Labem Region; L: Liberec Region; H: Hradec Kralove Region; E: Pardubice Region; J: Vysocina Region; B: South Moravian Region; M: Olomouc Region; T: Moravian-Silesian Region; Z: Zlin Region.

Table 3. The total number of participating laboratories, isolates and distribution of the major *spa* types and strains belonging to the different MLST CCs among the Czech regions.

Region	No. of Particip. Laboratories	No. of Isolates [1]	No. of spa Types	CC5					CC398	CC22	CC8	CC45	CC97	Other CCs
				t003	t586	t014	t002	Other						
Prague	9	180	29	56 (31.1)	46 (25.6)	30 (16.7)	6 (3.3)	18 (10)	4 (2.2)	3 (1.7)	6 (3.3)	1 (0.6)	2 (1.1)	8 (4.4)
Central Bohemian	4	40	8	7 (17.5)	10 (25)	8 (20)	10 (25)	3 (7.5)	1 (2.5)	0	0	0	0	1 (2.5)
South Bohemian	4	84	9	23 (27.4)	48 (57.1)	6 (7.1)	0	6 (7.1)	0	0	0	1 (1.2)	0	0
Pilsen	2	76	15	31 (40.8)	3 (3.9)	28 (36.8)	1 (1.3)	5 (6.6)	0	3 (3.9)	1 (1.3)	1 (1.3)	0	3 (3.9)
Karlovy Vary	1	25	7	16 (64)	3 (12)	2 (8)	0	1 (4)	2 (8)	1 (4)	0	0	0	0
Usti nad Labem	2	28	7	18 (64.2)	1 (3.6)	5 (17.8)	0	2 (7.1)	1 (3.6)	0	0	0	0	1 (3.6)
Liberec	1	13	5	2 (15.4)	5 (38.5)	3 (23)	1 (7.7)	2 (15.4)	0	0	0	0	0	0
Hradec Kralove	3	40	9	12 (30)	0	15 (37.5)	4 (10)	5 (12.5)	2 (5)	0	0	1 (2.5)	0	1 (2.5)
Pardubice	3	33	8	5 (15.2)	4 (12.1)	18 (54.5)	2 (6.06)	3 (9.1)	0	0	0	0	1 (3.0)	0
Vysocina	4	32	5	18 (56.3)	5 (15.6)	6 (18.8)	2 (6.2)	0	1 (3.1)	0	0	0	0	0
South Moravian	2	40	10	27 (67.5)	4 (10.0)	0	1 (2.5)	3 (7.5)	3 (7.5)	0	0	0	0	2 (5.0)
Olomouc	1	14	1	14 (100.0)	0	0	0	0	0	0	0	0	0	0
Zlin	1	11	2	10 (90.9)	0	0	0	1 (9.1)	0	0	0	0	0	0

CC: clonal complex; [1] number of isolates comprises only of *spa*-typeable isolates.

3. Discussion

In our study we analyzed genotypically and phenotypically 618 MRSA strains isolated from blood of patients hospitalized in the Czech Republic in period 2016–2018. It represents 75% of the Czech MRSA isolates submitted to the EARS-Net.

We demonstrate that the majority of MRSA strains in our study are resistant to erythromycin, clindamycin and ciprofloxacin. A recent study from the Czech Republic also confirmed the high frequency of MRSA isolates resistant to antibiotics from the same classes (erythromycin, clindamycin and ofloxacin); however, only 4.5% of the studied MRSA isolates were derived from bloodstream infections (BSI) [11]. The earlier study concerning the antibiotic resistance of blood isolates from the Czech Republic (collection of MRSA blood isolates from 20 hospitals from the 2000–2002 period) reported resistance to more antibiotics (also gentamicin and rifampicin) [6]. This shift in a resistance phenotype is a result of clonal displacement (from ST239 to ST225 and ST5) [6,9].

We detected 52 different *spa* types among 616 *spa*-typeable MRSA strains. The most common *spa* types included t003, t586, t014 and t002, respectively. Type t003 is the most prevalent *spa* type from blood isolates in the Czech Republic from 2004 [9]. Our result concerning the high abundance of t003, t002 and t014 is in concordance with the multicentric European study that *spa*-typed MRSA blood isolates collected in 25 European countries, where t003 was reported to be the second most common, t002 the fourth and t014 the twentieth most common *spa* type [3]. High prevalence of t003, t586 and t014 was also detected in a recent Czech study investigating MRSA strains originating from various infections [11]. Neradova et al. detected a high proportion of t003, t002 and t014 from BSI from the Czech university hospital [12]. Types t003 and t014 were also detected to be the dominant *spa* types in a study investigating MRSA outbreak in the intensive care unit in the Czech tertiary care hospital [13]. Interesting is the high proportion of t586 (20.9% of the isolates) in our study. According to the Ridom Spa server database [14], this *spa* type has been reported in many European countries (e.g., Germany, Netherlands, France, Belgium, Croatia, Norway, Spain); however, to our knowledge, there has not been any other country detecting such a high proportion of it. MRSA strains typed as t586 were isolated from blood of patients hospitalized in the Czech Republic [11]; however, this is the first study detecting it from blood on a nationwide scale.

The *spa* type distribution varied between the Czech regions. t003 was widespread, it was the most frequently isolated from the eastern part of the country. t586 isolates were frequently isolated from northwestern, southwestern and middle western part of the country (Liberec, Prague, Central Bohemian and South Bohemian regions). Our results corroborate the observation of the recent study conducted by Tkadlec et al. [11] They typed MRSA isolated from various infection sites (or asymptomatic colonization) from 11 Czech hospitals. It is important to note that the dominance of just one *spa* type (or few) in some regions (our study) does not mean that the other *spa* types are not present in these parts of the country. The number of participating laboratories from different regions should be taken into consideration. Some laboratories participating in EARS-Net send only data, thus NRL for ATB does not obtain strains for further typing. From some regions we obtain strains from laboratories belonging to small healthcare facilities rather than laboratories from big hospitals. This might underrepresent prevalence of different *spa* types among the Czech regions in our study.

spa-typeable strains were divided into 6 clusters. Representative strains of each *spa* CC differing in antibiograms were typed by MLST and SCC*mec* typing. Our data analysis shows that the clustering results of BURP analysis and results from Bionumerics software (MLST CCs) are comparable. Isolates were clustered in the same way with either of the two aforementioned methods, with the exception of two *spa* types, which were evaluated as singletons by BURP analysis. Strommenger et al. [15] showed 96.8% concordance between the two methods (*spa* typing/BURP and MLST/eBURST).

Altogether, 565 (91.7%) MRSA strains from our study belonged to CC5. CC5 was reported to be the most abundant MLST CC of staphylococcal isolates from invasive infections in Europe, of which 80% were MRSA [16]. According to the results of more detailed genotyping of the representative strains, we can say that the most common genotype (clone) in our study was ST225/SCC*mec*II. This correlates with the results of whole-genome sequencing data of MRSA from invasive infections from Aanensen et al. [16] The geographic origin of this clone was Middle Europe, more exactly the Czech Republic and Germany. The European clade of ST225 is the descendant of the American clade. It diverged around 1995 and spread to several European countries (Germany, the Czech Republic, Switzerland and Denmark) [17]. Another clone present in our study, ST5/SCC*mec*II, was previously characterized as a USA100 clone (New York/Japan Clone) [18–20]. ST5 is an ancestor of ST225 with the variation in one MLST locus [17]. ST5-SCC*mec*II was reported also in other European countries, e.g., Hungary, Portugal or Austria [21–23]. We might hypothesize that the strain of genotype ST5688/SCC*mec*IV was derived from the Pediatric clone, which is characterized as ST5/SCC*mec*IV [24]. The difference between ST5 and ST5688 is only a single nucleotide in the internal fragment of the *pta* gene.

Our study demonstrates that livestock-associated MRSA (LA-MRSA) were isolated from the human bloodstream infections. The majority of the strains (92.9%) in the second cluster (*spa* CC011–MLST CC398) were resistant to tetracycline, which is a common marker of LA-MRSA [25]. All the t011 (*spa* CC 011) strains and the majority of the t034 (*spa* CC 011) and t127 strains (singletons) (87.5% and 85.7%, respectively) were resistant to the aforementioned antibiotic. The t011 and t034 isolates were typed as ST398 and possessed SCC*mec*IV or V element. The presence of the ST398 LA-MRSA strains and related *spa* types in the Czech Republic was confirmed by several studies. Tegegne et al. [26] reported a wide geographical spread of these strains (isolated from bulk tank milk of cows, sheep and goats) throughout the country. These *spa* types were detected in more than 90% of the *spa*-typed MRSA strains from the Czech livestock animals (pigs, cattle, goats and sheep) as well as from food of animal origin and the environment [27]. A recent study [28] investigated nasal MRSA carriage among veterinary professionals from the Czech Republic. The majority of isolates belonged to ST398 and were clustered into *spa* CC011. Tkadlec et al. [11] showed that 2.5% of the MRSA strains isolated from the various infections were of CC398. The results of our study show that LA-MRSA are also able to cause serious infections (bloodstream); however, the prevalence of these strains among MRSA isolated from blood remains low (2.3%). LA-MRSA ST398 could be the cause of a hospital outbreak, as reported by Wulf et al. [29].

EMRSA-15 (ST22/SCC*mec*IV) strains appeared in the early nineties and subsequently spread to the various hospitals in the United Kingdom and gradually disseminated to other European countries [30]. After 2001, this epidemic clone was detected in hospitals in the Czech Republic [7]. Our study demonstrates the presence of this clone among the isolates from BSI. Strains typed as ST22/SCC*mec*IV (*spa* types t032 and t2436) were grouped in the *spa* CC2436 (MLST CC22). Faria et al. [31] characterized MRSA isolated from BSI from Portugal, when the majority of them were typed as EMRSA-15. Another study [32] detected the presence of this clone in intensive care units from five different countries (years 2008–2011).

t008, t024, t304 and t4000 strains in our study (*spa* CC 024 and one singleton) belong to MLST CC8. The presence of t008 and t024 MRSA *spa* types in BSI in Europe is quite frequent: Grundman et al. [3] showed that t008 is the third most common and t024 is the 15th most common MRSA *spa* type isolated from blood of patients. Tkadlec et al. [11] detected CC8 strains (t008, t024, *etc.*) to be the second most frequently isolated MLST CC from MRSA infections of various origin from the 11 Czech hospitals. More than 64% of them were reported to be community associated (CA-MRSA).

Two isolates of t015 and t1231 (*spa* cluster 5), one t026 isolate (excluded from BURP analysis) and one t330 isolate (singleton) belong to MLST CC45. In 2006, *S. aureus* isolated from BSI typed as CC45 was one of the predominant clones circulating in Europe [16]. In our study we demonstrate the presence of the "Berlin IV" clone, which is characterized as ST45/SCC*mec*IV [33]. All the four aforementioned isolates were of the same genotype.

This clone was also isolated from a nasal swab of the Czech MRSA carrier in 2008 [34]. This epidemic MRSA was initially isolated in Berlin hospitals in early nineties and subsequently disseminated to other areas of Germany [33,35]. A recent phylogenetic analysis proposes that acquisition of the SCC*mec*IV element occurred multiple times within the staphylococcal ST45 population [33].

The last *spa* cluster 6 in our study consisted of two t359 strains and one t267 strain. These isolates were typed as ST97 (MLST CC97). They possessed a SCC*mec*IV or SCC*mec*V element. CC97 MRSA strains were isolated from various infections (data from the Czech Republic, 0.9% of all the strains from the study) and their origin was CA-MRSA [11]. Studies have shown that ST97 MRSA are able to cause hospital outbreak [36,37].

Our study has typed a large collection of samples (75% of the Czech MRSA blood isolates submitted to EARS-Net in 2016–2018 period). Its limitation lies in a choice of the representative isolates belonging to the different *spa* CCs (for MLST analysis and SCC*mec* typing). Not all the *spa* types within some clonal complexes were further typed (for example, within the *spa* CC003 we further typed isolates belonging to the three most common *spa* types and no other rare *spa* types). This might underrepresent the presented diversity of genotypes.

Our study demonstrates that strains belonging to CC5 (ST225, ST5) are the most prevalent among MRSA isolated from the blood cultures from the Czech Republic. The majority of these strains confer a multidrug-resistant phenotype. Although other clones (e.g., EMRSA-15, Berlin IV) appear sporadically, CC5 clones remain the dominant MRSA bloodstream isolates from 2004.

4. Materials and Methods

4.1. Bacterial Strains

S. aureus strains isolated from blood of patients hospitalized in Czech hospitals in 2016–2018 were sent to the National Reference Laboratory for Antibiotics (NRL for ATB), National Institute of Public Health (Prague, the Czech Republic), by laboratories participating in EARS-Net, which is the largest publicly funded system for surveillance of antimicrobial resistance in Europe (https://www.ecdc.europa.eu/en/about-us/networks/disease-networks-and-laboratory-networks/ears-net-about, accessed on the 18 December 2020). At least two blood culture (BC) sets were taken and incubated in BC bottles in automatic systems for 5 days. Positive BC bottles were inoculated on blood agar plates and bacterial colonies were subsequently identified by Matrix—Assisted Laser Desorption Ionization—Time of Flight Mass Spectometry (MALDI-TOF) or other commonly used methods [38]. A total number of 1887 *S. aureus* isolates were reported to EARS-Net in 2016 (45 reporting laboratories), 1944 in 2017 (47 reporting laboratories) and 2244 in 2018 (48 reporting laboratories) (Table 4) [39]. Population sample representativeness, hospital sample representativeness and isolate representativeness was high during the studied period. Blood culture sets/1000 patient days was 18.0 in 2016 and 2017 and 17.0 in 2018 (Table 4) [39]. The staphylococcal isolates data are submitted into EARS-Net annually by the data manager on behalf of the participating laboratories, the majority of the isolates are regularly sent to NRL for ATB for confirmation and further typization. We obtained and analyzed 618 single-patient MRSA strains sent by 37 laboratories over the study period. This number represents 75% (n = 618/824) of all the MRSA strains submitted to the EARS-Net. In 2016 it was 69.2% (n = 182/263), 84% in 2017 (n = 216/257) and 72.4% in 2018 (n = 220/304) (Table 4) [39]. The estimated national population coverage included in the EARS-Net was 85% in 2016 and 2017. In 2018 it counted for 81% [39].

Isolates were inoculated on Nutrient Agar (OXOID, the Czech Republic) and cultivated overnight at 35 °C in aerobic atmosphere. Strain confirmation to the corresponding species was performed using MALDI-TOF (Microflex Bruker; Bremen, Germany) by flexControl software (Bruker Daltonics; Bremen, Germany).

Table 4. Number of reported isolates and data on the sample representativeness according to EARS-Net and number of MRSA strains sent to NRL for ATB from the participating laboratories in EARS-Net.

		Year of the Study			Reference
		2016	2017	2018	
No. of reported staphylococcal isolates	EARS-Net	1887	1944	2244	[39]
No. of MRSA (%)		263 (13.9)	257 (13.2)	304 (13.6)	
No. of single-patient MRSA strains sent to NRL for ATB from the laboratories participating in EARS-Net (% are calculated from the number of MRSA isolates reported in EARS-Net)	NRL for ATB	182 (69.2)	216 (84.0)	220 (72.4)	this study
Number of participating laboratories in our study		31	37	36	
Population sample representativeness	EARS-Net	high	high	high	[39]
Hospital sample representativeness		high	high	high	
Isolate sample representativeness		high	high	high	
Blood culture sets/1000 patient days		18.0	18.0	17.0	
Estimated national population coverage (%)		85	85	81	

4.2. Antibiotic Susceptibility Testing and MRSA Detection

Susceptibility to erythromycin, clindamycin, chloramphenicol, tigecycline, gentamicin, ciprofloxacin, trimethoprim/sulfamethoxazole, rifampicin, fusidic acid, vancomycin and linezolid was tested using broth microdilution method, while susceptibility to ceftaroline and tetracycline by disc diffusion method (according to the EUCAST methodology, breakpoints ver. 9.0—EUCAST 2019 [40]). Susceptibility to ceftaroline was tested using breakpoints for indications other than pneumonia (resistant <17mm, susceptible ≥20 mm). Inducible clindamycin resistance was tested by a broth microdilution method according to the CLSI methodology [41]. Methicillin resistance was screened using cefoxitine disc (30 µg). Strains with the zone diameter <22 mm were reported as MRSA.

4.3. Molecular Typing

4.3.1. mecA/mecC Detection

The presence of genes encoding alternative penicillin-binding proteins (methicillin resistance) was confirmed by polymerase chain reaction (PCR) screening for *mecA/mecC* genes. *mecA* was detected using P4 (5′-TCC AGA TTA CAA CTT CAC CAG G-3′) and P7 (5′-CCA CTT CAT ATC TTG TAA CG-3′) primers [42]. PCR conditions were 4 min at 94 °C, followed by 30 cycles of 45 s at 94 °C, 45 s at 50 °C and 1 min at 72 °C. The final elongation was 2 min at 72 °C (Bio-Rad, DNA Engine Dyad® Dual-Bay Thermal Cycler; Bio-Rad Laboratories, Hercules, California, USA). *mecC* gene was detected according to Stegger et al. [43]. All the primers used in our study are listed in the Supplementary Table S2.

4.3.2. *spa* Typing and Based Upon Repeat Analysis (BURP)

In all MRSA isolates, a single locus of the repeat region X of the *S. aureus* protein A gene (*spa*) was sequenced. DNA amplification and DNA preparation for Sanger sequencing were performed according to the protocol from the official Ridom Spa Server website [44] using primers 1113f (5′-TAA AGA CGA TCC TTC GGT GAG C-3′) and 1514r (5′-CAG CAG TAG TGC CGT TTG CTT-3′). Sequences were evaluated and *spa* types determined using Ridom StaphType software.

To infer the clonal relatedness based on *spa* polymorphisms (*spa* CCs), MRSA strains were clustered by BURP analysis using Ridom StaphType software. Clustering parameters were chosen according to the RidomStaph Type user guide [45]: *spa* types were clustered if cost was less or equal 6 (value defining cluster dimension, the default value was used) and *spa* types that were shorter than 4 repeats were excluded (to include the highest number of *spa* types, the least possible value recommended was used). The strains with inadequate number of repeats were excluded from BURP analysis.

Article

Clonal Diversity of *Klebsiella* spp. and *Escherichia* spp. Strains Isolated from Patients with Ventilator-Associated Pneumonia

Jan Papajk [1], Kristýna Mezerová [2,*], Radovan Uvízl [1], Taťána Štosová [3] and Milan Kolář [3]

1. Department of Anesthesiology, Resuscitation and Intensive Care Medicine, University Hospital Olomouc, 77900 Olomouc, Czech Republic; jan.papajk@fnol.cz (J.P.); radovan.uvizl@fnol.cz (R.U.)
2. Department of Microbiology, Faculty of Medicine and Dentistry, Palacký University Olomouc, 77515 Olomouc, Czech Republic
3. Department of Microbiology, University Hospital Olomouc, 77515 Olomouc, Czech Republic; tatana.stosova@fnol.cz (T.Š.); milan.kolar@fnol.cz (M.K.)
* Correspondence: kristyna.mezerova@upol.cz

Abstract: Ventilator-associated pneumonia (VAP) is one of the most severe complications affecting mechanically ventilated patients. The condition is caused by microaspiration of potentially pathogenic bacteria from the upper respiratory tract into the lower respiratory tract or by bacterial pathogens from exogenous sources such as healthcare personnel, devices, aids, fluids and air. The aim of our prospective, observational study was to confirm the hypothesis that in the etiology of VAP, an important role is played by etiological agents from the upper airway bacterial microflora. At the same time, we studied the hypothesis that the vertical spread of bacterial pathogens is more frequent than their horizontal spread among patients. A total of 697 patients required mechanical ventilation for more than 48 h. The criteria for VAP were met by 47 patients. Clonality of bacterial isolates from 20 patients was determined by comparing their macrorestriction profiles obtained by pulsed-field gel electrophoresis (PFGE). Among these 20 patients, a total of 29 PFGE pulsotypes of *Klebsiella* spp. and *Escherichia* spp. strains were observed. The high variability of clones proves that there was no circulation of bacterial pathogens among hospitalized patients. Our finding confirms the development of VAP as a result of bacterial microaspiration and therefore the endogenous origin of VAP.

Keywords: ventilator-associated pneumonia; *Klebsiella* spp.; *Escherichia* spp.; pulsed-field gel electrophoresis (PFGE); clonality; endogenous infection

1. Introduction

Ventilator-associated pneumonia (VAP) is one of the most severe complications affecting mechanically ventilated patients. VAP has a considerable impact on patient prognosis due to longer ventilation time and higher mortality. The incidence of VAP is reported to be 9–27% [1]. The risk of developing VAP is highest in the first five days of mechanical ventilation and then gradually decreases [2]. Mortality associated with VAP is 33–50%, depending on the bacterial pathogen, adequacy of the antibiotic therapy and comorbidities of the patient [1]. With strict preventive measures in place, the death rate may decrease to approximately 9–13% [3]. The incidence of VAP is influenced by a range of risk factors contributing to undesirable microaspiration of potentially pathogenic bacteria into the lower respiratory tract. Microaspirations occur not only due to respiratory invasive procedures, including intubation or bronchoscopy, but also passively due to leakage of pooled secretions (from the paranasal sinuses, nasopharynx, oropharynx or stomach) from the space above the endotracheal tube cuff. Even insertion of the tube itself disrupts the natural barrier protecting the airways [4] and a biofilm forming on its surface may become a source of bacterial contamination of the lower respiratory tract [5]. All these mechanisms, individually or together, participate in the endogenous origin of VAP. The independent risk factors for VAP are mainly previous administration of antibiotics and patient comorbidities [1]. The exogenous sources of bacterial pathogens responsible for VAP in the intensive care setting may include healthcare personnel, devices, aids, fluids or air [6].

The study aimed to confirm the hypothesis that in the etiology of VAP, an important role is played by etiological agents from the upper airway bacterial flora, and that vertical spread of bacterial pathogens is more common than their horizontal spread among patients.

2. Results

Patients over 18 years of age hospitalized at the Department of Anesthesiology, Resuscitation and Intensive Care Medicine, University Hospital Olomouc, Czech Republic, between 11 January 2018 and 22 May 2020 were involved in this prospective, observational study.

Over the study period, a total of 697 patients required mechanical ventilation for more than 48 h. The criteria for VAP were met by 47 patients. The clonality study included 20 patients (18 males, 2 females) whose VAP was caused by *Klebsiella* spp. and *Escherichia* spp. As for demographic data, only age was normally distributed (median 58, interquartile range, IQR, 23–83). The other parameters showed non-normal distribution. The mean body mass index was 28 ± 5 (median 28, IQR 19–48). The median Acute Physiology and Chronic Health Evaluation II (APACHE II) score on admission was 24 (IQR 14–32). The median duration of mechanical ventilation and intensive care unit (ICU) stay was 11 days (IQR 5–43) and 13 days (IQR 6–44), respectively. The patients had a 30-day mortality rate of 20%.

A total of 49 *Klebsiella* spp. and *Escherichia* spp. isolates were obtained from 20 patients. Of those, nine *Escherichia* spp. isolates came from five patients and 40 *Klebsiella* spp. isolates from 17 patients; the latter included four isolates from patients from whom *Klebsiella variicola* or *Escherichia* spp. isolates were also obtained.

2.1. PFGE Analysis of Klebsiella spp. Isolates

For 26 *Klebsiella pneumoniae* isolates from 12 patients, different restriction profiles obtained with SpeI digestion of DNAs were observed, resulting in 16 pulsotypes. Isolates with identical restriction profiles were documented among different types of samples collected from the patients (Figure 1). Additionally, more than one clone was observed among isolates coming from patients referred to as PAT 8, PAT 9 and PAT 12.

Clustering analysis of nine isolates identified as *Klebsiella variicola* coming from five patients contributed to our finding that there was no clonal spread among patients in the Department of Anesthesiology, Resuscitation and Intensive Care Medicine. Furthermore, more than one clone was observed in the patient PAT 2 (Figure 2). A dendrogram constructed for five *Klebsiella oxytoca* isolates coming from 2 patients supported clonal diversity among different patients (Figure 3). Nevertheless, the phylogenetic tree based on PFGE profiles revealed identical strains isolated from different types of samples collected from each patient.

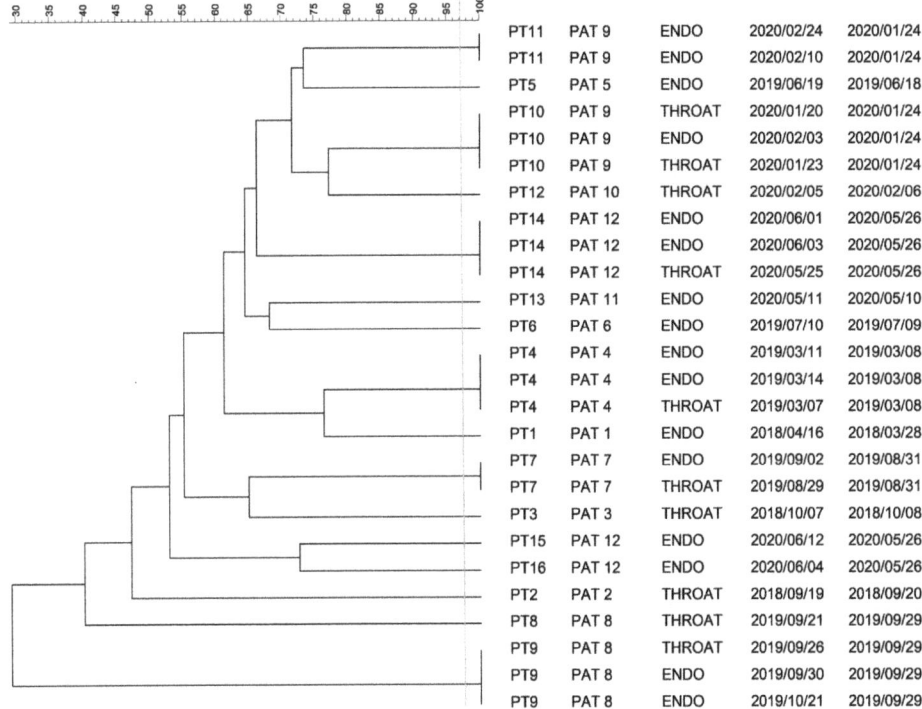

Figure 1. Dendrogram for restriction patterns of *K. pneumoniae* isolates. Legend: horizontal axis—similarity of isolates (%); vertical axis—pulsotype, patient code, type of sample, date of sample collection, date of VAP diagnosis; PT pulsotype, PAT patient, ENDO endotracheal aspirate sample, THROAT throat swab. The vertical line indicates the similarity threshold set at 97%.

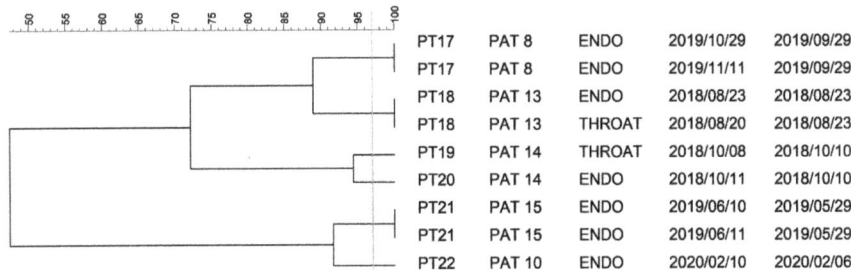

Figure 2. Dendrogram for restriction patterns of *K. variicola* isolates. Legend: horizontal axis—similarity of isolates (%); vertical axis—pulsotype, patient code, type of sample, date of sample collection, date of VAP diagnosis; PT pulsotype, PAT patient, ENDO endotracheal aspirate sample, THROAT throat swab. The vertical line indicates the similarity threshold set at 97%.

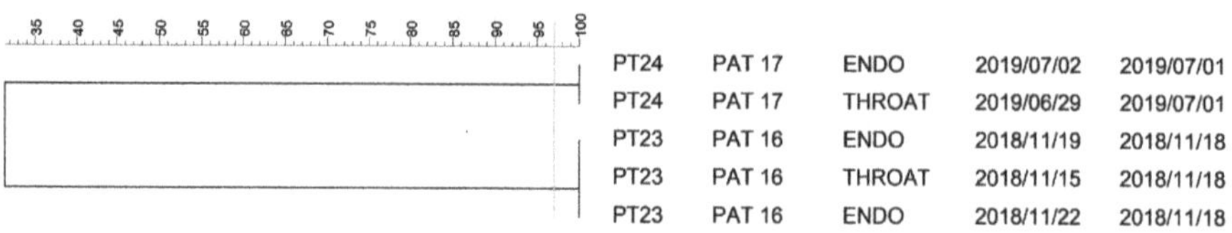

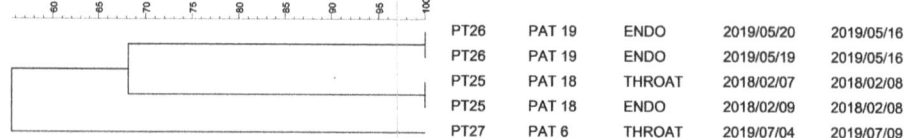

Figure 3. Dendrogram for restriction patterns of *K. oxytoca* isolates. Legend: horizontal axis—similarity of isolates (%); vertical axis—pulsotype, patient code, type of sample, date of sample collection, date of VAP diagnosis; PT pulsotype, PAT patient, ENDO endotracheal aspirate sample, THROAT throat swab. The vertical line indicates the similarity threshold set at 97%.

2.2. PFGE Analysis of Escherichia spp. Isolates

PFGE identified three pulsotypes among five *Escherichia coli* isolates belonging to three patients (Figure 4), supporting clonal diversity among different patients. The same results were obtained by restriction profiles of *Escherichia hermannii* DNA as four isolates were categorized to two phylotypes corresponding with patient codes (Figure 5).

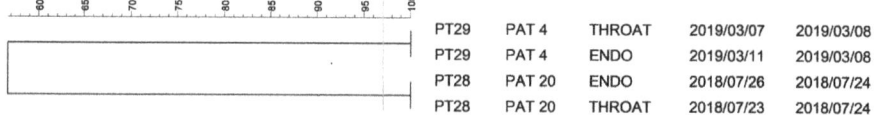

Figure 4. Dendrogram for restriction patterns of *E. coli* isolates. Legend: horizontal axis—similarity of isolates (%); vertical axis—pulsotype, patient code, type of sample, date of sample collection, date of VAP diagnosis; PT pulsotype, PAT patient, ENDO endotracheal aspirate sample, THROAT throat swab. The vertical line indicates the similarity threshold set at 97%.

Figure 5. Dendrogram for restriction patterns of *E. hermannii* isolates. Legend: horizontal axis—similarity of isolates (%); vertical axis—pulsotype, patient code, type of sample, date of sample collection, date of VAP diagnosis; PT pulsotype, PAT patient, ENDO endotracheal aspirate sample, THROAT throat swab. The vertical line indicates the similarity threshold set at 97%.

In 15 patients (75%), the bacterial pathogen that caused VAP was isolated from the upper respiratory tract before the development of VAP, or bacterial strains identified from the upper respiratory tract and endotracheal aspirate (ETA) samples showed identical restriction profiles in the same patient. In the remaining five patients, we confirmed the presence of the detected pathogen only in ETA samples after VAP had occurred.

3. Discussion

Over the study period, the incidence of VAP in the Department of Anesthesiology, Resuscitation and Intensive Care Medicine reached 7%, a lower rate compared to long-term reports [1]. The incidence was compared to 2018 data (1 January–31 December 2018) showing 20 cases of VAP among 291 patients mechanically ventilated for over 48 h (unpublished data). The 2018 rate was also 7%, suggesting a stable incidence of VAP in the department. In their comparison of data from the National Healthcare Safety Network, Dudeck et al. reported a downward trend in the incidence of VAP [7,8]. However, recent guidelines by the Infectious Diseases Society of America and the American Thoracic Society state a stable VAP rate (approx. 10%) in mechanically ventilated patients [9]. The present study found a mortality rate of 20% among VAP patients. A meta-analysis by Melsen et al. reported lower overall mortality (13%). However, the opposite was true for comparable patient subgroups (APACHE II score 20–29), with rates of 20% and 36%, respectively [3]. Mortality rates in different studies are also difficult to compare due to various methodologies. According to Forel et al., 28-day and 90-day mortality of patients with VAP was 27% and 42%, respectively [10]. While a study from Thailand documented 30-day mortality of 46% [11], Tejada et al. reported a rate of 44% without time specification [12]. A multi-center study by Herkel et al. assessed 30-day mortality with regard to adequate or inadequate empirical antibiotic therapy (27% vs. 45%) [13].

In the pathogenesis of VAP, microaspiration of bacteria from secretions in the space above the endotracheal tube cuff or the oropharynx plays the major role. Less frequently, the infection is caused by exogenously acquired pathogens. Thus, most VAP cases are of endogenous origin [6,14]. The risk factors for the development of VAP are mainly urgent tracheal intubation, reintubation, bronchoscopy and intolerance of enteral feeding, that is, situations representing a higher risk of microaspiration [15]. The introduction of routine assessment of the bacterial flora in both the upper and lower respiratory tract has allowed early identification of bacterial pathogens responsible for VAP. ETA sample collection results in more frequently detected pathogens (93%) compared to not only oropharyngeal swab (OS) and gastric aspiration samples (59% and 57%, respectively), but especially to protected specimen brushing (36%) [16]. The latter approach has the lowest sensitivity of all invasive techniques and is therefore not routinely performed, as stated in a meta-analysis by Fernando et al. [17]. Our results suggest that taking OS and ETA samples twice a week is sufficient.

To the best of our knowledge, this is the first study comparing the clonality of *Klebsiella* and *Escherichia* spp. strains isolated from different types of samples in each patient with VAP. Among 20 patients, a total of 29 PFGE pulsotypes were observed. Restriction profiles obtained from 26 *K. pneumoniae* isolates revealed 16 pulsotypes among 12 patients. *K. variicola* isolates also showed high variability of clones, as six pulsotypes were obtained from isolates belonging to five patients. Where *K. oxytoca*, *E. coli* and *E. hermannii* isolates were analyzed by PFGE, the number of pulsotypes always corresponded with the number of patients, proving that there was no circulation of pathogen among hospitalized patients.

Comparison of PFGE pulsotypes obtained in this study also showed high variability of bacterial clones among different patients, which correlates with a study by Hanulik et al. demonstrating clonal diversity among 23 *K. pneumoniae* isolates with only three pairs of clones belonging to six different patients [18]. A later study by Pudova et al. observed unique restriction profiles of analyzed isolates (74%) from hospital-acquired pneumonia (HAP) patients, suggesting only rare clonal spread of HAP bacterial pathogens among individual patients [19]. Unlike our study, circulation of multidrug-resistant *K. pneumoniae* isolates causing VAP in Egypt was confirmed by PFGE analysis. A study by Mohamed et al. included 19 clinical isolates from different patients and four environmental isolates, resulting in 17 pulsotypes. The restriction profiles of clinical and environmental isolates were similar, suggesting the exogenous origin of VAP infection [20]. Identical clones of *K. pneumoniae* were also detected in 29% of VAP patients in China. Clonal relationship of the *K. pneumoniae* strains was studied by random amplified polymorphic DNA (RAPD) and multilocus sequence typing, revealing 21 different RAPD patterns and 25 sequence types (ST) among 49 *K. pneumoniae* isolates. The most frequent clone, ST23 (43% prevalence) corresponding to hypervirulent *K. pneumoniae* (hvKP), evinced an identical RAPD pattern for all analyzed isolates, suggesting their epidemiological relationship [21]. According to a study by Tabrizi et al., hvKP isolated from mechanically-ventilated drug-poisoning patients was related to ST23 with the same PFGE pulsotype pattern, also underlining its epidemiological importance [22]. Based on our PFGE results, no epidemiologic strain was detected among the investigated patients.

In 75% of patients, the identified bacterial pathogen was first isolated from the upper respiratory tract as part of the bacterial flora. Subsequently, its presence in the endotracheal secretion of a patient with clinically expressed VAP was confirmed. This finding confirms the development of VAP resulting from bacterial microaspiration as reported by Pudova et al. [19].

The study limitations are its retrospective design, evaluation of only two bacterial species, and inclusion of only one center.

4. Materials and Methods

4.1. Patients and Clinical Material

All patients over 18 years of age who required mechanical ventilation for more than 48 h at the Department of Anesthesiology, Resuscitation and Intensive Care Medicine over the study period were involved in the study. Biological samples for microbiology testing, collected as described below, were a routine part of standard care for mechanically ventilated patients.

4.2. Sample Processing

The study included patients who met the clinical criteria for VAP caused by strains of *Klebsiella* spp. and *Escherichia* spp. The clinical signs of pneumonia are defined as the presence of newly developed or progressive infiltrates on chest radiographs plus at least two other signs of respiratory tract infection: temperature > 38 °C, purulent sputum, leukocytosis (white blood cell, WBC > $10 \times 10^3/mm^3$) or leukopenia (WBC < $4 \times 10^3/mm^3$), signs of inflammation on auscultation, cough and/or respiratory insufficiency with a PaO_2/FiO_2 ratio of ≤300 mm Hg that develop after more than 48 h of mechanical ventilation.

Excluded were patients with signs of pneumonia at the time of initiation of mechanical ventilation or with neutropenia, organ donors, those who later switched to withhold therapy or palliative care, and patients with VAP caused by bacterial pathogens other than *Klebsiella* spp. and *Escherichia* spp.

4.3. Collection of Samples for Microbiological Culture and Identification of Isolated Bacteria

In all patients, OS samples were taken on admission and then twice weekly, and ETA samples were taken twice weekly following the initiation of mechanical ventilation. OS samples were collected from the back wall of the oropharynx using a commercially available sample collection kit with a transport medium (Copan Diagnostics, Murrieta, CA, USA). ETA samples were collected by aspiration of secretions from an orotracheal tube using a sterile closed collecting system, with subsequent rinsing of the suction catheter with 10 mL of sterile saline and closing of the test tube with a sterile stopper. The identification of bacteria was performed by MALDI-TOF MS (Biotyper Microflex, Bruker Daltonics, Bremen, Germany) [23]. The study analyzed all *Escherichia* spp. and *Klebsiella* spp. strains isolated from OS and ETA collected from the enrolled patients. Table S1 in Supplementary data summarizes isolated bacterial species, dates of sample collection and VAP diagnosis of the enrolled patients.

4.4. Genotyping of Selected Bacterial Isolates

Clonal relationships of bacterial isolates were determined by comparing their macrorestriction profiles obtained by pulsed-field gel electrophoresis (PFGE). Bacterial DNA was isolated according to a protocol previously described in a study by Husickova et al. [24]. Briefly, DNA was isolated from a bacterial culture incubated at 37 °C for 16 h in Mueller–Hinton broth. The cells were washed three times with washing buffer followed by dilution of bacteria for optical density of 1.0–1.5 at 600 nm. The cells were subsequently mixed with 2% low melting point agarose (Bio-Rad, Hercules, CA, USA) to form blocks. The prepared agarose blocks were incubated at 37 °C in lysis buffer containing lysozyme. After 24 h, the blocks were transferred into deproteination buffer with proteinase K and incubated at 55 °C for another 24 h. The obtained blocks were finally washed in TE buffer and stored at 4 °C. According to manufacturer's instructions, enzymes XbaI and SpeI (New England Biolabs, Ipswich, MA, USA) were used for DNA restriction. *Escherichia* spp. isolates were digested by XbaI while SpeI-digested genomic DNA was used for obtaining restriction profiles of *Klebsiella* spp. isolates. The obtained DNA fragments were separated by PFGE, which was carried out in 1.2% agarose gel at 6 V cm^{-1} and pulse times of 2–35 s for 24 h. Thiourea (final concentration 50 μM) was added to an electrophoresis buffer in order to improve the typeability of the strains. Ethidium bromide was used for staining the gel, the obtained restriction profiles were documented by an imaging device and compared by the GelCompar II software (Applied Maths, Kortrijk, Belgium). Dendrograms were constructed by the unweighted pair group method with arithmetic mean combined with a hierarchical clustering method with Dice's coefficient. Optimization and band matching tolerance was set at 2%. Restriction profiles reaching 97% similarity were considered identical.

4.5. Statistical Analysis

Data were analyzed with IBM SPSS Statistics for Windows version 23.0 (IBM Corp., Armonk, NY, USA). Quantitative variables are presented as means and standard deviations (SD), minimum and maximum values and medians. The Shapiro–Wilk test for normality was used to verify that most data are not normally distributed (the only exception being age). Qualitative data (males/females, 30-day mortality) are presented as counts and percentages.

5. Conclusions

The results of this study, namely unique profiles confirming high variability of bacterial pathogens isolated from different patients, led us to conclude that the isolates did not spread among the hospitalized patients, suggesting that all VAP infections were endogenously acquired. At the same time, the results prove that strict adherence to hygiene and epidemiological precautions and careful surveillance of bacterial pathogens causing VAP, including assessment of the upper respiratory tract microflora, in clinical practice, may effectively prevent the horizontal spread of bacterial pathogens among mechanically ventilated patients. The observations of the study also indicate that bacterial microflora of the upper respiratory tract might predict the pathogens implicated in VAP. Thus, regular screening of a patient's oral microflora might guide empirical antibiotic treatment when the patient subsequently develops VAP, possibly increasing the rate of appropriate antibiotic treatment.

Supplementary Materials: The following are available online at https://www.mdpi.com/article/10.3390/antibiotics10060674/s1, Table S1: ENDO endotracheal aspirate sample, ESCO *E. coli*, ESHE *E. hermannii*, KLOX *K. oxytoca*, KLPN *K. pneumoniae*, KLVA *K. variicola*, PAT patient, THROAT throat swab.

Author Contributions: Conceptualization, M.K. and J.P.; Methodology, K.M., T.Š. and R.U.; Formal Analysis, K.M. and R.U.; Investigation, J.P.; Resources, J.P.; Data Curation, K.M., T.Š. and J.P.; Writing—original draft preparation, K.M., M.K. and J.P.; Writing—review and editing, K.M., M.K. and J.P.; Visualization, K.M. and J.P.; Supervision, M.K. and R.U. All authors have read and agreed to the published version of the manuscript.

Funding: This research was funded by the grant IGA_LF_2021_022 and project MH CZ—DRO (FNOL, 00098892).

Institutional Review Board Statement: This study was conducted according to the guidelines of the Declaration of Helsinki and approved by the Joint Institutional Ethics Committee of University Hospital Olomouc Ethics Committee (no. 173/2018).

Informed Consent Statement: Informed consent was obtained from all subjects involved in the study. (In case informed consent to participation in the study could not be obtained due to the provision of continuous analgesia/sedation to mechanically ventilated patients, close relatives were asked for it and properly informed).

Data Availability Statement: The data presented in this study are available on request from the corresponding author. The data are not publicly available due to protection of privacy of patients included in the study.

Acknowledgments: The authors are thankful to K. Langová for performing statistical analyses.

Conflicts of Interest: The authors declare no conflict of interest.

References

1. American Thoracic Society; Infectious Diseases Society of America. Guidelines for the Management of Adults with Hospital-acquired, Ventilator-associated, and Healthcare-associated Pneumonia. *Am. J. Respir. Crit. Care Med.* **2005**, *171*, 388–416. [CrossRef] [PubMed]
2. Chastre, J.; Fagon, J.-Y. Ventilator-associated Pneumonia. *Am. J. Respir. Crit. Care Med.* **2002**, *165*, 867–903. [CrossRef]
3. Melsen, W.G.; Rovers, M.M.; Groenwold, R.H.; Bergmans, D.C.; Camus, C.; Bauer, T.T.; Hanisch, E.; Klarin, B.; Koeman, M.A.; Krueger, W.; et al. Attributable mortality of ventilator-associated pneumonia: A meta-analysis of individual patient data from randomised prevention studies. *Lancet Infect. Dis.* **2013**, *13*, 665–671. [CrossRef]
4. Zolfaghari, P.S.; La Wyncoll, D. The tracheal tube: Gateway to ventilator-associated pneumonia. *Crit. Care* **2011**, *15*, 310. [CrossRef] [PubMed]
5. Hunter, J.D. Ventilator associated pneumonia. *BMJ* **2012**, *344*, e3325. [CrossRef] [PubMed]
6. Safdar, N.; Crnich, C.J.; Maki, D.G. The pathogenesis of ventilator-associated pneumonia: Its relevance to developing effective strategies for prevention. *Respir. Care* **2005**, *50*, 725–739.
7. Dudeck, M.A.; Weiner, L.M.; Allen-Bridson, K.; Malpiedi, P.J.; Peterson, K.D.; Pollock, D.A.; Sievert, D.M.; Edwards, J.R. National Healthcare Safety Network (NHSN) report, data summary for 2012, Device-associated module. *Am. J. Infect. Control* **2013**, *41*, 1148–1166. [CrossRef]
8. Dudeck, M.A.; Horan, T.C.; Peterson, K.D.; Allen-Bridson, K.; Morrell, G.; Pollock, D.A.; Edwards, J.R. National Healthcare Safety Network (NHSN) Report, data summary for 2010, device-associated module. *Am. J. Infect. Control* **2011**, *39*, 798–816. [CrossRef]
9. Kalil, A.C.; Metersky, M.L.; Klompas, M.; Muscedere, J.; Sweeney, D.A.; Palmer, L.B.; Napolitano, L.M.; O'Grady, N.P.; Bartlett, J.G.; Carratalà, J.; et al. Management of Adults With Hospital-acquired and Ventilator-associated Pneumonia: 2016 Clinical Practice Guidelines by the Infectious Diseases Society of America and the American Thoracic Society. *Clin. Infect. Dis.* **2016**, *63*, e61–e111. [CrossRef]
10. Forel, J.-M.; Voillet, F.; Pulina, D.; Gacouin, A.; Perrin, G.; Barrau, K.; Jaber, S.; Arnal, J.-M.; Fathallah, M.; Auquier, P.; et al. Ventilator-associated pneumonia and ICU mortality in severe ARDS patients ventilated according to a lung-protective strategy. *Crit. Care* **2012**, *16*, R65. [CrossRef]
11. Werarak, P.; Kiratisin, P.; Thamlikitkul, V. Hospital-acquired pneumonia and ventilator-associated pneumonia in adults at Siriraj Hospital: Etiology, clinical outcomes, and impact of antimicrobial resistance. *J. Med. Assoc. Thai.* **2010**, *93*, S126–S138.
12. Artigas, A.T.; Dronda, S.B.; Vallés, E.C.; Marco, J.M.; Usón, M.C.V.; Figueras, P.; Suarez, F.J.; Hernández, A. Risk factors for nosocomial pneumonia in critically ill trauma patients. *Crit. Care Med.* **2001**, *29*, 304–309. [CrossRef]
13. Herkel, T.; Uvizl, R.; Doubravska, L.; Adamus, M.; Gabrhelik, T.; Sedlakova, M.H.; Kolar, M.; Hanulik, V.; Pudova, V.; Langova, K.; et al. Epidemiology of hospital-acquired pneumonia: Results of a Central European multicenter, prospective, observational study compared with data from the European region. *Biomed. Pap.* **2016**, *160*, 448–455. [CrossRef]
14. Berthelot, P.; Grattard, F.; Mahul, P.; Pain, P.; Jospé, R.; Venet, C.; Carricajo, A.; Aubert, G.; Ros, A.; Dumont, D.; et al. Prospective study of nosocomial colonization and infection due to Pseudomonas aeruginosa in mechanically ventilated patients. *Intensiv. Care Med.* **2001**, *27*, 503–512. [CrossRef]
15. Uvizl, R.; Kolar, M.; Herkel, T.; Vobrova, M.; Langova, K. Possibilities for modifying risk factors for the development of hospital-acquired pneumonia in intensive care patients: Results of a retrospective, observational study. *Biomed. Pap.* **2017**, *161*, 303–309. [CrossRef]
16. Doubravská, L.; Uvízl, R.; Herkel', T.; Kolář, M.; Gabrhelík, T.; Röderová, M.; Htoutou Sedláková, M.; Langová, K.; Kolek, V.; Jakubec, P.; et al. Detection of the etiological agents of hospital-acquired pneumonia—Validity and comparison of different types of biological sample collection: A prospective, observational study in intensive care patients. *Epidemiol. Mikrobiol. Imunol.* **2017**, *66*, 155–162. [PubMed]
17. Fernando, S.M.; Tran, A.; Cheng, W.; Klompas, M.; Kyeremanteng, K.; Mehta, S.; English, S.; Muscedere, J.; Cook, D.J.; Torres, A.; et al. Diagnosis of ventilator-associated pneumonia in critically ill adult patients—A systematic review and meta-analysis. *Intensiv. Care Med.* **2020**, *46*, 1170–1179. [CrossRef] [PubMed]
18. Hanulík, V.; Uvízl, R.; Husičková, V.; Htoutou Sedláková, M.; Kolář, M. Pneumonia-causing bacterial pathogens in intensive care patients. *Klin. Mikrobiol. Infekc. Lek.* **2011**, *17*, 135–140.
19. Pudová, V.; Working Group; Sedláková, M.H.; Kolář, M. Clonality of Bacterial Pathogens Causing Hospital-Acquired Pneumonia. *Curr. Microbiol.* **2016**, *73*, 312–316. [CrossRef] [PubMed]
20. Mohamed, E.R.; Aly, S.A.; Halby, H.M.; Ahmed, S.H.; Zakaria, A.M.; El-Asheer, O.M. Epidemiological typing of multidrug-resistant Klebsiella pneumoniae, which causes paediatric ventilator-associated pneumonia in Egypt. *J. Med. Microbiol.* **2017**, *66*, 628–634. [CrossRef]
21. Yan, Q.; Zhou, M.; Liu, W.-E.; Zou, M. Hypervirulent Klebsiella pneumoniae induced ventilator-associated pneumonia in mechanically ventilated patients in China. *Eur. J. Clin. Microbiol. Infect. Dis.* **2016**, *35*, 387–396. [CrossRef] [PubMed]
22. Tabrizi, A.M.A.; Badmasti, F.; Shahcheraghi, F.; Azizi, O. Outbreak of hypervirulent Klebsiella pneumoniae harbouring blaVIM-2 among mechanically-ventilated drug-poisoning patients with high mortality rate in Iran. *J. Glob. Antimicrob. Resist.* **2018**, *15*, 93–98. [CrossRef]

23. Croxatto, A.; Prod'hom, G.; Greub, G. Applications of MALDI-TOF mass spectrometry in clinical diagnostic microbiology. *FEMS Microbiol. Rev.* **2012**, *36*, 80–407. [CrossRef] [PubMed]
24. Husickova, V.; Cekanova, L.; Chroma, M.; Htoutou-Sedlakova, M.; Hricova, K.; Kolář, M. Carriage of ESBL- and AmpC-positive Enterobacteriaceae in the gastrointestinal tract of community subjects and hospitalized patients in the Czech Republic. *Biomed. Pap.* **2012**, *156*, 348–353. [CrossRef] [PubMed]

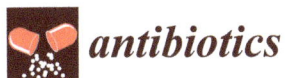

Article

Bacterial Pathogens and Evaluation of a Cut-Off for Defining Early and Late Neonatal Infection

Pavla Kucova [1], Lumir Kantor [2,*], Katerina Fiserova [1], Jakub Lasak [2], Magdalena Röderova [1] and Milan Kolar [1]

[1] Department of Microbiology, Faculty of Medicine and Dentistry, Palacky University Olomouc and University Hospital Olomouc, 779 00 Olomouc, Czech Republic; pavla.kucova@fnol.cz (P.K.); katerina.fiserova@fnol.cz (K.F.); magdalena.roderova@upol.cz (M.R.); milan.kolar@fnol.cz (M.K.)

[2] Neonatal Department, University Hospital Olomouc, 779 00 Olomouc, Czech Republic; jakub.lasak@fnol.cz

* Correspondence: kantorl@senat.cz

Abstract: Bacterial infections are an important cause of mortality and morbidity in newborns. The main risk factors include low birth weight and prematurity. The study identified the most common bacterial pathogens causing neonatal infections including their resistance to antibiotics in the Neonatal Department of the University Hospital Olomouc. Additionally, the cut-off for distinguishing early- from late-onset neonatal infections was assessed. The results of this study show that a cut-off value of 72 h after birth is more suitable. Only in case of early-onset infections arising within 72 h of birth, initial antibiotic therapy based on gentamicin with ampicillin or amoxicillin/clavulanic acid may be recommended. It has been established that with the 72-h cut-off, late-onset infections caused by bacteria more resistant to antibiotics may be detected more frequently, a finding that is absolutely crucial for antibiotic treatment strategy.

Keywords: newborn; infection; bacteria; antibiotic therapy

1. Introduction

Neonatal infections may be defined as infectious diseases occurring in newborns within 4 weeks after birth. They may be classified as early-onset or late-onset, with the cut-off for distinguishing early- from late-onset infections ranging between 72 h and 7 days.

Early-onset neonatal infections are caused by microorganisms transmitted in utero or as the baby moves down the birth passage (antepartum or intrapartum), with 85% of them occurring within 24 h from birth [1,2]. The most common etiologic agents are *Escherichia coli*, *Streptococcus agalactiae* (GBS), and *Listeria monocytogenes*. Less frequently, chlamydias and mycoplasmas are shown to play an etiologic role [3–5]. For initial antibiotic therapy, ampicillin or amoxicillin with clavulanic acid, combined with gentamicin are recommended [2,6,7]. In the literature, however, information is available about increasing resistance of *Escherichia coli* to antibiotics including aminopenicillins combined with inhibitors of bacterial beta-lactamases (ampicillin/sulbactam and amoxicillin/clavulanic acid) and potential failure of antibiotic therapy [8–11]. The risk factors for the development of early-onset infections include vaginal colonization with GBS, prelabor rupture of membranes, prematurity, multiple abortions, maternal malnutrition, and congenital abnormalities [12–14].

Late-onset neonatal infections are caused by bacteria associated with hospital care. Multidrug-resistant bacteria are frequently responsible for these infections. Important sources are artificial materials, in particular, cannulas or catheters [13,15]. The most common bacterial pathogens are *Staphylococcus aureus*, coagulase-negative staphylococci, *Klebsiella pneumoniae*, *Escherichia coli*, *Enterobacter* spp., *Serratia marcescens*, *Pseudomonas aeruginosa*, *Acinetobacter baumannii*, anaerobic bacteria, and yeasts [16–18]. The risk factors for acquiring infections include prematurity, congenital abnormalities, and invasive care such as central venous catheter placement or respiratory support [13,19]. In many cases,

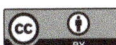

antibiotic therapy requires application of antibacterial drugs effective against multidrug-resistant bacteria such as carbapenems, glycopeptides, and aminoglycosides in relevant combinations [20].

A very important part of the overall therapeutic approach to neonatal infections is microbiological examination of adequate clinical materials, in particular, blood and cerebrospinal fluid cultures. The obtained results allow targeted antibiotic therapy based on identification of bacterial pathogens and determination of their susceptibility/resistance to antibiotics. Under defined conditions, nasopharyngeal and rectal swabs, pharyngeal aspirate, urine, and other specimens may also be of clinical importance if very carefully interpreted [21].

Our study aimed to assess the cut-offs for distinguishing early- from late-onset neonatal infections and determine the most frequent bacterial pathogens causing or suspected of causing neonatal infections, including their resistance to antibacterial drugs.

2. Results

Over a 3-year period, a total of 7221 newborns were either born or transported to the Neonatal Department of the University Hospital Olomouc. Neonatal infections were treated in 364 cases (5%), in whom 263 bacterial and 59 mycotic pathogens were isolated.

Clinical sepsis (72%) was most common in newborns, followed by bloodstream infections (13%) and pneumonia (9%); less frequent were meningitis (1%) and necrotizing enterocolitis (1%). In 4% of newborns treated for infections of unclear origin, no bacterial pathogens were isolated.

The sample consisted of the following gestational age subgroups: term 38%, moderate to late preterm 28%, very preterm 20% and extremely preterm newborns 14%. The birth weight subgroups were as follows: normal birth weight 41%, low birth weight 26%, very low birth weight 14% and extremely low birth weight 19%.

The most frequently isolated bacteria were *Escherichia coli* (22%), *Klebsiella pneumoniae* (12%), coagulase-negative staphylococci (12%), and *Staphylococcus aureus* (10%) (Table 1). The results show that Enterobacterales accounted for more than half (56%) of all bacterial pathogens. *Streptococcus agalactiae* caused infection in only nine newborns and *Listeria monocytogenes* was detected in a single infant. Besides bacterial pathogens, *Candida* spp. were responsible for 59 cases of infections (majority of which was treated topically), with *Candida albicans* causing infections in 47 (<1%) newborns. *Candida parapsilosis* and *Candida tropicalis* were confirmed as etiologic agents in only 7 and 5 neonatal infections, respectively.

Overall, 6% of newborns in 2015 and 5% in both 2016 and 2017 were treated with antibiotics for confirmed or suspected early- or late-onset infection. Table 2 shows bacterial pathogens causing early- and late-onset infections as defined by the two cut-offs (72 h and 7 days).

Table 1. Bacteria isolated from newborns prior to initiation of antibiotic therapy.

Bacterial Species	No. of Isolates	Percentage
Escherichia coli	57	22
Klebsiella pneumoniae	31	12
Coagulase-negative staphylococci	31	12
Staphylococcus aureus	25	10
Enterobacter cloacae	16	6
Klebsiella oxytoca	16	6
Stenotrophomonas maltophilia	15	6
Pseudomonas aeruginosa	14	5
Enterococcus faecalis	11	4
Streptococcus agalactiae	9	3
Burkholderia cepacia complex	8	3
Citrobacter freundii	4	2
Ralstonia picketii/insidiosa	4	2
Pseudomonas putida	2	1

Table 1. Cont.

Bacterial Species	No. of Isolates	Percentage
Acinetobacter baumannii	2	1
Klebsiella aerogenes	2	1
Enterobacter kobei	2	1
Serratia marcescens	2	1
Haemophilus influenzae type b	2	1
Enterobacter asburiae	2	1
Others	8	3

Legend: others—bacteria isolated only once (*Salmonella* Enteritidis, *Providencia rettgeri*, *Proteus mirabilis*, *Morganella morganii*, *Listeria monocytogenes*, *Streptococcus anginosus*, *Streptococcus intermedius*, and *Enterococcus faecium*).

Table 2. Numbers of bacterial/mycotic pathogens from newborns treated with antibiotics with regard to different cut-offs for distinguishing between early- and late-onset infections.

Bacterial Pathogen	Early-Onset (Absolute No.)		Late-Onset (Absolute No.)		
	≤72 h	≤7 days	>72 h	>7 days	*p*-Value
Escherichia coli	15	26	42	31	<0.001
Klebsiella pneumoniae	10	19	21	12	0.002
Coagulase-negative staphylococci	4	15	27	16	<0.001
Staphylococcus aureus	3	12	22	13	0.002
Enterobacter cloacae	5	9	11	7	0.063
Klebsiella oxytoca	2	7	14	9	0.031
Stenotrophomonas maltophilia	1	7	14	8	0.016
Pseudomonas aeruginosa	1	8	13	6	0.008
Enterococcus faecalis	3	7	8	4	0.063
Streptococcus agalactiae	8	9	1	0	0.500
Burkholderia cepacia complex	0	3	8	5	0.125
Citrobacter freundii	1	3	3	1	
Ralstonia picketii/insidiosa	0	3	4	1	
Pseudomonas putida	0	0	2	2	
Acinetobacter baumannii	0	1	2	1	
Klebsiella aerogenes	0	1	2	1	
Enterobacter kobei	0	0	2	2	
Serratia marcescens	0	0	2	2	
Haemophilus influenzae type b	1	2	1	0	
Enterobacter asburiae	0	1	2	1	
Other bacteria	3	6	5	2	
Mycotic pathogen	≤72 h	≤7 days	>72 h	>7 days	
Candida albicans	3	24	44	23	<0.001
Candida parapsilosis	0	3	7	4	0.125
Candida tropicalis	0	2	5	3	

Legend: *p*-values are given for bacterial and *Candida* species with a number of isolates > 5.

When the 72-h cut-off for developing symptoms of early-onset infection was applied, a total of 57 pathogens were isolated, mostly enterobacteria (58%). The most frequently isolated species were *Escherichia coli* (26%) and *Klebsiella pneumoniae* (18%). The use of the other cut-off, i.e., early-onset infections in the first 7 days of life, resulted in isolation of 139 pathogenic bacteria. The most common organisms were enterobacteria (47%), mainly *Escherichia coli* (19%) and *Klebsiella pneumoniae* (14%), followed by Gram-positive bacteria (31%), mainly coagulase-negative staphylococci (11%) and *Staphylococcus aureus* (9%).

In case of late-onset infections defined by the 72-h cut-off, a total of 206 bacterial pathogens were isolated. The most common were enterobacteria (48%), in particular, *Escherichia coli* (20%), followed by *Klebsiella pneumoniae* (10%) and *Enterobacter cloacae* (5%). Further, there were 28% of Gram-positive bacteria (coagulase-negative staphylococci in 13% and *Staphylococcus aureus* in 11%). When late-onset neonatal infections were defined by symptoms occurring from the eighth day, 124 bacterial pathogens were identified; the most frequent species were *Escherichia coli* (25%) and *Klebsiella pneumoniae* (10%).

Assessment of the two cut-offs (i.e., ≤72 h and ≤7 days of life) showed that the presence changed for most bacterial species. This was obvious in case of coagulase-negative staphylococci; when the 72-h cut-off was applied, only 4 out of 31 cases could be characterized as early-onset, as compared with 15 cases when using the 7-day cut-off. Similar differences were observed for *Staphylococcus aureus*, *Escherichia coli*, and *Klebsiella pneumoniae* (Figure 1). Yet another example may be non-fermenting Gram-negative bacteria. Out of 14 cases with *Pseudomonas aeruginosa* infection, 1 and 8 were interpreted as early-onset according to the 72-h and 7-day cut-offs, respectively. Similarly, among 15 cases in which *Stenotrophomonas maltophilia* was isolated, only 1 was early-onset when the 72-h cut-off was used, as compared with 7 cases when applying the other cut-off. In case of *Candida albicans* infections, it is clear that according to the 72-h cut-off, only 3 out of 47 cases could be defined as early-onset, while with the 7-day cut-off, it was 24 cases (Figure 1).

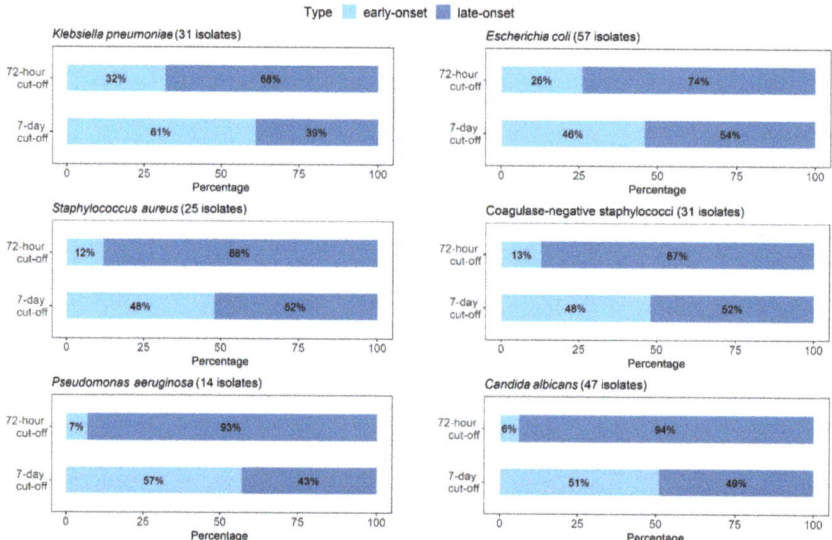

Figure 1. Proportional representation of early- and late-onset infections with regard to both cut-offs (72-h and 7-day) shown for *Klebsiella pneumoniae*, *Escherichia coli*, *Staphylococcus aureus*, coagulase-negative staphylococci, *Pseudomonas aeruginosa*, and *Candida albicans*.

Table 3 shows the numbers of suspected or confirmed causative bacteria isolated from newborns treated with antibiotics as well as the numbers of newborns in whom no bacterial pathogen was detected. According to the results, only one bacterial species was isolated in 76% of newborns, more than one microorganisms were isolated in 9% and no etiologic agent was identified in 15% of infants with clinical sepsis.

Table 3. Identification of etiologic agents causing/suspected of causing neonatal infections.

Etiology of Confirmed or Suspected Infections	2015 (Absolute No.)	2016 (Absolute No.)	2017 (Absolute No.)
No identified pathogen	19	23	14
Monomicrobial etiology	101	81	94
Polymicrobial etiology	12	9	11
Total	132	113	119

The results suggest relatively good susceptibility of the most frequently isolated enterobacteria (*Escherichia coli*, *Klebsiella pneumoniae*, *Enterobacter cloacae*, and *Klebsiella oxytoca*) to antibacterial drugs with the exception of ampicillin and cefazolin. Production of broad-spectrum beta-lactamases (only ESBL and AmpC types) was confirmed in eight strains, i.e., 6% of isolated enterobacteria (Table 4). All those strains were isolated from neonates who developed infection from day 4 of life onwards. Resistance to meropenem was not noted.

Table 4. Broad-spectrum beta-lactamase (ESBL- and AmpC only)-positive enterobacteria.

Species	No. of Strains	Type of Broad-Spectrum Beta-Lactamase
Klebsiella pneumoniae	3	ESBL—CTX-M-15
Klebsiella pneumoniae	1	ESBL—CTX-M-9
Escherichia coli	2	ESBL—CTX-M-15
Enterobacter cloacae	1	AmpC—EBC
Citrobacter freundii	1	AmpC—CIT

Pulsed-field gel electrophoresis (PFGE) of 3 CTX-M-15-positive *Klebsiella pneumonia* and 2 CTX-M-15-positive *Escherichia coli* strains showed that those were strains with unique restriction genetic profiles. Therefore, clonal horizontal transmission was ruled out (Figures 2 and 3).

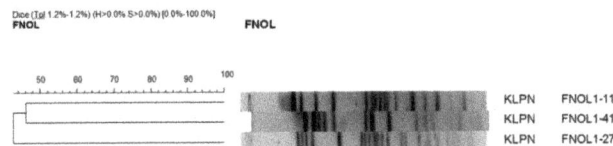

Figure 2. Pulsed-field gel electrophoresis (PFGE) of 3 CTX-M-15-positive *Klebsiella pneumonia* strains.

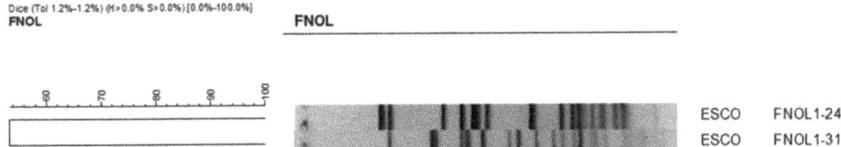

Figure 3. PFGE of 2 CTX-M-15-positive *Escherichia coli* strains.

The most frequently isolated Gram-positive bacteria, *Staphylococcus aureus*, was 100% susceptible to oxacillin. It means that methicillin-resistant *Staphylococcus aureus* (MRSA) was not detected. Very high susceptibility was found to ciprofloxacin, erythromycin, clindamycin, gentamicin, and glycopeptides (vancomycin and teicoplanin). Higher resistance levels were documented in coagulase-negative staphylococci, but vancomycin and teicoplanin were found to be very effective. Isolated strains of *Enterococcus faecalis* and *Streptococcus agalactiae* were 100% susceptible to ampicillin and glycopeptides (vancomycin and teicoplanin).

Susceptibility of the most frequently isolated bacterial pathogens to antibiotics is illustrated in Tables 5 and 6.

Table 5. Susceptibility of enterobacteria to selected antibiotics (percentages).

Antibiotic/Pathogen	Escherichia coli	Klebsiella pneumoniae	Klebsiella oxytoca	Enterobacter cloacae
AMI	95	100	100	100
AMP	28	0	0	0
AMS	84	90	100	0
CIP	98	90	100	100
COL	100	87	94	81
CPM	98	90	100	94
CRX	95	90	100	0
CTX	95	90	100	81
CTZ	98	90	100	81
CZL	77	77	44	0
GEN	88	90	100	100
MER	100	100	100	100
PPT	96	90	100	81
TOB	88	90	100	100

Legend: AMI—amikacin, AMP—ampicillin, AMS—ampicillin/sulbactam, CIP—ciprofloxacin, COL—colistin, CPM—cefepime, CRX—cefuroxime, CTX—cefotaxime, CTZ—ceftazidime, CZL—cefazolin, GEN—gentamicin, MER—meropenem, PPT—piperacillin/tazobactam, TOB—tobramycin.

Table 6. Susceptibility of *Staphylococcus aureus* and coagulase-negative staphylococci to selected antibiotics (percentages).

Antibiotic/Pathogen	Staphylococcus aureus	Coagulase-Negative Staphylococci
OXA	100	28
CIP	100	57
CLI	80	51
TEI	100	93
VAN	100	93
ERY	80	30
GEN	80	45

Legend: OXA—oxacillin, CLI—clindamycin, TEI—teicoplanin, VAN—vancomycin, ERY—erythromycin.

3. Discussion

An indispensable part of the therapeutic approach to neonatal infections is application of antibacterial drugs immediately after establishing the diagnosis or as soon as strong suspicion arises. Antibiotic regimens should consider microbiological examinations of the newborn and its mother as well as local results of surveillance of the most common bacterial pathogens and their resistance to antibiotics. Based on microbiology test results, an integral part of the overall therapeutic approach, targeted antibiotic therapy should be administered.

Over the study period, a total of 7221 newborns were hospitalized in the Neonatal Department of the University Hospital Olomouc, with bacterial infections being treated in 5% of them. This percentage is very high for several reasons. Some of the neonates were transported to our tertiary neonatal unit due to serious health complications. As some preterm neonates were treated more than once, the percentage reflects the number of treated cases rather than the number of treated children. Therefore, the rate is not the incidence of neonatal infections, but the incidence of antibiotic treatment, preemptive in some cases. The study results suggest that the most common bacterial agents causing or suspected of causing neonatal infections were enterobacteria (52% of all isolated pathogens) and staphylococci (21%). The most frequent causative species were *Escherichia coli* (22%), *Klebsiella pneumoniae* (12%), coagulase-negative staphylococci (12%), and *Staphylococcus aureus* (10%). *Candida* spp. infections were caused by *Candida albicans* in the vast majority of cases (80%). These results are consistent with those published by Russell who found that in neonatal infections, the most common isolates were *Escherichia coli*, coagulase-negative staphylococci, *Staphylococcus aureus*, and *Enterococcus* spp. [22]. Shane et al. reported that in neonatal infections, *Streptococcus agalactiae* (43%) and *Escherichia coli* (29%) were most frequently isolated. These species belong to the most important pathogens contributing to the development of early-onset neonatal infections. According to the authors, late-onset infections were caused by *Staphylococcus aureus*, coagulase-negative staphylococci, enterococci, enterobacteria, and *Streptococcus pyogenes* [23]. In a study by Bulkowstein et al., the most common pathogens causing early-onset infections were *Escherichia coli* (34%), *Streptococcus agalactiae* (22%), *Klebsiella pneumoniae* (13%), *Enterococcus faecalis* (9%), and *Staphylococcus aureus* (5%). The spectrum of pathogens was similar for late-onset infections; most frequently, the authors isolated *Escherichia coli* (29%), *Streptococcus pneumoniae* (13%), *Staphylococcus aureus* (9%), and *Klebsiella pneumoniae* (7%) [24].

Given the present results, the 72-h cut-off appears to be more suitable for distinguishing early- from late-onset neonatal infections. Therefore, the use of a different antibiotics could be advised. Within 72 h of birth, microorganisms transmitted from the mother in utero or during birth were isolated more frequently. However, when infections developing in the first 7 days of life were considered as early-onset, more bacteria associated with nosocomial infections were isolated. Our results indicate that with the 72-h cut-off, bacteria originating from the mother (mainly *Streptococcus agalactiae*) were detected. At the same time, the frequency of non-fermenting bacteria (e.g., *Stenotrophomonas maltophilia* and *Pseudomonas aeruginosa*) was very low. With the 7-day cut-off for early neonatal infections, almost a double number of bacterial pathogens was identified. These bacteria show higher levels of resistance to antibiotics, and they are very often associated with hospital care and nosocomial infections. It should be emphasized that infections caused by enterobacteria producing broad-spectrum beta-lactamases would also fall into the category of early-onset infections if the 7-day cut-off was used. However, if the 72-h cut-off was applied, all these infections would be characterized as late-onset. Alternatively, bacterial strains were detected that tend to be related to the use of long-term central venous catheters, in particular coagulase-negative staphylococci. It has been established that with the 72-h cut-off, late-onset infections caused by bacteria more resistant to antibiotics may be detected more frequently, a finding that is absolutely crucial for antibiotic treatment strategy.

Infections caused by *Candida* spp. are associated with significant morbidity and mortality in infants. As with bacterial infections, premature babies with extremely low birth weight (less than 1000 g) are most at risk of mycotic infections [25]. A rather serious disease of premature neonates is candidiasis, which can manifest as candidemia, urinary tract infection, or as impairment of any tissue or structure. The risk factors for developing candidiasis include prematurity, central vascular catheterization, abdominal surgery, necrotizing enterocolitis, exposure to broad-spectrum antibacterial agents (e.g., third-generation cephalosporins and carbapenems), parenteral nutrition, antacid use, and endotracheal intubation [26]. The use of catheters or endotracheal tubes destroys the body's natural barriers, allowing yeasts to penetrate, multiply, and invade sterile body areas. It is, therefore, clear that mycotic infection would not be possible without prior colonization. According to Roilides, the species most commonly occurring in pediatric patients are *Candida albicans* (50%), *Candida parapsilosis* (21%), and *Candida tropicalis* (10%) [27]. The same species were also most frequent in the present study. The highest rates of yeasts were noted after the first 72 h of life. In these cases, it is more preferable to use the 72-h cut-off for early neonatal infections, since almost 10 times less yeasts were detected compared to the 7-day cut-off.

In the present study, GBS accounted for a very small proportion (3%) of bacterial pathogens identified over the 3-year period. This species mainly plays a role in early-onset infections. This fact was confirmed by the present study, with 8 out of 9 GBS strains being isolated in the first 72 h of life. It may be calculated that GBS neonatal infection affected 1.2 newborns per 1000 live births. According to Strakova et al., the incidence of invasive streptococcal neonatal infections ranged from 0.7 to 1.0 cases per 1000 live births in 2001 and 2002 [28]. Simetka et al. reported early-onset GBS infections in 1.2 newborns per 1000 live births in 2003–2005 [29]. These findings may be explained by very effective prophylaxis as early as in the prenatal period, that is screening of all pregnant women between 35 and

37 weeks of gestation, early laboratory diagnosis and relevant prepartum/intrapartum antibiotic prophylaxis [30–32].

In the present study, antimicrobial susceptibility testing showed relatively high efficacy of antibiotics. No MRSA strains or vancomycin-resistant enterococci were detected. Production of broad-spectrum beta-lactamases (CTX-M-15, CTX-M-9, EBC, and CIT) was confirmed in only 6% of enterobacteria with unique genetic profiles; no clonal spread was confirmed. On the other hand, a considerable therapeutic problem is posed by multidrug-resistant strains of *Stenotrophomonas maltophilia* and *Burkholderia cepacia* complex susceptible to antibiotics contraindicated in neonatal care.

The main limitation of the study is its retrospective character. In addition, data from only one neonatal center were processed. It is most crucial to follow local antimicrobial resistance surveillance results when choosing initial antibiotic treatment.

4. Material and Methods

The primary outcome of the study is to evaluate the cut-offs for distinguishing early- from late-onset neonatal infections. In neonatology, there are two most used cut-offs. They are 72 h of life and 7 days of life [1,2,6,11,13]. The aim of the study was to evaluate these existing and widely used cut-offs, based on bacteria isolated in specific postnatal age. We did not want to suggest a new cut-off. The secondary outcome can be characterized as the determination of the most frequent bacterial/mycotic pathogens causing or suspected of causing neonatal infections, including resistance to antibacterial drugs.

Biological samples (urine, stools, blood cultures, venous cannulas, cerebrospinal fluid, bronchoalveolar lavage fluid, axillary, throat, nasal, ear, conjunctival, and wound swabs) were obtained from newborns before antibiotic treatment. All biological samples were collected only as part of standard clinical care and active bacterial surveillance program.

Patients' parents gave informed consent to hospitalization, sample collection, and anonymous enrollment in the study. Ethics committee approval was not required as the study did not interfere with the diagnostic and therapeutic process.

The case inclusion criterion was antibiotic treatment, irrespective of infection type, provided to newborns staying in the Neonatal Department of the University Hospital Olomouc in 2015–2017. No patient treated with antibiotics was excluded from the study. To define infections, the modified NEO-KISS criteria were used for early- as well as late-onset sepsis.

Bacterial isolates were identified by MALDI-TOF MS (Biotyper Microflex, Bruker Daltonics, Bremen, Germany) [33]. Each identified strain was included only once in the database.

Bacteria isolated from blood or cerebrospinal fluid were considered to be etiologic agents. If a newborn was treated with antibiotics and bacteria were isolated from other samples, the bacteria were identified as a suspected etiologic agent.

Susceptibility to antibiotics was determined by using the microdilution method in accordance with the EUCAST recommendations [34]. Production of ESBLs and AmpC-type beta-lactamases was detected by relevant phenotypic tests and confirmed by PCR detecting genes specific for particular beta-lactamase types [35].

The similarity of 3 CTX-M-15-positive *Klebsiella pneumoniae* and 2 CTX-M-15-positive *Escherichia coli* isolates was assessed with PFGE. Bacterial DNA was isolated using a technique described by Husickova et al. and digested by the *Xba*I restriction endonuclease (New England Biolabs, Ipswich, MA, USA) for 24 h at 37 °C [36]. The obtained DNA fragments were separated by PFGE on 1.2% agarose gel for 24 h at 6 V/cm and pulse times of 2–35 s. Subsequently, the gel was stained with ethidium bromide. The resulting restriction profiles were analyzed with the GelCompar II software (Applied Maths, Kortrijk, Belgium) using the Dice coefficient (1.2%) for comparing similarity and unweighted pair group method with arithmetic means for cluster analysis. The results were interpreted according to criteria described by Tenover et al. [37].

Statistical analyses were conducted using IBM SPSS Statistics version 22 (IBM, New York City, NY, USA) and the statistical environment R, version 4.0.2. The presence of bacteria assessed according to both cut-offs was compared with the McNemar's one-sided test. The tests were performed at a 0.05 level of significance.

5. Conclusions

The results clearly show that the therapeutic approach to neonatal infections must be based on their character including classification as early-/late-onset. As a cut-off value, 72 h after birth are more suitable. At the same time, it must be stressed that microbiological tests are necessary to allow targeted antibiotic therapy including application of adequate antibiotics if multidrug-resistant bacterial pathogens are detected. The results of this study confirm that only in case of early-onset infections arising within 72 h of birth, initial antibiotic therapy based on gentamicin with ampicillin or amoxicillin/clavulanic acid may be recommended. It is also clear that initial antibiotic treatment must be based on local surveillance of the most common bacterial pathogens and their resistance to antibiotics.

Author Contributions: Conceptualization, P.K. and M.K.; methodology, M.K. and L.K.; validation, M.K., L.K., and J.L.; formal analysis, P.K. and K.F.; investigation, P.K., K.F., M.R., and J.L.; resources, J.L. and P.K.; writing-original draft preparation, M.K.; writing-review and editing, P.K.; supervision, M.K.; project administration, M.K. and L.K.; funding acquisition, M.K. All authors have read and agreed to the published version of the manuscript.

Funding: This research was funded by the Czech Health Research Council (project no. NV18-05-00340), grant IGA_LF_2021_022, project LO1304, and by MH CZ—DRO (FNOL, 00098892).

Institutional Review Board Statement: The study was conducted according to the guidelines of the Declaration of Helsinki. Ethics committee approval was not required as the study did not interfere with the diagnostic and therapeutic process.

Informed Consent Statement: Patients' parents gave written informed consent to sample collection, anonymous enrollment in the study and publication of the results.

Data Availability Statement: The support data are not publicly available due to privacy issues.

Acknowledgments: The authors thank Michaela Varejkova (Department of Probability and Mathematical Statistics, Faculty of Mathematics and Physics, Charles University, Prague, Czech Republic) for help in the statistical processing of the results and Pavel Kurfürst for proofreading.

Conflicts of Interest: The authors declare no conflict of interest. The funders had no role in the design of the study; in the collection, analyses, or interpretation of data; in the writing of the manuscript; or in the decision to publish the results.

References

1. Shah, B.A.; Padbury, J.F. Neonatal sepsis. *Virulence* **2014**, *5*, 170–178. [CrossRef] [PubMed]
2. Cortese, F.; Scicchitano, P.; Gesualdo, M.; Filaninno, A.; De Giorgi, E.; Schettini, F.; Laforgia, N.; Ciccone, M.M. Early and Late Infections in Newborns: Where Do We Stand? A Review. *Pediatr. Neonatol.* **2016**, *57*, 265–273. [CrossRef]
3. Tzialla, C.; Borghesi, A.; Pozzi, M.; Stronati, M. Neonatal infections due to multi-resistant strains: Epidemiology, current treatment, emerging therapeutic approaches and prevention. *Clin. Chim. Acta* **2015**, *451*, 71–77. [CrossRef] [PubMed]
4. McMillan, J.A.; Weiner, L.B.; Lamberson, H.V.; Hagen, J.H.; Aubry, R.H.; Abdul-Karim, R.W.; Sunderji, S.G.; Higgins, A.P. Efficacy of maternal screening and therapy in the prevention of chlamydia infection of the newborn. *Infection* **1985**, *13*, 263–266. [CrossRef] [PubMed]
5. Darville, T. Chlamydia trachomatis Infections in Neonates and Young Children. *Semin. Pediatr. Infect. Dis.* **2005**, *16*, 235–244. [CrossRef]
6. Santos, R.P.; Tristram, D. A Practical Guide to the Diagnosis, Treatment, and Prevention of Neonatal Infections. *Pediatr. Clin. N. Am.* **2015**, *62*, 491–508. [CrossRef]
7. Mukhopadhyay, S.; Wade, K.C.; Puopolo, K.M. Drugs for the Prevention and Treatment of Sepsis in the Newborn. *Clin. Perinatol.* **2019**, *46*, 327–347. [CrossRef]
8. Poirel, L.; Madec, J.-Y.; Lupo, A.; Schink, A.-K.; Kieffer, N.; Nordmann, P.; Schwarz, S. Antimicrobial Resistance in Escherichia coli. *Microbiol. Spectr.* **2018**, *6*, 289–316. [CrossRef]

9. European Centre for Disease Prevention and Control. Data from the ECDC Surveillance Atlas—Antimicrobial resistance. Available online: https://www.ecdc.europa.eu/en/antimicrobial-resistance/surveillance-and-disease-data/data-ecdc (accessed on 5 May 2020).
10. Paitan, Y. Current Trends in Antimicrobial Resistance of Escherichia coli. *Curr. Top. Microbiol. Immunol.* **2018**, *416*, 181–211. [CrossRef]
11. Stoll, B.J.; Hansen, N.I.; Sánchez, P.J.; Faix, R.G.; Poindexter, B.B.; Van Meurs, K.P.; Bizzarro, M.J.; Goldberg, R.N.; Frantz, I.D.; Hale, E.C.; et al. Early Onset Neonatal Sepsis: The Burden of Group B Streptococcal and *E. coli* Disease Continues. *Pediatrics* **2011**, *127*, 817–826. [CrossRef]
12. Ocviyanti, D.; Wahono, W.T. Risk Factors for Neonatal Sepsis in Pregnant Women with Premature Rupture of the Membrane. *J. Pregnancy* **2018**, *2018*, 1–6. [CrossRef]
13. Camacho-Gonzalez, A.; Spearman, P.W.; Stoll, B.J. Neonatal Infectious Diseases. *Pediatr. Clin. N. Am.* **2013**, *60*, 367–389. [CrossRef] [PubMed]
14. Shane, A.L.; Stoll, B.J. Neonatal sepsis: Progress towards improved outcomes. *J. Infect.* **2014**, *68*, S24–S32. [CrossRef]
15. Cho, H.J.; Cho, H.-K. Central line-associated bloodstream infections in neonates. *Korean J. Pediatr.* **2019**, *62*, 79–84. [CrossRef] [PubMed]
16. Dong, H.; Cao, H.; Zheng, H. Pathogenic bacteria distributions and drug resistance analysis in 96 cases of neonatal sepsis. *BMC Pediatr.* **2017**, *17*, 1–6. [CrossRef] [PubMed]
17. Cohen-Wolkowiez, M.; Moran, C.; Benjamin, D.K.; Cotten, C.M.; Clark, R.H.; Smith, P.B. Early and Late Onset Sepsis in Late Preterm Infants. *Pediatr. Infect. Dis. J.* **2009**, *28*, 1052–1056. [CrossRef] [PubMed]
18. Hornik, C.; Fort, P.; Clark, R.; Watt, K.; Benjamin, D.; Smith, P.; Manzoni, P.; Jacqz-Aigrain, E.; Kaguelidou, F.; Cohen-Wolkowiez, M. Early and late onset sepsis in very-low-birth-weight infants from a large group of neonatal intensive care units. *Early Hum. Dev.* **2012**, *88*, S69–S74. [CrossRef]
19. Alcock, G.; Liley, H.G.; Cooke, L.; Gray, P.H. Prevention of neonatal late-onset sepsis: A randomised controlled trial. *BMC Pediatr.* **2017**, *17*, 98. [CrossRef]
20. Folgori, L.; Bielicki, J. Future Challenges in Pediatric and Neonatal Sepsis: Emerging Pathogens and Antimicrobial Resistance. *J. Pediatr. Intensiv. Care* **2019**, *8*, 17–24. [CrossRef] [PubMed]
21. Zea-Vera, A.; Ochoa, T.J. Challenges in the diagnosis and management of neonatal sepsis. *J. Trop. Pediatr.* **2015**, *61*, 1–13. [CrossRef] [PubMed]
22. Russell, A.R.B. Neonatal sepsis. *Paediatr. Child Health* **2011**, *21*, 265–269. [CrossRef]
23. Shane, A.L.; Sánchez, P.J.; Stoll, B.J. Neonatal sepsis. *Lancet* **2017**, *390*, 1770–1780. [CrossRef]
24. Bulkowstein, S.; Ben-Shimol, S.; Givon-Lavi, N.; Melamed, R.; Shany, E.; Greenberg, D. Comparison of early onset sepsis and community-acquired late onset sepsis in infants less than 3 months of age. *BMC Pediatr.* **2016**, *16*, 1–8. [CrossRef] [PubMed]
25. Greenberg, R.G.; Benjamin, D.K. Neonatal candidiasis: Diagnosis, prevention, and treatment. *J. Infect.* **2014**, *69*, S19–S22. [CrossRef]
26. Hope, W.; Castagnola, E.; Groll, A.; Roilides, E.; Akova, M.; Arendrup, M.; Arikan-Akdagli, S.; Bassetti, M.; Bille, J.; Cornely, O.; et al. ESCMID* guideline for the diagnosis and management of Candida diseases 2012: Prevention and management of invasive infections in neonates and children caused by Candida spp. *Clin. Microbiol. Infect.* **2012**, *18*, 38–52. [CrossRef]
27. Roilides, E. Invasive candidiasis in neonates and children. *Early Hum. Dev.* **2011**, *87*, S75–S76. [CrossRef]
28. Straková, L.; Motlová, J. Active surveillance of early onset disease due to group B streptococci in newborns. *Indian J. Med. Res.* **2004**, *119*, 205–207. [PubMed]
29. Simetka, O.; Petros, M.; Podesvová, H. Prevention of early-onset neonatal group B streptococcal infection: Neonatal outcome after introduction of national screening guideline. *Ceska Gynekol.* **2010**, *75*, 41–46.
30. Van Dyke, M.K.; Phares, C.R.; Lynfield, R.; Thomas, A.R.; Arnold, K.E.; Craig, A.S.; Mohle-Boetani, J.; Gershman, K.; Schaffner, W.; Petit, S.; et al. Evaluation of Universal Antenatal Screening for Group B Streptococcus. *New Engl. J. Med.* **2009**, *360*, 2626–2636. [CrossRef]
31. Boyer, K.M.; Gotoff, S.P. Prevention of Early-Onset Neonatal Group B Streptococcal Disease with Selective Intrapartum Chemoprophylaxis. *N. Engl. J. Med.* **1986**, *314*, 1665–1669. [CrossRef]
32. American Academy of Pediatrics Committee on Infectious Diseases and Committee on Fetus and Newborn. Revised guidelines for prevention of early-onset group B streptococcal (GBS) infection. *Pediatrics* **1997**, *99*, 489–496. [CrossRef] [PubMed]
33. Croxatto, A.; Prod'hom, G.; Greub, G. Applications of MALDI-TOF mass spectrometry in clinical diagnostic microbiology. *FEMS Microbiol. Rev.* **2012**, *36*, 380–407. [CrossRef] [PubMed]
34. The European Committee on Antimicrobial Susceptibility Testing—EUCAST. Available online: https://www.eucast.org/ (accessed on 10 January 2015).
35. Röderova, M.; Halova, D.; Papousek, I.; Dolejska, M.; Masarikova, M.; Hanulik, V.; Pudova, V.; Broz, P.; Htoutou-Sedlakova, M.; Sauer, P.; et al. Characteristics of Quinolone Resistance in Escherichia coli Isolates from Humans, Animals, and the Environment in the Czech Republic. *Front. Microbiol.* **2017**, *7*, 2147. [CrossRef]

36. Husickova, V.; Cekanova, L.; Chroma, M.; Htoutou-Sedlakova, M.; Hricova, K.; Kolář, M. Carriage of ESBL- and AmpC-positive Enterobacteriaceae in the gastrointestinal tract of community subjects and hospitalized patients in the Czech Republic. *Biomed. Pap.* **2012**, *156*, 348–353. [CrossRef] [PubMed]
37. Tenover, F.C.; Arbeit, R.D.; Goering, R.V.; Mickelsen, P.A.; Murray, B.E.; Persing, D.H.; Swaminathan, B. Interpreting chromosomal DNA restriction patterns produced by pulsed-field gel electrophoresis: Criteria for bacterial strain typing. *J. Clin. Microbiol.* **1995**, *33*, 2233–2239. [CrossRef]

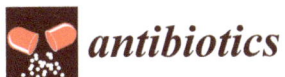

Article

Spread of Linezolid-Resistant *Enterococcus* spp. in Human Clinical Isolates in the Czech Republic

Lucia Mališová [1,2], Vladislav Jakubů [1,2,3], Katarína Pomorská [1], Martin Musílek [4] and Helena Žemličková [1,2,3,*]

1. National Reference Laboratory for Antibiotics, Centre for Epidemiology and Microbiology, National Institute of Public Health, 10000 Prague, Czech Republic; lucia.malisova@szu.cz (L.M.); vladislav.jakubu@szu.cz (V.J.); katarina.pomorska@szu.cz (K.P.)
2. Department of Microbiology, 3rd Faculty of Medicine Charles University, University Hospital Kralovske Vinohrady and National Institute of Public Health, 10000 Prague, Czech Republic
3. Department of Clinical Microbiology, Faculty of Medicine and University Hospital, Charles University, 53002 Hradec Kralove, Czech Republic
4. National Reference Laboratory for Meningococcal Infections, Centre for Epidemiology and Microbiology, National Institute of Public Health, 10000 Prague, Czech Republic; martin.musilek@szu.cz
* Correspondence: hzemlickova@szu.cz

Abstract: The aim of this study was to map and investigate linezolid resistance mechanisms in linezolid-resistant enterococci in the Czech Republic from 2009 to 2019. Altogether, 1442 isolates of *Enterococcus faecium* and *Enterococcus faecalis* were examined in the National Reference Laboratory for Antibiotics. Among them, 8% of isolates ($n = 115$) were resistant to linezolid (*E. faecium*/$n = 106$, *E. faecalis*/$n = 9$). Only three strains of *E. faecium* were resistant to tigecycline, 72.6% of isolates were resistant to vancomycin. One isolate of *E. faecium* harbored the *cfr* gene. The majority (87%, $n = 11$) of *E. faecium* strains were resistant to linezolid because of the mutation G2576T in the domain V of the 23S rRNA. This mutation was detected also in two strains of *E. faecalis*. The presence of the *optrA* gene was the dominant mechanism of linezolid resistance in *E. faecalis* isolates. None of enterococci contained *cfrB*, *poxtA* genes, or any amino acid mutation in genes encoding ribosomal proteins. No mechanism of resistance was identified in 4 out of 106 *E. faecium* linezolid resistant isolates in this study. Seventeen sequence types (STs) including four novel STs were identified in this work. Clonal complex CC17 was found in all *E. faecium* isolates.

Keywords: *Enterococcus faecium*; *Enterococcus faecalis*; linezolid resistance; 23S rRNA; optrA

1. Introduction

Enterococci are Gram-positive bacteria, commensals of the gastrointestinal tract and opportunistic pathogens able to cause community-acquired and nosocomial infections. Two species, *Enterococcus faecium* and *Enterococcus faecalis*, are considered to be one of the most important nosocomial pathogens worldwide [1]. They cause life-threatening infections especially in elderly, polymorbid and immunocompromised patients [2]. Increasing resistance of enterococci to penicillin, aminoglycosides, glycopeptides or to the last resort antibiotics (daptomycin, tigecycline, linezolid) prevents these drugs from being effective in the treatment of infections caused by these bacteria [3].

Linezolid is a bacteriostatic antibiotic efficient only against Gram-positive bacteria including methicillin-resistant *Staphylococcus aureus* (MRSA) and vancomycin resistant enterococci [4]. It inhibits the accuracy of the protein translation by binding to the peptidyl transferase centrum (PTC) in the V domain of the 23S rRNA inside the 50S ribosomal subunit [5]. Since the introduction of linezolid into clinical use in 2000 (USA) [4], seven mechanisms have been described as related to the linezolid resistance in enterococci: Mutations in the 23S rRNA and genes encoding ribosomal proteins L3, L4, and L22, the

Citation: Mališová, L.; Jakubů, V.; Pomorská, K.; Musílek, M.; Žemličková, H. Spread of Linezolid-Resistant *Enterococcus* spp. in Human Clinical Isolates in the Czech Republic. *Antibiotics* **2021**, *10*, 219. https://doi.org/10.3390/antibiotics10020219

Academic Editor: Jeffrey Lipman

Received: 27 January 2021
Accepted: 20 February 2021
Published: 22 February 2021

Publisher's Note: MDPI stays neutral with regard to jurisdictional claims in published maps and institutional affiliations.

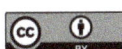

Copyright: © 2021 by the authors. Licensee MDPI, Basel, Switzerland. This article is an open access article distributed under the terms and conditions of the Creative Commons Attribution (CC BY) license (https://creativecommons.org/licenses/by/4.0/).

acquisition of plasmid carrying genes *cfr* (chloramphenicol-florfenicol) [6], *optrA* (ABC transporter that confers resistance to oxazolidinones and phenicols) [7] and *poxtA* (ABC transporter; resistance to oxazolidinones, phenicols and tetracyclines) [8]. The most common mechanism of linezolid resistance in enterococci is the conversion of G to T at position 2576 in the 23S rRNA [9]. Ribosomal proteins L3, L4, L22 play an important role in the stabilization and conformation of the ribosome (PTC). Therefore, mutations in genes (*rplC*, *rplD*, and *rplV*) encoding these proteins lead to the amino acid changes followed by disruption of translation. This type of mechanism is predominantly linked with linezolid resistance in *Staphylococcus epidermidis* [10].

The gene *cfr* encodes a methyltransferase that catalyzes the posttranscriptional methylation of nucleotide A2503 in the 23S rRNA [10]. It has been described for the first time in *S. aureus* in 2005 [11], and it can be transferred across different bacterial species and genera [12]. New mechanisms, *optrA* (China, 2015) [7] and *poxtA* [8], belonging to the ABC-F family of ATP-binding cassette (efflux pump genes) were revealed recently. Comparative analysis at the protein levels in the genome of linezolid resistant *S. aureus* revealed 32% protein homology between them [8]. Gene *optrA* has been more often detected in livestock than in humans and its occurrence is more associated with *E. faecalis* than *E. faecium* strains [1]. *PoxtA* was originally identified in Italian isolate MRSA in 2018 [8] and its prevalence amongst the enterococcal population is still under investigation.

The purpose of this study was to investigate the spread of linezolid resistant enterococci acquired from human clinical specimens in the Czech Republic over the period of 10 years, and to analyze molecular mechanisms of their resistance to linezolid.

2. Results

2.1. Antibiotic Susceptibility of Linezolid Resistant Isolates of E. faecium and E. faecalis

Altogether, 1442 enterococcal isolates (791/58.5%/*E. faecium*, 651/45%/*E. faecalis*) were examined in the National Reference Laboratory for Antibiotics from 2009 to 2019. Of them, 115 strains (8%) were resistant to linezolid: 106 isolates (13.4%) of *E. faecium* and 9 strains (1.4%) of *E. faecalis*. The number of linezolid resistant enterococci increased from 2009 to 2019 (*E. faecium*; from 2009/0 to 2019/32, *E. faecalis*; from 2009/0 to 2019/4, Supplementary Figure S1). Resistance to vancomycin was confirmed in 72.6% ($n = 77$) of *E. faecium* strains. Resistance to teicoplanin was detected in 70% ($n = 74$) of isolates, 2.8% ($n = 3$) of strains were resistant to tigecycline. The majority of linezolid resistant *E. faecium* isolates were resistant also to gentamicin (76.5%, $n = 89$) and streptomycin (69%, $n = 79$). None of linezolid resistant *E. faecalis* strains was resistant to ampicillin, teicoplanin, vancomycin and tigecycline. All of them were resistant to gentamicin, 4 isolates also to streptomycin (Table 1, Supplementary Table S1).

2.2. Mechanisms of Linezolid and Vancomycin Resistance

Altogether, 93.4% ($n = 99$) of *E. faecium* isolates harbored the point mutation G2576T in the V domain of the 23S rRNA, two strains of *E. faecium* were positive for the presence of *optrA* gene, one isolate was *cfr* positive. There was not revealed the mechanism of linezolid resistance in four isolates. In 7 out of 9 *E. faecalis* isolates, the presence of *optrA* gene was confirmed, the mutation G2576T was revealed in two samples. Resistance to vancomycin was detected only in *E. faecium* strains. The presence of *vanA* (92%, $n = 71$), and *vanB* ($n = 2$) genes was confirmed. Four isolates were resistant to vancomycin due to the combination of *vanA*, *vanB* ($n = 4$) genes (Table 1, Supplementary Table S1).

Table 1. Molecular characteristics and antibiotic susceptibility of 115 human clinical isolates of *Enterococcus faecium* (n = 106) and *Enterococcus faecalis* (n = 9) analyzed in the study. Absolute numbers are expressed in % (number of isolates) and depict the number of resistant population in the group.

ST	CC	Number of Isolates	AMP	LNZ	TEI	VAN	GEN	STR	TGC	Mechanism of LNZ-R	Van Genotype
							E. faecium				
ST80	17	53	100(53)	100(53)	94 (50)	94(50)	98(52)	85(45)	5.6 (3)	ΔG2576T (53)	vanA (50)
ST117	17	24	100(24)	100(24)	45.8 (11)	54(13)	75(18)	83(20)	0	ΔG2576T (22) / cfr (1) / * (1)	vanA (10) / vanB (2) / vanA,vanB (1)
ST18	17	13	100(13)	100(13)	46(6)	53.8(7)	84.6(11)	38.4(5)	0	ΔG2576T (12) / * (1)	vanA (5) / vanA,vanB (2)
ST761	17	4	100(4)	100(4)	25(1)	25(1)	75(3)	75(3)	0	ΔG2576T (3) / cfrB (1)	vanA (1)
ST78	17	3	100(3)	100(3)	33.3(1)	33.3(1)	33.3(1)	66.6(2)	0	ΔG2576T (3)	vanA,vanB (1)
ST17	17	2	100(2)	100(2)	50(1)	50(1)	0	0	0	ΔG2576T (2)	vanA (1)
ST203	17	1	100(1)	100(1)	100(1)	100(1)	0	100(1)	0	ΔG2576T (1)	vanA (1)
ST552	17	1	100(1)	100(1)	0	0	100(1)	0	0	ΔG2576T (1)	-
ST262	17	1	100(1)	100(1)	0	0	0	100(1)	0	optrA (1)	-
ST1487 †	17	1	100(1)	100(1)	100(1)	100(1)	100(1)	100(1)	0	* (1)	vanA (1)
ST3501 †	17	2	100(2)	100(2)	100(2)	100(2)	100(2)	0	0	ΔG2576T (2)	vanA (2)
ST3502 †	17	1	0	100(1)	0	0	0	100(1)	0	optrA (1)	-
							E. faecalis				
ST6	2	1	0	100(1)	0	0	100(1)	100(1)	0	ΔG2576T (1)	-
ST476	476	3	0	100(3)	0	0	100(3)	0	0	optrA (3)	-
ST480	480	2	0	100(2)	0	0	100(2)	50(1)	0	optrA (2)	-
ST858	unknown	2	0	100(2)	0	0	100(2)	100(2)	0	optrA (2)	-
ST1982 †	unknown	1	0	100(1)	0	0	100(1)	0	0	ΔG2576T (1)	-

ST, sequence type; CC, clonal complex; AMP, ampicillin; LNZ, linezolid; TEI, teicoplanin; VAN, vancomycin; GEN, gentamicin; STR, streptomycin; TGC, tigecycline; *, unknown mechanism of linezolid resistance; LNZ-R, linezolid resistance; -, wild type; †, novel sequence types.

2.3. Molecular Typing-MLST Analysis

Altogether, 12 different sequence types (STs) were found in linezolid resistant *E. faecium* strains. The most frequent STs detected were ST80 ($n = 53$) and ST117 ($n = 24$), followed by ST18 ($n = 13$), ST761 ($n = 4$), ST78 ($n = 3$). Other STs were represented by a single or two isolates: ST17 ($n = 2$), ST203 ($n = 1$), ST552 ($n = 1$), ST262 ($n = 1$). Due to the new type of *gyd* allele, three novel STs were identified in the study: ST1487 ($n = 1$), ST3501 ($n = 2$), ST3502 ($n = 1$) (Supplementary Figure S2). Almost all strains of *E. faecium* (97%, $n = 103$) belonged to the same clonal complex, CC17 (Table 1, Supplementary Table S1). MLST typing revealed a high genetic variability within the group of *E. faecalis* strains. Altogether, there were confirmed 5 STs: ST6/CC2 ($n = 1$)/, ST476/CC476 ($n = 3$), ST480 ($n = 2$), ST858 ($n = 2$) and a new ST1982 ($n = 1$) (Supplementary Figure S3).

3. Discussion

This is the first study mapping linezolid resistant enterococci acquired from human clinical specimen in the Czech Republic. Enterococci have become one of the most prevalent (nosocomial) pathogens over the past decades and linezolid provides one of the therapeutic options for infections caused by this bacteria.

Among 1442 enterococci sent to the National Reference Laboratory for Antibiotics from 2009 to 2019, 8% of them were resistant to linezolid. Congruently with other European countries, the pattern of occurrence of linezolid resistant enterococci increased from year to year (0/2009-36/2019) [9,13]. Except for 3 strains (2.6%) almost all analyzed enterococci were susceptible to tigecycline, an alternative option in the treatment of enterococcal infections. In accordance with this observation, the majority of the European countries reports generally low prevalence (<1%) of isolates resistant to last-resort antibiotics (daptomycin, tigecycline, linezolid) [14]. A lower rate of linezolid resistance in enterococci could be explained by lower selection pressure of this antibiotic or by its mechanism. The substitution of G to T in the position 2576 in the 23S rRNA develops as a spontaneous mutation. It was reported that the frequency of the spontaneous resistance to linezolid (in enterococci) is lower than to other antibiotics [15]. This statement has been confirmed also in this work, 87.8% (101/115) of linezolid resistant enterococci contained the mutation G2576T in the 23S rRNA [16]. Mutations in *rplC*, *rplD*, and *rplV* genes were not observed in this work. Mutations in genes encoding ribosomal proteins (L3, L4, L22) were more commonly seen in coagulase-negative staphylococci (preferentially *S. epidermidis*) than in enterococci [17].

The rate of *E. faecium* isolates harboring gene *optrA* was negligible. Altogether, only two isolates (ST262, ST3502) were positive for the *optrA* gene. This result is not surprising, the occurrence of *optrA* has been associated more with *E. faecalis* than *E. faecium* species [18,19]. The presence of the gene *optrA* was the dominant mechanism responsible for the linezolid resistance in *E. faecalis* strains. It is worth noting, that *optrA* positive linezolid resistant enterococci can confer MICs of linezolid different than other linezolid resistant enterococci [20]. All enterococci positive for the gene *optrA* were associated with MICs for linezolid up to the level up to 8 mg/L. The majority of enterococci harboring the G2576T mutation had MICs $\geq$ 16 mg/L.

None from enterococci analyzed in this work harbored the gene *poxtA*. This, a novel antibiotic resistance determinant, was until now identified only in one clinical isolate of *E. faecium* in Greece in 2018 [21]. Despite the sporadic occurrence of the *poxtA*, the scattered distribution of this gene among the different Gram-positive species (e.g., *S. aureus*, *Enterococcus* spp., etc.) deserves an attention [22].

At present, eight different types of *van* genes conferring vancomycin resistance mechanisms are known. The *vanA* and *vanB* resistance genotypes are the most frequently detected variants in clinical isolates of *E. faecium* and *E. faecalis* worldwide [14]. Vancomycin resistance caused by the presence of gene *vanA* was a dominant mechanism in the group of vancomycin resistant enterococci in the Czech Republic. Due to the location of the gene *vanA* on plasmid, this fragment of DNA can spread easier than *vanB*, which is usually a part of the bacterial chromosome [23]. Based on the global spread of enterococci resistant to the different kinds of antibiotics (including the last resort antibiotics), a molecular epidemiology studies are performed to obtain insights into the dissemination of these strains. MLST is a molecular typing method with suitable discriminatory power [23] very often used for this purpose. One pandemic clone of CC17 was detected in linezolid resistant *E. faecium* isolates in the Czech Republic from 2009 to 2019. The enterococcal lineage of CC17 is responsible for the spread of linezolid and vancomycin resistance in hospitals all around the world [1]. Moreover, strains belonging to this clonal complex show persistence in the environment and high colonization capability [24]. In this study, linezolid resistant enterococci belonged to 12 different STs, but a majority (50%) of isolates typed as ST80 was observed [25]. ST80 was described for the first time in blood of Israeli patient in 1997 (unpublished data, the source: pubmlst.org). Since then it has been detected all over the world. ST18, ST78, and ST117 were associated with enterococci also in other European countries [24,25]. ST17, ST203, and ST552 were observed earlier by Egan et al. in Ireland [26]. In concordance with others, a high risk STs associated with linezolid resistance in enterococci involved also ST262 [27], ST761 [28] and newly identified STs 3501, 3502, 1487 and 1982. A classical hospital-associated CC2 (ST6) of *E. faecalis* has been already detected in Spain and Poland [29,30]. STs 585 and 476 have been observed in overall diverse population of *optrA*-positive *E. faecalis* strains in Portugal [31].

Inability to infer the linezolid resistance mechanism in three *E. faecium* isolates suggests the possibility of presence of additional mechanisms of resistance. It is supported by results of studies on enterococci with a silent mechanism of resistance, but still exhibiting linezolid resistance [32]. Enterococci are adaptable bacteria characterized by a high plasticity of genome (a high rate of DNA recombination). Therefore, novel mechanisms of resistance to different kinds of antibiotics have emerged relatively rapidly. Efflux pumps, cell wall thickness and biofilm formation are still discussed as putative alternative pathways of linezolid resistance [33,34].

In conclusion, this study provided the first insight into the population structure of linezolid resistant enterococci in the Czech Republic within the period of 10 years. It showed that the rate of linezolid resistant enterococci was comparable with other European countries and it increased in both groups of examined enterococci. The main mechanism of linezolid resistance among clinical *E. faecium* isolates was the G2576T mutation in the domain V of the 23S rRNA. The presence of gene *optrA* was the major cause of linezolid resistance in *E. faecalis* strains. A high risk clone CC17 was the only CC detected in linezolid resistant *E. faecium* strains in the Czech Republic within last decade.

Still increasing prevalence of enterococci resistant to the last resort antibiotics as well as their ability to acquire novel DNA fragments encoding (new) resistance determinants predestine these bacteria to even more successful spreading. Therefore, enterococci resistant to linezolid represents a public health concern and monitoring the spread of these bacteria is necessary.

4. Materials and Methods

4.1. Bacterial Isolates

Screening of *E. faecium*/*E. faecalis* strains is performed as a part of European Antimicrobial Resistance Surveillance Network (EARS-Net) and the study of Monitoring of Antibiotic Resistance in the National Reference Laboratory for Antibiotics (National Institute of Public Health, Prague, Czech Republic). Enterococci presented in this study were acquired from 40 laboratories in the period from 2009 to 2019. The majority of strains, 61% ($n = 875$), was of invasive origin (blood; $n = 873$, cerebrospinal fluid; $n = 2$). The rest of isolates was acquired form non-invasive clinical specimens, and involved surgical wound, urine, pus, sputum, catheter, aspirate, bile, and swab (mouth, throat, nose, and vagina). Altogether, 5% ($n = 70$) of enterococci were isolated from rectal swab and stool sample. One isolate was of unknown origin. Characteristics of linezolid resistant strains are given in the Supplementary Table S1. Enterococci resistant to linezolid are further examined to reveal the mechanism of linezolid resistance and their epidemiological relationship

(MLST). Resistance to linezolid (≥4 mg/L) was defined according to the European Committee on Antimicrobial Susceptibility Testing (EUCAST) breakpoint (www.eucast.org). All strains were routinely cultivated on Columbia blood agar (Oxoid, Brno, Czech Republic) aerobically at 36 ± 1 °C. Identification of strains was performed by Matrix-Assisted Laser Desorption Ionization-Time of Flight Mass Spectrometry (MALDI-TOF MS; Microflex Bruker, Bremen, Germany) according to the manufacturer's protocol (www.bruker.com).

4.2. Susceptibility Testing

Minimal inhibitory concentrations (MICs) of ampicillin, linezolid, teicoplanin, vancomycin, gentamicin, streptomycin, and tigecycline were determined by broth microdilution method according to ISO 20776-1. Interpretation of susceptibility testing results was performed as recommended by EUCAST, version according to a corresponding year (last used version 9.0). Strains ATCC 29212 and ATCC 51299 were used as quality control in this study (both strains recommended by EUCAST; www.eucast.org).

4.3. Detection of Determinants of Linezolid Resistance

Mechanism of resistance to linezolid was determined by PCR (*cfr*, *cfrB*, *oprA*, and *poxtA*) and Sanger sequencing (23S rRNA, *rplC*, *rplD*, and *rplV*). DNA extraction was obtained from a fresh culture (24 hours) according to the manufacturer's protocol (GenElute TM Bacterial Genomic DNA Kits, Sigma Aldrich, St. Louis, MO, USA). The list of enterococcal specific primers and settings of PCR used in the study are given in the Supplementary Table S2. PCR products of *cfr*, *oprA* were resolved in 1.5% agarose (TopVision Agarose, Thermo Scientific, St. Louis, MO, USA) in electrophoresis (5 V/cm) for 45 minutes. NCTC13923 was used as control strain for *optrA* detection in this study. The detection of *cfr*, *poxtA*, and *cfrB* was performed according to procedures as described previously [8,12,35]. The amplified fragments of the 23S rRNA, *rplC*, *rplD*, and *rplV* were sequenced by analyzer Applied Biosystems 3130xL. Point mutation/s associated with linezolid resistance were analyzed using software Bionumerics 7.6.2 (Applied Maths, Ghent, East Flanders, Belgium).

4.4. Detection of Mechanism of Vancomycin Resistance

Isolates resistant to linezolid and simultaneously resistant to vancomycin were further examined. The mechanism of resistance to vancomycin was screened by PCR using primers under conditions that are listed in the Supplementary Table S2. Electrophoresis was carried out as described above.

4.5. MLST Typing of Linezolid Resistant Strains of E. faecium, E. faecalis

Epidemiology of enterococci was investigated by the multilocus sequence typing (MLST) analysis as described earlier [36]. Seven primers targeting *adk* (adenylate kinase), *atpA* (ATP synthase, alpha subunit), *ddl* (d-alanine:d-alanine ligase), *gyd* (glyceraldehyde-3-phosphate dehydrogenase), *gdh* (glucose-6-phosphate dehydrogenase), *purK* (phosphoribosylaminoimidazol carboxylase ATPase subunit) and *pstS* (phosphate ATP-binding cassette transporter) alleles were used to amplify target region in *E. faecium* isolates. *PstS* (phosphate ATP binding cassette transporter), *gki* (putative glucokinase), *aroE* (shikimate 5-dehydrogenase), *xpt* (shikimate 5-dehydrogenase), *gyd*, *gdh*, and *yiqL* (acetyl-coenzyme A acetyltransferase) were used for MLST analysis of *E. faecalis* strains. Alleles *gyd* and *gdh* were amplified using the same primers for both species. The list of primers used for MLST analysis of enterococci is given in the Supplementary Table S3. All sequences were processed by analyser (Applied Biosystems 3130xL, Foster City, CA, USA). Allelic profiles, sequence types (STs) and clonal complexes (CC) of enterococci were determined using Bionumerics 7.6.2 (Applied Maths, Ghent, East Flanders, Belgium) and free available website pubmlst.org (https://pubmlst.org/organisms).

Supplementary Materials: The following are available online at https://www.mdpi.com/2079-6382/10/2/219/s1, Figure S1: Detection of linezolid resistant enterococci acquired from human clinical specimen in the Czech Republic from 2009 to 2019, Figure S2: STs occurrence in the group of linezolid resistant *E. faecium* (n = 106) strains from 2009 to 2019, Figure S3: STs occurrence in the group of linezolid resistant *E. faecalis* (n = 9) isolates from 2009 to 2019, Table S1: Phenotypic and genotypic characteristics of the 115 linezolid-resistant enterococcal isolates examined in the NRL for ATB between 2009 and 2019, Table S2: Primers used in the study, Table S3: Primers used in the MLST analysis of *E. faecium* and *E. faecalis* isolates.

Author Contributions: L.M. methodology, data analysis, witting—original draft preparation; V.J. writing—review and editing; K.P. writing—review and editing; M.M. methodology; H.Ž. writing—review and editing, project administration. All authors have read and agreed to the published version of the manuscript.

Funding: This research was funded by Ministry of Health, Czech Republic-conceptual development of research organization the National Institute of Public Health–NIPH, 75010330.

Data Availability Statement: The data presented in this study are available on request from the corresponding author.

Acknowledgments: Authors appreciate technical assistance of Jiří Kašík and Markéta Čechová. We would like to thank all EARS-Net participating laboratories for sending strains to the National Reference Laboratory for Antibiotics.

Conflicts of Interest: The authors declare no conflict of interest.

References

1. Prieto, A.M.; van Schaik, W.; Rogers, M.R.C.; Coque, T.M.; Baquero, F.; Corander, J.; Willems, R.J.L. Global Emergence and Dissemination of Enterococci as Nosocomial Pathogens: Attack of the Clones? *Front. Microbiol.* **2016**, *26*, 788.
2. Arias, C.A.; Murray, B.E. The rise of the *Enterococcus*: Beyond vancomycin resistance. *Nat. Rev. Microbiol.* **2012**, *10*, 266–278. [CrossRef] [PubMed]
3. Murray, B.E. The life and times of the *Enterococcus*. *Clin. Microbiol. Rev.* **1990**, *3*, 46–65. [CrossRef]
4. Mendes, R.E.; Deshpande, L.M.; Jones, R.N. Linezolid update: Stable in vitro activity following more than a decade of clinical use and summary of associated resistance mechanisms. *Drug Resist. Updates* **2014**, *17*, 1–12. [CrossRef]
5. Bourgeois-Nicolaos, N.; Massias, L.; Couson, B.; Butel, M.J.; Andremont, A.; Doucet-Populaire, F. Dose Dependence of Emergence of Resistance to Linezolid in *Enterococcus faecalis* In Vivo. *J. Infect. Dis.* **2007**, *10*, 1480–1488. [CrossRef] [PubMed]
6. Diaz, L.; Kiratisin, P.; Mendes, R.E.; Panesso, D.; Singh, K.V.; Arias, C.A. Transferable plasmid-mediated resistance to linezolid due to cfr in a human clinical isolate of *Enterococcus faecalis*. *Antimicrob. Agents Chemother.* **2012**, *56*, 3917–3922. [CrossRef]
7. Wang, Y.; Lv, Y.; Cai, J.; Schwarz, S.; Cui, L.; Hu, Z.; Zhang, R.; Li, J.; Zhao, Q.; He, T.; et al. A novel gene, optrA that confers transferable resistance to oxazolidinones and phenicols and its presence in *Enterococcus faecalis* and *Enterococcus faecium* of human and animal origin. *J. Antimicrob. Chemother.* **2015**, *70*, 2182–2190. [CrossRef]
8. Antonelli, A.; D'Andrea, M.M.; Brenciani, A.; Galeotti, C.L.; Morroni, G.; Pollini, S.; Varaldo, P.E.; Rossolini, G.M. Characterization of poxtA, a novel phenicol–oxazolidinone–tetracycline resistance gene from an MRSA of clinical origin. *J. Antimicrob. Chemother.* **2018**, *73*, 1763–1769. [CrossRef] [PubMed]
9. Klare, I.; Fleige, C.; Geringer, U.; Thurmer, A.; Bender, J.; Mutters, N.T.; Mischnik, A.; Werner, G. Increased frequency of linezolid resistance among clinical *Enterococcus faecium* isolates from German hospital patients. *J. Glob. Antimicrob. Resist.* **2015**, *3*, 128–131. [CrossRef] [PubMed]
10. Patel, S.N.; Memari, N.; Shahinas, D.; Toye, B.; Jamieson, F.B.; Farrell, D.J. Linezolid resistance in *Enterococcus faecium* isolated in Ontario, Canada. *Diagn. Microbiol. Infect. Dis.* **2013**, *77*, 350–353. [CrossRef] [PubMed]
11. Rossney, A.S.; Shore, A.C.; Morgan, P.M.; Fitzgibbon, M.M.; O'Connell, B.; Coleman, D.C. The emergence and importation of diverse genotypes of methicillin-resistant Staphylococcus aureus (MRSA) harboring the Panton-Valentine leukocidin gene (pvl) reveal that pvl is a poor marker for community-acquired MRSA strains in Ireland. *J. Clin. Microbiol.* **2007**, *45*, 2554–2563. [CrossRef]
12. Bender, J.K.; Fleige, C.; Klare, I.; Fiedler, S.; Mischnik, A.; Mutters, N.T.; Dingle, K.E.; Werner, G. Detection of a cfr(B) Variant in German *Enterococcus faecium* Clinical Isolates and the Impact on Linezolid Resistance in *Enterococcuss* pp. *PLoS ONE* **2016**, *11*, e0167042. [CrossRef] [PubMed]
13. Moure, Z.; Lara, N.; Marín, M.; Sola-Campoy, P.J.; Bautista, V.; Gómez-Bertomeu, F.; Gómez-Dominguez, C.; Pérez-Vázquez, M.; Aracil, B.; Campos, J.; et al. Spanish Linezolid-Resistant Enterococci Collaborating Group, Interregional spread in Spain of linezolid-resistant *Enterococcus* spp. isolates carrying the optrA and poxtA genes. *Int. J. Antimicrob. Agents* **2020**, *55*, 105977. [CrossRef] [PubMed]
14. Bender, J.K.; Cattoir, V.; Hegstad, K.; Sadowy, E.; Coque, T.M.; Westh, H.; Hammerum, A.M.; Schaffer, K.; Burns, K.; Murchan, S.; et al. Update on prevalence and mechanisms of resistance to linezolid, tigecycline and daptomycin in enterococci in Europe: Towards a common nomenclature. *Drug Resist. Updates* **2018**, *40*, 25–39. [CrossRef]

15. Prystowsky, J.; Siddiqui, F.; Chosay, J.; Shinabarger, D.L.; Millichap, J.; Peterson, L.R.; Noskin, G.A. Resistance to linezolid: Characterization of mutations in rRNA and comparison of their occurrences in vancomycin-resistant enterococci. *Antimicrob. Agents Chemother.* 2001, *45*, 2154–2156. [CrossRef] [PubMed]
16. Ntokou, E.; Stathopoulos, C.; Kristo, I.; Dimitroulia, E.; Labrou, M.; Vasdeki, A.; Makris, D.; Zakynthinos, E.; Tsakris, A. Intensive care unit dissemination of multiple clones of linezolid-resistant *Enterococcus faecalis* and *Enterococcus faecium*. *J. Antimicrob. Chemother.* 2012, *67*, 1819–1823. [CrossRef]
17. Mendes, R.E.; Deshpande, L.M.; Costello, A.J.; Farrell, D.J. Molecular epidemiology of Staphylococcus epidermidis clinical isolates from U.S. hospitals. *Antimicrob. Agents Chemother.* 2012, *56*, 4656–4661. [CrossRef]
18. Cavaco, L.M.; Bernal, J.F.; Zankari, E.; Le'on, M.; Hendriksen, R.S.; Perez-Gutierrez, E.; Aarestrup, F.M.; Donado-Godoy, P. Detection of linezolid resistance due to the optrA gene in *Enterococcus faecalis* from poultry meat from the American continent (Colombia). *J. Antimicrob. Chemother.* 2017, *72*, 678–683. [PubMed]
19. Vorobieva, V.; Roer, L.; Justesen, U.S.; Hansen, F.; Frimodt-Moller, N.; Hasman, H.; Hammerum, A.M. Detection of the optrA gene in a clinical ST16 *Enterococcus faecalis* isolate in Denmark. *J. Glob. Antimicrob. Resist.* 2017, *10*, 12–13. [CrossRef]
20. Ruiz-Ripa, L.; Feßler, A.T.; Hanke, D.; Eichhorn, I.; Azcona-Gutiérrez, J.M.; Pérez-Moreno, M.O.; Seral, C.; Aspiroz, C.; Alonso, C.A.; Torres, L.; et al. Mechanisms of Linezolid Resistance Among Enterococci of Clinical Origin in Spain-Detection of optrA- and cfr(D)-Carrying *E. faecalis*. *Microorganisms* 2020, *8*, 1155. [CrossRef]
21. Papagiannitsis, C.C.; Tsilipounidaki, K.; Malli, E.; Petinaki, E. Detection in Greece of a clinical *Enterococcus faecium* isolate carrying the novel oxazolidinone resistance gene poxtA. *J. Antimicrob. Chemother.* 2019, *8*, 2461–2462. [CrossRef] [PubMed]
22. Wu, Y.; Fan, R.; Wang, Y.; Lei, L.; Feßler, A.T.; Wang, Z.; Wu, C.; Schwarz, S.; Wang, Y. Analysis of combined resistance to oxazolidinones and phenicols among bacteria from dogs fed with raw meat/vegetables and the respective food items. *Sci. Rep.* 2019, *1*, 15500. [CrossRef] [PubMed]
23. Werner, G.; Fleige, C.; Neumanna, B.; Bender, J.K.; Layer, F.; Klare, I. Evaluation of DiversiLab®, MLST and PFGE typing for discriminating clinical *Enterococcus faecium* isolates. *J. Microbiol. Methods* 2015, *118*, 81–84. [CrossRef] [PubMed]
24. Werner, G. Molecular Typing of Enterococci/VRE. Werner. *J. Bacteriol. Parasitol.* 2013, *10*, 2155–9597. [CrossRef]
25. Kerschner, H.; Cabal, A.; Hartl, R.; Machherndl-Spandl, S.; Allerberger, F.; Ruppitsch, W.; Apfalter, P. Hospital outbreak caused by linezolid resistant *Enterococcus faecium* in Upper Austria. *Antimicrob. Resist. Infect. Control* 2019, *8*, 150. [CrossRef]
26. Egan, S.A.; Shore, A.C.; O'Connell, B.; Brennan, G.I.; Coleman, D.C. Linezolid resistance in *Enterococcus faecium* and Enterococcus faecalis from hospitalized patients in Ireland: High prevalence of the MDR genes optrA and poxtA in isolates with diverse genetic backgrounds. *J. Antimicrob. Chemother.* 2020, *75*, 1704–1711. [CrossRef]
27. Quiñones, D.; Aung, M.S.; Martins, J.P.S.; Urushibara, N.; Kobayashi, N. Genetic characteristics of VanA-type vancomycin-resistant *Enterococcus faecalis* and *Enterococcus faecium* in Cuba. *New Microbes New Infect.* 2018, *21*, 125–127. [CrossRef] [PubMed]
28. Wang, S.; Guo, Y.; Lv, J.; Qi, X.; Li, D.; Chen, Z.; Zhang, X.; Wang, L.; Yu, F. Characteristic of *Enterococcus faecium* clinical isolates with quinupristin/dalfopristin resistance in China. *BMC Microbiol.* 2016, *16*, 246. [CrossRef]
29. Kawalec, M.; Pietras, Z.; Danilowicz, E.; Jakubczak, A.; Gniadkowski, M.; Hryniewicz, W.; Willems, R. Clonal structure of *Enterococcus faecalis* isolated from Polish hospitals: The characterization of epidemic clones. *J. Clin. Microbiol.* 2007, *1*, 147–153. [CrossRef]
30. Ruiz-Garbajosa, P.; Bonten, M.J.; Robinson, D.A.; Top, J.; Nallapareddy, S.R.; Torres, C.; Coque, T.M.; Canton, R.; Baquero, F.; Murray, B.E.; et al. Multilocus sequence typing scheme for *Enterococcus faecalis* reveals hospital-adapted genetic complexes in a background of high rates of recombination. *J. Clin. Microbiol.* 2006, *44*, 2220–2228. [CrossRef]
31. Freitas, A.R.; Tedim, A.P.; Novais, C.; Lanza, V.L.; Peixe, L. Comparative genomics of global optrA-carrying Enterococcus faecalis uncovers a common chromosomal hotspot for optrA acquisition within a diversity of core and accessory genomes. *Microb. Genom.* 2020, *6*, e000350. [CrossRef] [PubMed]
32. Brenciani, A.; Morroni, G.; Vincenzi, C.; Manso, E.; Mingoia, M.; Giovanetti, E.; Varaldo, P.E. Detection in Italy of two clinical *Enterococcus faecium* isolates carrying both the oxazolidinone and phenicol resistance gene optrA and a silent multiresistance gene cfr. *J. Antimicrob. Chemother* 2016, *71*, 1118–1129. [CrossRef] [PubMed]
33. Tian, Y.; Li, T.; Zhu, Y.; Wang, B.; Zou, X.; Li, M. Mechanisms of linezolid resistance in staphylococciand enterococci isolated from two teaching hospitals in Shanghai, China. *BMC Microbiol.* 2014, *14*, 292. [CrossRef] [PubMed]
34. Hua, R.; Xia, Y.; Wu, W.; Yan, J.; Yang, M. Whole transcriptome analysis reveals potential novel mechanisms of low-level linezolid resistance in *Enterococcus faecalis*. *Gene* 2018, *647*, 143–149. [CrossRef]
35. Morales, G.; Picazo, J.J.; Baos, E.; Candel, F.J.; Arribi, A.; Peláez, B.; Andrade, R.; de la Torre, M.A.; Fereres, J.; Sánchez-García, M. Resistance to Linezolid Is Mediated by the cfr Gene in the First Report of an Outbreak of Linezolid-Resistant Staphylococcus aureus. *Clin. Inf. Dis.* 2010, *50*, 821–825. [CrossRef]
36. Belén, A.; Pavón, I.; Maiden, M.C.J. Multilocus Sequence Typing. *Methods Mol. Biol.* 2009, *551*, 129–140.

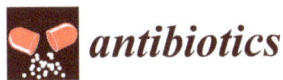

Article

Clinical Implication of the Relationship between Antimicrobial Resistance and Infection Control Activities in Japanese Hospitals: A Principal Component Analysis-Based Cluster Analysis

Tomokazu Shoji [1,2], Natsu Sato [1], Haruhisa Fukuda [3], Yuichi Muraki [4], Keishi Kawata [2] and Manabu Akazawa [1,*]

[1] Department of Public Health and Epidemiology, Meiji Pharmaceutical University, Noshio, Kiyose 204-8588, Tokyo, Japan; tshohji@yamanashi.ac.jp (T.S.); y161154@std.my-pharm.ac.jp (N.S.)
[2] Department of Pharmacy, University of Yamanashi Hospital, Shimokato, Chuo 409-3898, Yamanashi, Japan; kkawata@yamanashi.ac.jp
[3] Department of Health Care Administration and Management, Graduate School of Medical Sciences Kyushu University, Maidashi, Higashi, Fukuoka 812-8582, Japan; h_fukuda@hcam.med.kyushu-u.ac.jp
[4] Department of Clinical Pharmacoepidemiology, Kyoto Pharmaceutical University, Yamashina, Kyoto 607-8414, Japan; y-muraki@mb.kyoto-phu.ac.jp
* Correspondence: makazawa@my-pharm.ac.jp; Tel.:+81-42-495-8932

Abstract: There are few multicenter investigations regarding the relationship between antimicrobial resistance (AMR) and infection-control activities in Japanese hospitals. Hence, we aimed to identify Japanese hospital subgroups based on facility characteristics and infection-control activities. Moreover, we evaluated the relationship between AMR and hospital subgroups. We conducted a cross-sectional study using administrative claims data and antimicrobial susceptibility data in 124 hospitals from April 2016 to March 2017. Hospitals were classified using cluster analysis based the principal component analysis-transformed data. We assessed the relationship between each cluster and AMR using analysis of variance. Ten variables were selected and transformed into four principal components, and five clusters were identified. Cluster 5 had high infection control activity. Cluster 2 had partially lower activity of infection control than the other clusters. Clusters 3 and 4 had a higher rate of surgeries than Cluster 1. The methicillin-resistant *Staphylococcus aureus* (MRSA)/*S. aureus* detection rate was lowest in Cluster 1, followed, respectively, by Clusters 5, 2, 4, and 3. The MRSA/*S. aureus* detection rate differed significantly between Clusters 4 and 5 ($p = 0.0046$). Our findings suggest that aggressive examination practices are associated with low AMR whereas surgeries, an infection risk factor, are associated with high AMR.

Keywords: antimicrobial resistance; infection prevention and control; antimicrobial stewardship; hospital; cluster analysis; principal component analysis

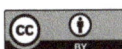

1. Introduction

Antimicrobial resistance (AMR) is an emerging global public health crisis. In Japan, the National Action Plan on AMR 2016–2020 issued in 2016, demanded medical institutions to promote comprehensive AMR control, linking the efforts of the existing infection control team (ICT) at the field level with those of the antimicrobial stewardship program (ASP) [1]. Methicillin-resistant *Staphylococcus aureus* (MRSA) is the most common AMR and should be monitored by each institution [2]. One of the goals of the action plan was to reduce the MRSA resistance rate to 20% by 2020 [1]. In 2020, the MRSA resistance rate decreased; however, it is still much higher than the corresponding outcome indices [3].

Quality indicators (QIs) related to infection control and the proper use of antibacterial agents including hand disinfection compliance rates, implementation of facility guidelines [4] and the implementation rate of Therapeutic Drug Monitoring (TDM), have been proposed [5]. In Japan, a surveillance system called Japan Surveillance for Infection Prevention and Healthcare Epidemiology (J-SIPHE) is in operation, and clinical indicators (e.g., antibacterial drug usage, blood culture collection rate, etc.) of participating institutions were collected [6]. In this way, various Qis have been proposed as infection control indicators, but implementing them remains difficult as there is no clear benchmark. Individual indicators are intricately intertwined and should be evaluated comprehensively [7].

The Japanese Ministry of Health, Labour and Welfare (MHLW) incorporated the medical fee for infection prevention and control (IPC), which is classified into two types (IPC type 1 or IPC type 2) [8]. Type 1 applies to physicians or nurses with >0.8 full-time equivalent (FTE), while type 2 applies to each member with >0.5 FTE [9,10]. However, some facilities had difficulties claiming the IPC medical fee because of shortages in infection control supply materials, as well as human resources and facility equipment [11,12]. Therefore, we believe that it is necessary to evaluate not only IPC and ASP but also the status of the facility when considering the relationship with AMR.

The optimal Qis for evaluating IPC are unclear. Additionally, there are differences in medical care, human resources, and physical resources even in facilities with a similar type of IPC medical fee. Thus, it is difficult to distinguish between facilities based on specific QI or medical fee. A more practical approach to understanding individual IPC and its underlying mechanism is to consider the specific facility factors and infection control measures. Furthermore, there is a need to evaluate the factors that may be related to AMR.

In this study, we aimed to objectively summarize the variables associated with infection control and identify facility clusters based on structure and process factors. Moreover, we assessed the relationships between AMR and these clusters to clarify the factors that may affect AMR. The conceptual framework that guided our study was the quality of care model developed by Donabedian [13]. This conceptual framework comprises the following three domains: structure factors, process factors, and AMR (Figure 1). We conducted a principal component analysis to transform the selected variables included in the cluster analysis [14].

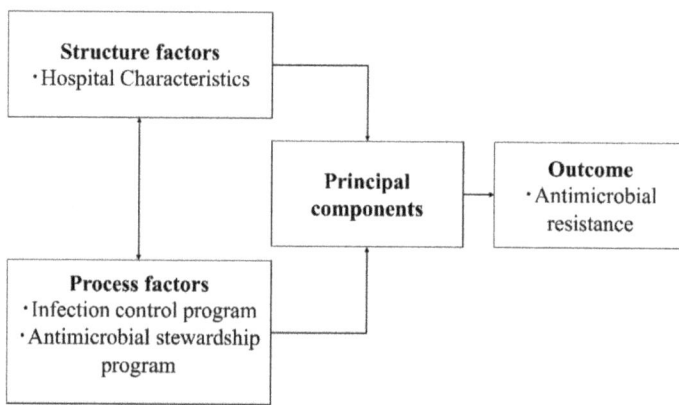

Figure 1. Conceptual framework.

2. Results

A total of 124 hospitals were analyzed, excluding 21 hospitals from 145 participating hospitals in this study. Data from these 21 hospitals were missing the following variables: the diagnostic procedure combination/per-diem payment system (DPC/PDPS) data file (4), the Japan Nosocomial Infections Surveillance (JANIS) specimen data (n = 10), JANIS patient age data (n = 6), and JANIS microbial susceptibility data (n = 1). Characteristics of the 124 analyzed hospitals are described in Table 1. The structure factors represented by the median number of beds in the facilities was 330 (interquartile range [IQR]: 223–478) beds; the median length of hospital stay was 12.4 (IQR: 11.1–14.1) days; the rate of surgeries for surgical site infection (SSI) surveillance among all surgeries was 26.5% ± 5.6%; 59.7% of the facilities were located in the eastern region of Japan; and 92.7% claimed IPC type 1 medical fee. The process-related factors were represented by the TDM implementation rate for vancomycin (79.2%), multiple sets of blood culture (81.1%), blood culture contamination (3.1%), number of Clostridioides difficile (CD) detection tests (4.2/1000 bed days), blood culture collected prior to broad spectrum antibiotic therapy (60.1%), and the number of bacterial tests (9.8/100 bed days). The median MRSA/Staphylococcus aureus (S. aureus) detection rate was 42.3% (IQR: 33.3–52.5).

Table 1. Hospital baseline characteristics for principal component analysis: median (interquartile range) or %.

Characteristics	Hospital Baseline (n = 124)
Structure factors	
Number of beds (beds) [a]	330 (223–478)
Number of patients admissions per year (patients) [a]	7099 (4576–11284)
Average length of stay (days)	12.4 (11.1–14.1)
Rate of surgeries (%) [b]	26.5 (5.6)
ICU patient admissions (%) [a]	0.3 (0–4.9)
CVC use patients (%) [a]	6.0 (4.6–8.5)
UC use patients (%) [a]	12.2 (9.4–15.1)
Region (East Japan: %)	59.7
Medical fee for IPC type 1 (%)	92.7
Teaching Hospital (%) [a]	87.1
7:1 hospital charge index (%) [a]	96.0
Pharmaceutical service (%) [a]	65.3
Process factors	
TDM implementation rate for vancomycin (%)	79.2 (67.0–84.9)
Multiple sets of blood cultures (%)	81.1 (68.7–88.5)
Contamination of blood cultures (%)	3.1 (1.9–4.6)
Number of CD detected test (/1000 bed days)	4.2 (2.6–5.4)
Blood culture collected prior to broad spectrum antibiotic therapy (%) [c]	60.1 (40.8–71.5)
Specimens for culture prior to broad spectrum antibiotic therapy (%) [a,c]	82.4 (72.6–88.4)
Number of bacterial tests (/100 bed days)	9.8 (6.7–12.9)
AUD of antibiotic injection (/100 bed days) [a]	15.8 (12.8–19.1)
DOT of antibiotic injection (/100 bed days) [a]	26.3 (22.4–30.3)
Antimicrobial resistance	
MRSA/*S. aureus* detection rate [a]	42.3 (33.3–52.5)

ICU, Intensive care unit; CVC, Central venous catheter; UC, Urinary catheter; IPC, Infection Prevention and Control; TDM, Therapeutic Drug Monitoring; CD, *Clostridioides difficile*; AUD, Antimicrobial Use Density; DOT, Days of Therapy; MRSA, Methicillin-resistant *Staphylococcus aureus*. [a] Variables not used for the principal component analysis. [b] Values are expressed as mean (SD, standard deviation). [c] Highly correlated was computed (γ = 0.76). Correlation of variation (CV) was calculated for both blood culture collected prior to broad spectrum antibiotic therapy (CV = 34.3) and specimens for culture prior to broad spectrum antibiotic therapy (CV = 18.2); the former was used.

We performed a principal component analysis based on an optimal subset of ten selected variables (in the first principal component created with all variables, there were no variables with eigenvectors >0.4, when eleven variables were selected, the cumulative eigen-value was less than 60%). Four structure factors including average length of stay, rate of surgeries, region, and IPC type were selected. By contrast, six process factors including the TDM implementation rate for vancomycin, multiple sets of blood cultures, blood culture contamination, the number of bacterial tests, the number of CD-detected tests, and blood culture collected prior to broad spectrum antibiotic therapy were selected. The first four principal components with eigenvalues >1 explained 63.0% of the variance and were therefore retained for further cluster analysis (Table A1). The first principal component accounted for 24.9% of variance for which the three factor scores with the largest eigenvectors were the number of bacterial tests, blood culture collected prior to broad spectrum antibiotic therapy, and number of CD detected tests. Therefore, the first principal component was characterized as the component for "bacterial test". Likewise, the second principal component, accounting for 14.8% of variance, was characterized as "surgeries", because the components were the rate of surgery, average length of stay, and region. The third principal component, which accounted for 12.9% of variance, was characterized as the "ability of infection control team", as the components were the TDM implementation rate for vancomycin, medical fee for IPC type, and rate of blood culture contamination. The fourth principal component, which accounted for 10.8% of variance, was characterized as "skill in performing blood cultures", as the components were multiple sets of blood cultures performed and blood culture contamination.

A hierarchical cluster analysis was performed among the 124 facilities based on the four principal components derived from the principal component analysis, and six distinct clusters were obtained (Figure 2). Cluster 6 included only one facility with data on the number of bacterial tests (52.0/100 bed days) and the number of CD detected tests (27.0/1000 bed days), and those values were considered outliers because they were significantly different from those of the other clusters. Therefore, we excluded this Cluster from further analysis. Cluster 1 (n = 25; 20%), Cluster 2 (n = 13; 11%), Cluster 3 (n = 5; 4%), Cluster 4 (n = 49; 40%), and Cluster 5 (n = 31; 25%) were established.

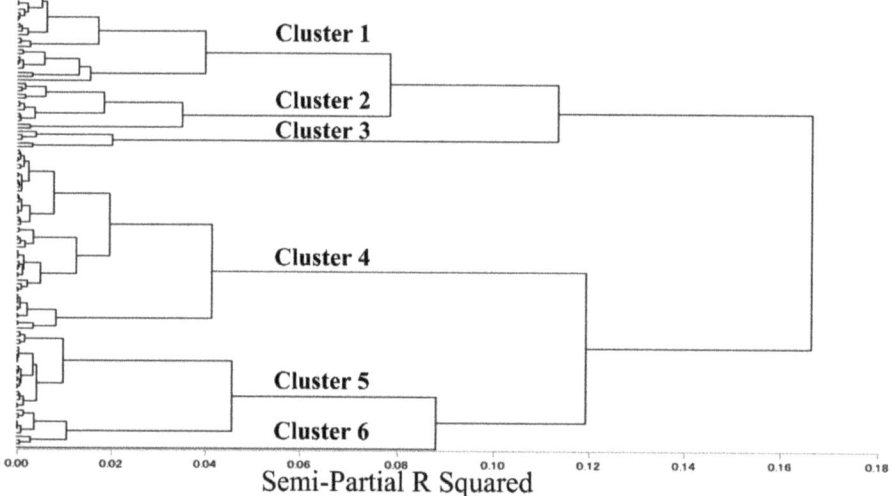

Figure 2. Dendrogram illustrating the results of the cluster analysis. Cluster 1 (n = 25), Cluster 2 (n = 13), Cluster 3 (n = 5), Cluster 4 (n = 49), Cluster 5 (n = 31), Cluster 6 (n = 1). Cluster 6 only had one facility, thus, it was considered an outlier and was excluded in the subsequent analyses.

Table 2 shows the clinical characteristics of the five clusters. The median number of beds decreased from the highest to lowest, as follows: Cluster 5, Cluster 4, Cluster 2, Cluster 1, and Cluster 3. Cluster 2, Cluster 4, and Cluster 5 included almost all facilities with IPC type 1. Cluster 5 had the shortest average length of stay (10.9 days) and the highest number of bacterial tests (14.6/100 bed days). Cluster 4 had the highest rate of surgeries (29.3%) and second longest average length of stay (13.2 days). Additionally, Cluster 4 had a lower number of blood cultures collected prior to broad spectrum antibiotic therapy (59.2%) and a lower number of bacterial tests (8.5/100 bed days) than Cluster 5. All facilities in Cluster 2 claimed IPC type 1. Meanwhile, Cluster 2 had the lowest number of multiple sets of blood cultures (46.3%) and the highest rate of contaminated blood cultures (4.1%). Cluster 1 was composed of facilities with both IPC types 1 and 2 and the lowest rate of surgeries (22.1%), while the number of blood cultures collected prior to broad spectrum antibiotic therapy (40.6%) was lower than for Cluster 2 and Cluster 5. Cluster 1 also had the second lowest number of bacterial tests (6.8/100 bed days). Cluster 3 was composed of facilities with IPC type 2 only. The average length of stay in Cluster 3 was longer than that in other clusters (14.9 days), and it had the lowest TDM implementation rate for vancomycin (9.7%), the lowest rate for blood culture collected prior to broad spectrum antibiotic therapy (30.1%), and the lowest number of bacterial tests (6.7/100 bed days). Table A2 shows more detailed data.

Table 2. Hospital characteristics according to the five clusters identified using principal component analysis-based cluster analysis: median or %.

	Cluster 1 (n = 25)	Cluster 2 (n = 13)	Cluster 3 (n = 5)	Cluster 4 (n = 49)	Cluster 5 (n = 31)	Overall p-Value
Structure factors						
Number of beds (beds)	269	275	106 [e]	304 [e]	466 [c,d]	0.0002
Number of patients admissions per year (patients)	6303	5789 [c]	2587 [b,d,e]	6184 [c]	11,046 [c,d]	<0.001
Average length of stay (days)	12.5	13.4	14.9 [e]	13.2 [e]	10.9 [c,d]	<0.001
Rate of surgeries (%) [f]	22.1 ± 4.8	25.3 ± 4.7	29.1 ± 6.3	29.3 ± 5.4 [a,e]	25.3 ± 3.7 [d]	0.0055 [g]
ICU patient admissions (%)	3.0	0	0	0	3.7	0.0365
CVC use patients (%)	6.1	8.0 [c]	3.1 [b,e]	5.6	6.4 [c]	0.0159
UC use patients (%)	13.3	12.3	14.2	12.1	12.0	0.3219
Region (East Japan: %)	92.0	84.6	0	36.7	70.9	
Medical fee for IPC type 1 (%)	84.0	100	0	100	100	
Teaching Hospital (%)	76.0	92.3	60.0	87.8	96.7	
7:1 hospital charge index (%)	92.0	100	100	94.0	100	
Pharmaceutical service (%)	64.0	76.9	40.0	65.3	64.5	
Process factors						
TDM implementation rate for vancomycin (%)	64.3 [b,d,e]	82.1 [a]	9.7 [d,e]	80.0 [a,c]	80.8 [a,c]	<0.001
Multiple sets of blood cultures (%)	80.6 [b]	46.3 [a,c,d,e]	78.0 [b]	82.3 [b]	85.0 [b]	<0.001
Contamination of blood cultures (%)	4.0	4.1	3.5	3.0	2.4	0.0988
Number of CD detected test (/1000 bed days)	3.8	3.7	4.4	3.8 [e]	5.4 [d]	0.0114
Blood culture collected prior to broad spectrum antibiotic therapy (%)	40.6 [d,e]	60.9	30.1 [e]	59.2 [a,e]	72.3 [a,c,d]	<0.001
Specimens for culture prior to broad spectrum antibiotic therapy (%)	72.8 [d,e]	87.3	63.0 [e]	81.8 [a,e]	85.9	<0.001
Number of bacterial tests (/100 bed days)	6.8 [e]	10.3 [e]	6.7 [e]	8.5 [e]	14.6 [a,b,c,d]	<0.001
AUD of antibiotic injection (/100 bed days)	15.4 [e]	18.3	12.8	14.5 [e]	19.1 [a,d]	<0.001
DOT of antibiotic injection (/100 bed days)	25.6 [e]	28.3 [d]	24.9	23.5 [b,e]	30.1 [a,d]	<0.001

ICU, Intensive care unit; CVC, Central venous catheter; UC, Urinary catheter; IPC, Infection Prevention and Control; TDM, Therapeutic Drug Monitoring; CD, Clostridioides difficile; AUD, Antimicrobial Use Density; DOT, Days of Therapy; MRSA, Methicillin-resistant *Staphylococcus aureus*. [a] different form Cluster 1 ($p < 0.05$), [b] different form Cluster 2 ($p < 0.05$), [c] different form Cluster 3 ($p < 0.05$), [d] different form Cluster 4 ($p < 0.05$), [e] different form Cluster 5 ($p < 0.05$). [f] mean ± SD. [g] ANOVA/Tukey–Kramer test.

Figure 3 shows a summary of the characteristics of the five clusters (based on Tables 1 and 2) in addition to the relationship between clusters and the MRSA/*S. aureus* detection rate. The MRSA/*S. aureus* detection rate ranked from the lowest to highest as follows: Cluster 1, Cluster 5, Cluster 2, Cluster 4, and Cluster 3 (36.8%, 37.3%, 40.6%, 47.0%, and 50.0%, respectively). The Kruskal–Wallis test followed by the Steel–Dwass test revealed significant differences between Cluster 4 and Cluster 5 ($p = 0.0046$).

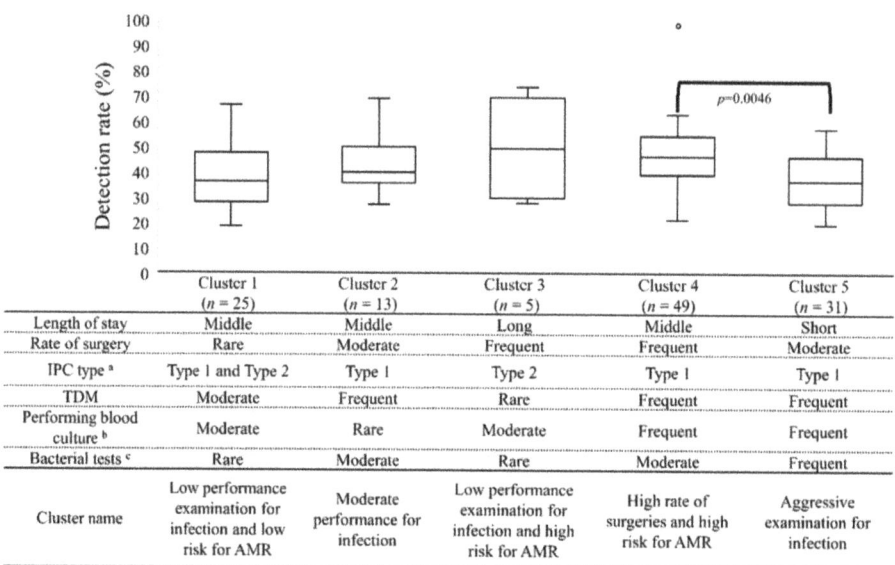

Figure 3. MRSA/*S. aureus* detection rate and summary of cluster characteristics. Each box plot is composed of five horizontal lines that display the minimum and maximum values and the 25th, 50th, and 75th percentiles of the corresponding variable. The cluster summary was categorized into three levels (Frequently, Moderate, Rare) or (Long, Middle, Short) based on the median value at hospital baseline (Table 1) and the comparison of that variable with each cluster (Table 2). [a] Medical fee for IPC type 1 or type 2. [b] Taking into account multiple sets of blood cultures and contamination of blood cultures. [c] Taking into account the number of CD detected test, blood cultures collected prior to broad spectrum antibiotic therapy, and number of bacterial tests. *S. aureus*, *Staphylococcus aureus*; MRSA, methicillin-resistant *S. aureus*; IPC, Infection Prevention and Control; TDM, Therapeutic Drug Monitoring.

3. Discussion

In this study, we implemented a principal component analysis-based cluster analysis of structure and process factors, which eventually resulted in the identification of five clusters. Our results indicate that when evaluating the MRSA detection rate for each facility, consideration should be paid to not only process factors but also structure factors including resources (e.g., number of medical staff) or risk factors (e.g., surgery), as these are also related with AMR.

We conducted multicenter analyses by principal component analysis-based cluster analysis. This method required many samples, which were not only useful in reducing dimensionality but also in detecting the key features of the data. This method has been applied to common diseases, such as chronic obstructive pulmonary disease, dermatomyositis, and chronic heart failure [15–18]. However, it has scarcely been used in evaluating infection control in health facilities.

This study showed the need to consider AMR in terms of infection control and facility characteristics, especially the number of bacterial examinations and surgeries related to SSI. For instance, the MRSA/*S. aureus* ratio between Cluster 4 and Cluster 5 had significant differences. In this study, Cluster 5 had the highest rate of activity for infection control. International guidelines demonstrate the detection of bacterial species, followed by optimization of antimicrobial stewardship, and prevention of growing AMR [19]. In our study, Cluster 4 had the highest rate of surgeries. The National Healthcare Safety Network reported that *S. aureus* is the most common pathogen of SSIs and that the proportion of SSIs caused by *S. aureus* increased to 30%, with MRSA comprising 49.2% [20]. Many surgeries for SSI surveillance may have reflected the high detection rate of AMR. Cluster 2 showed a higher MRSA/*S. aureus* detection rate than Cluster 5. A previous descriptive study reported by a Japanese university hospital showed that ICT recommendation improved the ratio of multiple sets of blood culture, similarly, affecting AMR [21]. Partial infection control activities may be insufficient (e.g., education of blood culture for medical staff) and may represent poor ICT activity, thereby affecting AMR. Cluster 3 was composed of facilities collecting IPC type 2 medical fees. These facilities did not have enough human resources, medical resources, and stratified facilities, as reported in previous studies [9,10]. In this study, the MRSA/*S. aureus* rate was the highest in Cluster 3, which suggests that IPC type 2 facilities require national level support for better implementation of infection control. Cluster 1 had low rates of infection control activities, surgeries, and MRSA/*S. aureus* detection. A recent retrospective study of one small-sized and eleven medium-sized hospitals (range: 73–354 number of beds) reported that these hospitals had a low number of bacterial tests, which meant that patients with serious infections were likely to be transferred to an acute care hospital. Therefore, AMR-isolation rates were reflected as lower in these hospitals [22]. Cluster 1 may reflect only a few incidents of encountering AMR, and infection-control activity could also possibly be low.

Nevertheless, there are also several limitations to our study. First, various factors that may affect resource use were not considered in our study because of the lack of available data. For example, a previous study reported that compliance with hand hygiene reduced nosocomial infections and MRSA transmission [23]. However, the usage of alcohol disinfection in the hospital is not recorded in the administrative data, and hence could not be used. These data may influence the MRSA/*S. aureus* detection rate. Second, as participation in this study was voluntary, the participating hospitals may not be representative of all hospitals in Japan. Moreover, a project managed by Kyushu University believes that the hospitals that participated in JANIS and participated in this study were already highly conscious of infection control; however, we were not able to evaluate associated biases. Future studies should evaluate not only the recruited hospitals but also all hospitals in Japan. Third, our two sets of data were not linked by individual patient identification. This limitation meant that patients in the DPC data cannot be linked with the JANIS data. Therefore, it was not possible to directly evaluate the medical procedures of patients with submitted bacterial tests. As an alternative, facility-level variables were obtained from the data to achieve our purpose. Our conceptual model showed that AMR is affected by the activity of the facilities; hence, we found the evaluation of variables at the facility-level to be appropriate. In the future, more detailed analyses may be possible if databases containing the provided medical care data and detected bacterial data at the individual patient-level are constructed.

4. Materials and Methods

4.1. Data Source

The administrative claims data were based on the DPC/PDPS, which is a national administrative claims database for acute inpatient care in Japan. Nationally uniform electronic DPC data include facility information (e.g., number of beds), patient clinical information (e.g., age, sex, disease, and admission and discharge date), and information on medical procedures (e.g., drug administration, surgery, examination, procedure, their codes, and cost) [24,25] used for patient classification and the DPC-based reimbursement system. They are used to improve systems and policies, including hospital management and service reimbursement. The JANIS data, which include microbiological data, provide information regarding patient demographics, specimen reception dates, specimen sources, types of bacteria, and susceptibility test results [26]. Moreover, the JANIS data encompass all testing results regardless of characteristics, such as infection status, colonization, or carrier status. JANIS has been launched as a voluntary AMR surveillance funded by the MHLW and managed by the National Institute of Infectious Diseases. JANIS clinical laboratory division collects comprehensive specimen-based data, which comply with JANIS data format, from participating hospitals each month.

We conducted a cross-sectional database analysis. We used both administrative claims data and microbiological data obtained from a research project managed by Kyu-shu University [27]. The project aimed to analyze the association between infection control, including antimicrobial consumption, and AMR. Kyushu University collected two sets of data from 145 acute care Japanese hospitals, which responded to the call for voluntary study participation.

The DPC/PDPS data and the JANIS data have different datasets. These data have common facility identifications, but not common patient identifications. Furthermore, our research objective was at the facility-level and not at the patient-level. Therefore, the variables collected and calculated were based on the identification of each facility.

4.2. Study Inclusion and Exclusion Criteria

This study included patients who had been admitted and included in the DPC data in each facility as well as those with specimen reception dates as indicated in the JANIS data between 1 April 2016, and 31 March 2017. Facilities without records of patient characteristics, hospitalizations, procedures, drugs, surgeries, or microbial susceptibility data were excluded because these variables were necessary for the principal component analysis and cluster analysis.

4.3. Variable Definitions and Facility Categories

Variables from the DPC data and JANIS data were obtained, calculated, and summarized at the facility-level and were evaluated as potential candidate variables for the following three domains: structure factor, process factor, and outcome. These definitions are presented in Table A3. The region and number of hospital beds were obtained from the DPC data. The following variables were also calculated from the DPC data: number of patient admissions per year, average length of stay, rate of surgeries, intensive care unit patient admissions, central venous catheter use, urinary catheter use, medical fee for IPC type (type 1 or type 2), hospital status (teaching or non-teaching), hospital charge index (7:1 or 10:1), and pharmaceutical services (claimed or non-claimed). Process factors included the following variables calculated from the JANIS data: multiple sets of blood cultures and contamination of blood cultures. Moreover, the following variables were calculated from DPC data: TDM implementation rate for vancomycin, number of CD detected tests, blood culture collected prior to broad spectrum antibiotic therapy, specimens for culture prior to broad spectrum antibiotic therapy, number of bacterial tests, antimicrobial use density (AUD) of antibiotic injections, and days of therapy (DOT) of antibiotic injections. AMR included the MRSA/*S. aureus* detection rate calculated from the JANIS data.

4.4. Principal Component Analysis and Cluster Analysis

Principal component analysis is a dimension-reducing method that replaces the variables in a dataset with a smaller number of derived variables. Dimension reduction may help to remove redundant variables that could possibly hinder the clustering process [18,28]. The goal of the principal component analysis was to extract a number of principal components to be used as clustering variables. One way to perform principal component analysis is by selecting a subset of variables that best approximates all the variables [29]. During variable selection for principal component analysis, we performed the following steps: first, we selected variables that can be considered resources for hospital infection control and excluded similar variables that reflect the size of the hospitals. In this study, medical fee for IPC type had been selected. The AMR domain was also selected for the outcome measure. Second, for the independent variables, correlations between survey variables were computed. Variables that were highly correlated ($\gamma > 0.70$) were avoided for simultaneous use in the principal component analysis and only either one was used. The coefficient of variation (CV) was calculated for highly correlated variables, and those with the largest CVs were selected for principal component analysis. Third, the optimal variable subset was explored in performing principal component analysis following these criteria: (1) greater number of variables, (2) fewer number of principal components with an eigenvalue >1, and (3) cumulative eigenvalue >60%. Variables with eigenvectors >0.4 were considered principal components.

A hierarchical cluster analysis was performed based on the Euclidean distances among the principal components [30]. We implemented the Ward method to minimize the total variance within clusters [31]. The number of clusters were based on the distribution of variables among the clusters.

4.5. Statistical Analyses

After performing the cluster analysis and choosing the number of clusters, each variable was compared among the clusters, and each cluster was labeled. We then compared the outcome measure (MRSA/*S. aureus* detection rate), which was the parameter that had not been used for the principal component analysis and cluster analysis. Continuous variables are expressed as means (standard deviation [SD]) or medians (interquartile range [IQR]) depending on whether their distributions are normal or skewed. Categorical variables are expressed as numbers (percentages) and binary variables are coded as 0/1 forms. Differences in characteristics between the clusters were assessed using an analysis of variance for continuous normally distributed variables, and non-parametric Kruskal–Wallis tests were used for non-normally distributed variables. All statistical analyses were performed with SAS 9.4 (SAS Institute, Cary, NC, USA), and $p < 0.05$ was defined as statistically significant.

5. Conclusions

We established a novel exploratory statistical methodology for multicenter Japanese hospitals, which led to the identification of subgroups based on structure and infection control factors. Our results suggest the importance of a multidimensional assessment of AMR, involving structure and infection control factors. Antimicrobial stewardship, including aggressive examination, is associated with low AMR while surgeries, an infection risk factor, are associated with high AMR. For more detailed research, it would be desirable to establish a database associating patient information with microbiological detection.

Author Contributions: Conceptualization, M.A. and T.S.; methodology, M.A. and T.S.; statistical analysis, N.S. and T.S.; resources, H.F.; data curation, H.F.; writing—original draft preparation, T.S.; writing—review and editing, K.K., Y.M.; M.A., supervision, M.A. All authors have read and agreed to the published version of the manuscript.

Funding: This research was funded by Grant-in-Aid for Scientific Research (KAKENHI), grant numbers JP17H04144 and JP19K22781.

Institutional Review Board Statement: The study was conducted according to the guidelines of the Declaration of Helsinki and was approved by the Institutional Review Board of the Meiji Pharmaceutical University (Protocol Code No. 202030).

Informed Consent Statement: Written informed consent was waived because of the retrospective design of the study.

Data Availability Statement: The data are not publicly available as the participants of this study did not agree for their data to be shared publicly.

Conflicts of Interest: The authors declare no conflict of interest.

Appendix A

Table A1. Principal component analysis.

	Eigenvalue	% of Variance	Eigenvector
Principal component 1: "Bacterial tests"	2.49	24.9	
Number of bacterial tests			0.52
Blood culture collected prior to broad spectrum antibiotic therapy			0.49
Number of CD detected test			0.42
Principal component 2: "Operations"	1.47	14.8	
Rate of surgeries			0.53
Region			−0.58
Average length of stay			0.44
Principal component 3: "Ability of ICT"	1.29	12.9	
TDM implementation rate for vancomycin			0.41
Medical fee for IPC type 1			0.60
Contamination of blood cultures			−0.4
Principal component 4: "Skill in performing blood cultures"	1.08	10.8	
Multiple sets of blood culture			−0.7
Contamination of blood cultures			0.51

CD, *Clostridioides difficile*; ICT, Infection Control Team; TDM, Therapeutic Drug Monitoring; IPC, Infection Prevention and Control.

Table A2. Hospital characteristics according to the five clusters identified using principal component analysis-based cluster analysis: median (interquartile range), or %.

	Cluster 1 (n = 25)	Cluster 2 (n = 13)	Cluster 3 (n = 5)	Cluster 4 (n = 49)	Cluster 5 (n = 31)	Overall p-Value [g]
Structure factors						
Number of beds (beds)	269 (190–490)	275 (218–559)	106 (100–163) [e]	304 (210–377) [e]	466 (337–505) [c,d]	0.0002
Number of patients admissions per year (patients)	6303 (4291–11901)	5789 (3952–12,996) [c]	2587 (1919–2962) [b,d,e]	6184 (4429–9231) [c]	11,046 (8988–13,612) [c,d]	<0.001
Average length of stay (days)	12.5 (11.2–13.4)	13.4 (10.7–14.8)	14.9 (13.2–20.4) [e]	13.2 (11.7–15) [e]	10.9 (9.9–11.8) [c,d]	<0.001
Rate of surgeries (%) [f]	22.1 ± 4.8 [d]	25.3 ± 4.7	29.1 ± 6.3	29.3 ± 5.4 [a,e]	25.3 ± 3.7 [d]	0.0055 [g]
ICU patient admissions (%)	3.0 (0–9.5)	0 (0–5.5)	0 (0–0)	0 (0–4.6)	3.7 (0–4.9)	0.0365
CVC use patients (%)	6.1 (4.7–9.6)	8.0 (5.0–9.7) [c]	3.1 (1.7–4.7) [b,e]	5.6 (3.9–8.0)	6.4 (4.7–8.1) [c]	0.0159
UC use patients (%)	13.3 (9.2–18.7)	12.3 (9.4–14.4)	14.2 (11.2–21.6)	12.1 (9.8–13.4)	12.0 (8.6–15.1)	0.3219
Region (East Japan: %)	92.0	84.6	0	36.7	70.9	
Medical fee for IPC type 1 (%)	84.0	100	0	100	100	
Teaching Hospital (%)	76.0	92.3	60.0	87.8	96.7	
7:1 hospital charge index (%)	92.0	100	100	94.0	100	
Pharmaceutical service (%)	64.0	76.9	40.0	65.3	64.5	
Process factors						
TDM implementation rate for vancomycin (%)	64.3 (40.3–73.0) [b,d,e]	82.1 (60.5–86.8) [a]	9.7 (4.9–61.5) [d,e]	80.0 (71.4–87.3) [a,c]	80.8 (76.3–88.7) [a,c]	<0.001
Multiple sets of blood cultures (%)	80.6 (66.5–86.5) [b]	46.3 (13.7–51.5) [a,c,d,e]	78.0 (74.5–88.5) [b]	82.3 (75.2–87.3) [b]	85.0 (74.0–92.4) [b]	<0.001
Contamination of blood cultures (%)	4.0 (2.5–4.9)	4.1 (1.3–9.2)	3.5 (2.6–5.3)	3.0 (1.8–4.2)	2.4 (1.9–3.7)	0.0988
Number of CD detected test (/1000 bed-days)	3.8 (1.5–5.1)	3.7 (2.5–4.9)	4.4 (1.6–8.2)	3.8 (2.5–4.6) [e]	5.4 (4–6.1) [d]	0.0114
Blood culture collected prior to broad spectrum antibiotic therapy (%)	40.6 (34.8–53.6) [d,e]	60.9 (37.7–74.8)	30.1 (21.4–45.1) [e]	59.2 (41.8–64.6) [a,e]	72.3 (66.3–79.6) [a,c,d]	<0.001
Specimens for culture prior to broad spectrum antibiotic therapy (%)	72.8 (63.4–80.4) [d,e]	87.3 (72.3–90.2)	63.0 (43.9–68.4) [e]	81.8 (74.6–85.7) [a,e]	85.9 (83.5–92.3) [a,c,d]	<0.001
Number of bacterial tests (/100 bed-days)	6.8 (5.6–9.4) [e]	10.3 (7.2–11.1) [e]	6.7 (2.4–9.3) [e]	8.5 (6.5–10.5) [e]	14.6 (11.6–19.0) [a,b,c,d]	<0.001

Table A2. Cont.

	Cluster 1 (n = 25)	Cluster 2 (n = 13)	Cluster 3 (n = 5)	Cluster 4 (n = 49)	Cluster 5 (n = 31)	Overall p-Value [g]
AUD of antibiotic injection (/100 bed-days)	15.4 (12.1–17.4) [e]	18.3 (14.1–20.2)	12.8 (10.5–16.7)	14.5 (11.1–16.0) [e]	19.1 (17.2–21.9) [a,d]	<0.001
DOT of antibiotic injection (/100 bed-days)	25.6 (21.7–28.4) [e]	28.3 (26.1–31.4) [d]	24.9 (16.7–26.3)	23.5 (19.6–26.8) [b,e]	30.1 (26.6–32.3) [a,d]	<0.001

ICU, Intensive care unit; CVC, Central venous catheter; UC, Urinary catheter; IPC, Infection Prevention and Control; TDM, Therapeutic Drug Monitoring; CD, *Clostridioides difficile*; AUD, Antimicrobial Use Density; DOT, Days of Therapy; MRSA, Methicillin-resistant *Staphylococcus aureus*. [a] different form Cluster 1 ($p < 0.05$), [b] different form Cluster 2 ($p < 0.05$), [c] different form Cluster 3 ($p < 0.05$), [d] different form Cluster 4 ($p < 0.05$), [e] different form Cluster 5 ($p < 0.05$). [f] mean ± SD. [g] ANOVA/Tukey–Kramer test.

Table A3. Definition of variables.

Name	Units	Definition
Structure factors		
Number of beds	Beds	Number of hospital beds
Number of admissions patients per year	Patients	
Average length of stay	Days	
Rate of surgeries	%	Number of JANIS SSI surveillance/Number of all surgeries × 100
ICU admission patients	%	ICU admission patients/Number of admission patients per year
CVC patients	%	Number of Central Venous Catheter used patients/Number of admission patients per year × 100
UC patients	%	Number of urinary Catheter used patients/Number of admission patients per year × 100
Region	%	West Japan = 0, East Japan = 1
Medical fee for IPC type 1	%	Medical fee for IPC type 2 = 0, Medical fee for IPC type 1 = 1
Teaching Hospital	%	Non-Teaching Hospital = 0, Teaching Hospital = 1
7:1 hospital charge index	%	10:1 hospital charge index = 0, 7:1 hospital charge index = 1
Pharmaceutical service	%	Non-Pharmaceutical service = 0, Pharmaceutical service = 1
Process factors		
TDM implementation rate for vancomycin	%	TDM performed patients in denominator/Patient treatment duration >3 days for vancomycin
Multiple sets of blood culture	%	Number of patients in whom multiple blood cultures were taken/Total number of patients who blood cultures were taken
Contamination of blood cultures	%	Number of contaminated cultures/Number of patients in whom multiple blood cultures were taken
Number of CD detected tests	/1000 bed-days	Number of CD detected tests/length of hospital stay for inpatients × 1000
Blood culture collected prior to broad spectrum antibiotic therapy	%	Before starting broad spectrum systemic antibiotic therapy in hospitalized adults with at least one blood culture/Admitted broad spectrum systemic antibiotic therapy
Specimens for culture prior to broad spectrum antibiotic therapy	%	Before starting broad spectrum systemic antibiotic therapy in hospitalized adults with bacterial culture/Admitted broad spectrum systemic antibiotic therapy
Number of bacterial tests	/100 bed-days	Number of bacterial tests/length of hospital stay for inpatients × 100
AUD of antibiotic injection	/100 bed-days	Antimicrobial consumptions (g)/(DDD [a] × length of hospital stay for inpatients) × 100
DOT of antibiotic injection	/100 bed-days	DOT/length of hospital stay for inpatients × 100
Antimicrobial resistance		
MRSA/*S. aureus* detection rate	%	MRSA detected patients/Number of MRSA + MSSA detected patients × 100

[a] Used WHO ATC/DDD index ver.2016. JANIS: Japan Nosocomial Infections Surveillance; SSI: Surgical site infection ICU, Intensive care unit; CVC, Central venous catheter; UC, Urinary catheter; IPC, Infection Prevention and Control; TDM, Therapeutic Drug Monitoring; CD, *Clostridioides difficile*; AUD, Antimicrobial Use Density; DOT, Days of Therapy; *S. aureus*, *Staphylococcus aureus*; MRSA, Methicillin-resistant *S. aureus*; MSSA, Methicillin-susceptible *S. aureus*.

References

1. The Government of Japan. National Action Plan on Antimicrobial Resistance (AMR), 2016–2020. Available online: http://www.mhlw.go.jp/file/06-Seisakujouhou-10900000-Kenkoukyoku/0000138942.pdf (accessed on 28 November 2021).
2. Japan Nosocomial Infections Surveillance, Ministry of Health, Labour and Welfare. JANIS Open Report. Available online: https://janis.mhlw.go.jp/english/report/index.html (accessed on 28 November 2021).
3. Gu, Y.; Fujitomo, Y.; Ohmagari, N. Outcomes and Future Prospect of Japan's National Action Plan on Antimicrobial Resistance (2016–2020). *Antibiotics* **2021**, *10*, 1293. [CrossRef] [PubMed]
4. Chou, A.F.; Yano, E.M.; McCoy, K.D.; Willis, D.R.; Doebbeling, B.N. Structural and process factors affecting the implementation of antimicrobial resistance prevention and control strategies in U.S. hospitals. *Health Care Manag. Rev.* **2008**, *33*, 308–322. [CrossRef] [PubMed]
5. Arcenillas, P.; Boix-Palop, L.; Gómez, L.; Xercavins, M.; March, P.; Martinez, L.; Riera, M.; Madridejos, R.; Badia, C.; Nicolás, J.; et al. Assessment of Quality Indicators for Appropriate Antibiotic Use. *Antimicrob. Agents Chemother.* **2018**, *62*, e00875-18. [CrossRef] [PubMed]
6. National Center for Global Health and Medicine. The Japan Surveillance for Infection Prevention and Healthcare Epidemiology System (J-SIPHE). Available online: https://j-siphe.ncgm.go.jp/ (accessed on 28 November 2021).
7. Brotherton, A.L. Metrics of Antimicrobial Stewardship Programs. *Med. Clin. N. Am.* **2018**, *102*, 965–976. [CrossRef]
8. Morikane, K. Infection Control in Healthcare Settings in Japan. *J. Epidemiol.* **2012**, *22*, 86–90. [CrossRef]
9. Maeda, M.; Muraki, Y.; Kosaka, T.; Yamada, T.; Aoki, Y.; Kaku, M.; Kawaguchi, T.; Seki, M.; Tanabe, Y.; Fujita, N.; et al. The first nationwide survey of antimicrobial stewardship programs conducted by the Japanese Society of Chemotherapy. *J. Infect. Chemother.* **2019**, *25*, 83–88. [CrossRef]
10. Maeda, M.; Muraki, Y.; Kosaka, T.; Yamada, T.; Aoki, Y.; Kaku, M.; Seki, M.; Tanabe, Y.; Fujita, N.; Niki, Y.; et al. Impact of health policy on structural requisites for antimicrobial stewardship: A nationwide survey conducted in Japanese hospitals after enforcing the revised reimbursement system for antimicrobial stewardship programs. *J. Infect. Chemother.* **2021**, *27*, 1–6. [CrossRef]
11. Maezawa, T.T.K.; Kuroda, Y.; Hori, S.; Kizu, J. Changes in infection control in medical facilities after the revision of medical fees. *Jpn. J. Infect. Prev. Control* **2014**, *29*, 429–436. [CrossRef]
12. Kobayashi, Y.Y.Y.; Yamada, M.; Asai, M.; Oda, H.; Ikuta, K. Changes in the cost of items for infection control and the MRSA infection incidence density rate in before and after "Additional Reimbursement for Infection Prevention 1". *Jpn. J. Infect. Prev. Control* **2016**, *31*, 370–377. [CrossRef]
13. Donabedian, A. Evaluating the quality of medical care. 1966. *Milbank Q.* **2005**, *83*, 691–729. [CrossRef]
14. Izenman, A.J. *Modern Multivariate Statistical Techniques: Regression, Classification, and Manifold Learning*; Springer: New York, NY, USA, 2008.
15. Burgel, P.-R.; Paillasseur, J.-L.; Caillaud, D.; Tillie-Leblond, I.; Chanez, P.; Escamilla, R.; Court-Fortune, I.; Perez, T.; Carré, P.; Roche, N. Clinical COPD phenotypes: A novel approach using principal component and cluster analyses. *Eur. Respir. J.* **2010**, *36*, 531–539. [CrossRef] [PubMed]
16. Zhu, H.; Wu, C.; Jiang, N.; Wang, Y.; Zhao, J.; Xu, D.; Wang, Q.; Li, M.; Zeng, X. Identification of 6 dermatomyositis subgroups using principal component analysis-based cluster analysis. *Int. J. Rheum. Dis.* **2019**, *22*, 1383–1392. [CrossRef] [PubMed]
17. Ahmad, T.; Desai, N.; Wilson, F.; Schulte, P.; Dunning, A.; Jacoby, D.; Allen, L.; Fiuzat, M.; Rogers, J.; Felker, G.M.; et al. Clinical Implications of Cluster Analysis-Based Classification of Acute Decompensated Heart Failure and Correlation with Bedside Hemodynamic Profiles. *PLoS ONE* **2016**, *11*, e0145881. [CrossRef] [PubMed]
18. Vavougios, G.D.; George, D.G.; Pastaka, C.; Zarogiannis, S.G.; Gourgoulianis, K.I. Phenotypes of comorbidity in OSAS patients: Combining categorical principal component analysis with cluster analysis. *J. Sleep Res.* **2016**, *25*, 31–38. [CrossRef]
19. Rhodes, A.; Evans, L.E.; Alhazzani, W.; Levy, M.M.; Antonelli, M.; Ferrer, R.; Kumar, A.; Sevransky, J.E.; Sprung, C.L.; Nunnally, M.E.; et al. Surviving Sepsis Campaign: International Guidelines for Management of Sepsis and Septic Shock: 2016. *Crit. Care Med.* **2017**, *45*, 486–552. [CrossRef]
20. Hidron, A.I.; Edwards, J.R.; Patel, J.; Horan, T.C.; Sievert, D.M.; Pollock, D.A.; Fridkin, S.K. NHSN annual update: Antimicrobial-resistant pathogens associated with healthcare-associated infections: Annual summary of data reported to the National Healthcare Safety Network at the Centers for Disease Control and Prevention, 2006–2007. *Infect. Control Hosp. Epidemiol.* **2008**, *29*, 996–1011. [CrossRef]
21. Shigemura, K.; Osawa, K.; Mukai, A.; Ohji, G.; Lee, J.J.; Yoshida, H.; Fujisawa, M.; Arakawa, S. Infection control team activity and recent antibiograms in the Kobe University Hospital. *J. Antibiot. (Tokyo)* **2013**, *66*, 511–516. [CrossRef]
22. Mitsuboshi, S.; Tsugita, M. Impact of alcohol-based hand sanitizers, antibiotic consumption, and other measures on detection rates of antibiotic-resistant bacteria in rural Japanese hospitals. *J. Infect. Chemother.* **2019**, *25*, 225–228. [CrossRef]
23. Pittet, D.; Hugonnet, S.; Harbarth, S.; Mourouga, P.; Sauvan, V.; Touveneau, S.; Perneger, T.V. Effectiveness of a hospital-wide programme to improve compliance with hand hygiene. Infection Control Programme. *Lancet* **2000**, *356*, 1307–1312. [CrossRef]
24. Uematsu, H.; Yamashita, K.; Kunisawa, S.; Fushimi, K.; Imanaka, Y. Estimating the disease burden of methicillin-resistant Staphylococcus aureus in Japan: Retrospective database study of Japanese hospitals. *PLoS ONE* **2017**, *12*, e0179767. [CrossRef]
25. Tanaka, S.; Seto, K.; Kawakami, K. Pharmacoepidemiology in Japan: Medical databases and research achievements. *J. Pharm. Health Care Sci.* **2015**, *1*, 16. [CrossRef] [PubMed]

26. Tsutsui, A.; Suzuki, S. Japan nosocomial infections surveillance (JANIS): A model of sustainable national antimicrobial resistance surveillance based on hospital diagnostic microbiology laboratories. *BMC Health Serv. Res.* **2018**, *18*, 799. [CrossRef] [PubMed]
27. Mimura, W.; Fukuda, H.; Akazawa, M. Antimicrobial utilization and antimicrobial resistance in patients with haematological malignancies in Japan: A multi-centre cross-sectional study. *Ann. Clin. Microbiol. Antimicrob.* **2020**, *19*, 7. [CrossRef] [PubMed]
28. Valletta, J.J.; Torney, C.; Kings, M.; Thornton, A.; Madden, J. Applications of machine learning in animal behaviour studies. *Anim. Behav.* **2017**, *124*, 203–220. [CrossRef]
29. Kuroda, M.; Masaya, I.; Yuichi, M.; Sakakihara, M. Principal components based on a subset of qualitative variables and its accelerated computational algorithm. In Proceedings of the ISI 58th World Statistics Congress of the International Statistical Institute, Dublin, Ireland, 21–26 August 2011.
30. Der, G.; Everitt, B.S. *A Handbook of Statistical Analyses Using SAS*, 3rd ed.; Chapman & Hall/CRC: New York, NY, USA, 2008; pp. 295–317.
31. Ward, J.H. Hierarchical Grouping to Optimize an Objective Function. *J. Am. Stat. Assoc.* **1963**, *58*, 236–244. [CrossRef]

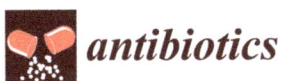

Article

Molecular and Anti-Microbial Resistance (AMR) Profiling of Methicillin-Resistant *Staphylococcus aureus* (MRSA) from Hospital and Long-Term Care Facilities (LTCF) Environment

Bing-Mu Hsu [1,2,†], Jung-Sheng Chen [3], I-Ching Lin [4,5,†], Gwo-Jong Hsu [6,†], Suprokash Koner [1,7,†], Bashir Hussain [1,7], Shih-Wei Huang [8,9] and Hsin-Chi Tsai [10,11,*]

1. Department of Earth and Environmental Sciences, National Chung Cheng University, Chiayi County 621, Taiwan; bmhsu@ccu.edu.tw (B.-M.H.); suprokashkoner@alum.ccu.edu.tw (S.K.); bashir@alum.ccu.edu.tw (B.H.)
2. Center for Innovative on Aging Society, National Chung Cheng University, Chiayi County 621, Taiwan
3. Department of Medical Research, E-Da Hospital, Kaohsiung City 824, Taiwan; ed113187@edah.org.tw
4. Department of Family Medicine, Asia University Hospital, Taichung City 413, Taiwan; D52282@auh.org.tw
5. Department of Kinesiology, Health and Leisure, Chienkuo Technology University, Chenghua County 500, Taiwan
6. Division of Infectious Diseases, Ditmanson Medical Foundation, Chia-Yi Christian Hospital, Chiayi City 600, Taiwan; 01347@cych.org.tw
7. Department of Biomedical Sciences, National Chung Cheng University, Chiayi County 621, Taiwan
8. Center for Environmental Toxin and Emerging Contaminant Research, Cheng Shiu University, Kaohsiung City 830, Taiwan; envhero@gcloud.csu.edu.tw
9. Super Micro Research and Technology Center, Cheng Shiu University, Kaohsiung City 830, Taiwan
10. Department of Psychiatry, School of Medicine, Tzu Chi University, Hualien County 970, Taiwan
11. Department of Psychiatry, Tzu-Chi General Hospital, Hualien County 970, Taiwan
* Correspondence: hsinchi@tzuchi.com.tw; Tel.: +88-638-561-825
† These authors contributed equally to this work.

Abstract: To provide evidence of the cross-contamination of emerging pathogenic microbes in a local network between long-term care facilities (LTCFs) and hospitals, this study emphasizes the molecular typing, the prevalence of virulence genes, and the antibiotic resistance pattern of methicillin-resistant *Staphylococcus aureus*. MRSA isolates were characterized from 246 samples collected from LTCFs, medical tubes of LTCF residents, and hospital environments of two cities, Chiayi and Changhua. Species identification, molecular characterization, and drug resistance analysis were performed. Hospital environments had a higher MRSA detection rate than that of LTCF environments, where moist samples are a hotspot of MRSA habitats, including tube samples from LTCF residents. All MRSA isolates in this study carried the exfoliative toxin *eta* gene (100%). The majority of MRSA isolates were resistant to erythromycin (76.7%), gentamicin (60%), and ciprofloxacin (55%). The percentage of multidrug-resistant MRSA isolates was approximately 50%. The enterobacterial repetitive intergenic consensus polymerase chain reaction results showed that 18 MRSA isolates belonged to a specific cluster. This implied that genetically similar isolates were spread between hospitals and LTCFs in Changhua city. This study highlights the threat to the health of LTCFs' residents posed by hospital contact with MRSA.

Keywords: methicillin-resistant *Staphylococcus aureus* (MRSA); long term care facilities (LTCF); multidrug resistance (MDR); *SCCmec* typing; enterobacterial repetitive intergenic consensus-polymerase chain reaction (ERIC-PCR)

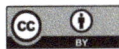

1. Introduction

In the past few decades, long-term care facilities (LTCFs) have faced an extreme threat from multidrug resistant (MDR) infectious pathogens [1,2]. The most abundant opportunistic pathogen is methicillin-resistant *Staphylococcus aureus* (MRSA), which not only affects healthcare centers, but is also associated with community and livestock infections [3–5]. The presence of *SCCmec* elements, consisting of *mecA* and *psm-mec* genes, enables resistance to various antibiotics including cephalosporins, oxacillin, imipenem, nafcillin, and p-lactam [6–8]. The most common molecular mechanism that enables resistance to these kinds of antibiotics is the *mecA* gene, which can synthesize PBP2A (a low-affinity penicillin-binding protein) and enables the continued synthesis of staphylococcal cell wall peptidoglycan through peptidoglycan transpeptidation when a high amount of beta-lactam antibiotics is present [9]. The *mecA* gene is situated on the staphylococcal cassette chromosome *mec* (*SCCmec*). Depending on the position of the *mec* and *ccr* complex sequences, *SCCmec* can be divided into I-to-VII types [10]. Globally, hospital-associated MRSA infections have been shown to be highly related to types I, II, and III of *SCCmec* and are sometimes enhanced by *SCCmec* IV. Moreover, community-associated MRSA infections commonly have a relationship with *SCCmec* type IV, V, or VII [10–12]. In Asia, there is strong evidence that the above-mentioned strains of MRSA generate ubiquitous epidemic nosocomial infections for health care and LTCF residents [13,14]. The previous study highlighted the presence of various virulence factors such as toxic shock syndrome toxin-1 (*tsst-1*), Panton–Valentine leukocidine (PVL), enterotoxins (*entA-E*), and exfoliative toxin (*eta, etb*) in MRSA isolates. These could enhance the severity of the infection during the pathogenesis process [15].

Continued spreading of infection-related diseases in hospitals and LTCF environments through these pathogens is not only hard to control but also requires proper surveillance, since they are not susceptible to antibiotic treatment [16–18]. Polymerase chain reaction (PCR)-based tools are commonly specific, low-cost methods to identify MDR and virulence genes, providing significant data during surveillance in hospital and LTCF environments [19,20]. For example, enterobacterial repetitive intergenic consensus sequence targeted PCR (ERIC-PCR) enables strain-level identification of these pathogens at the molecular level to categorize their genotyping in a range of evolutionary and epidemiological aspects [21]. Moreover, antibiotic susceptibility tests against largely populated antibiotics for these bacteria [22]. The distribution of these bacteria in hospital or LTCF environments has been well reported, although there is poor documentation of the pattern of distribution in terms of the infected hosts moving between these environments [23–26].

MRSA cross-contamination between hospitals and LTCFs is an important issue for public health, and most related research has focused on patients. In this study, our objectives were to classify molecular patterns and provide hotspot information on the environmental MRSA in a hospital and an affiliated LTCF. ERIC-PCR and *SCCmec* typing were performed for epidemiological typing of MRSA. Moreover, as the antibiotic resistance of MRSA is an urgent problem for public health, virulence gene profiling and antibiotic resistance were also conducted in this study.

2. Results

2.1. Detecting Rates of MRSA from LTCFs and Hospitals in Two Cities

A total of 246 LTCFs and hospital samples were collected to quantify the detection rate of MRSA. The overall percentage of MRSA prevalence in Changhua was 23.8% (39/164), and was 23.2% (19/82) in Chiayi (Table 1). The rate of MRSA in Changhua from LTCF (25%, 33/132) was higher than that from hospital samples (18.8%, 6/32). For Chiayi, samples from the hospital environment (25%, 8/32) contributed a higher rate than LTCF environment samples (22%, 11/50). For categorical division between arid versus moist samples, MRSA was detected in 22.2% (10/45) and 18.4% (7/38) of moist samples in the LTCF environments at Changhua and Chiayi, respectively; no MRSA was found in arid samples of LTCF from Changhua, although for Chiayi, 33.3% (4/12) were from arid samples. Thus, moist samples from Changhua and Chiayi hospitals accounted for 30% ($n = 20$) and 31.3% ($n = 16$) of the MRSA detection rate, respectively. Although the Changhua hospital arid samples had a detection rate of zero, this reached 18.3% ($n = 16$) for Chiayi hospital. The relative rate of MRSA detection included hospital environment samples for the outpatient floor (0%,

n = 18, vs. 14.3% n = 7), inpatient floor (28.6%, n = 7, vs. 50%, n = 6), and used ward area (57.1%, n = 7, vs. 30%, n = 10) for Changhua versus Chiayi, respectively. In addition, the detection rate of MRSA in mild area samples was less frequent than that in the severe area in the LTCF environment of Chiayi (11.5%, n = 26; 33.3%, n = 24). In the Chiayi City hospital environment, the used ward samples had a higher prevalence rate of MRSA than the vacant ward samples (30%, n = 10 and 11.1%, n = 9, respectively). In addition, 63 indwelling medical tubes from LTCF residents of Changhua were tested for MRSA. The highest detection rate was obtained from nasogastric tubes, at 60% (n = 15), followed by tracheostomy tubes at 38.9% (n = 18), whereas the lowest detection rate was from Foley catheter-balloon samples (23.3%, n = 30).

Table 1. Prevalence of MRSA from various samples.

Sampling Locations	Sampling Sources	Sample Types	Number (%)
Changhua city	LTCF environment	Moist samples (n = 45)	10 (22.2%)
		Arid samples (n = 24)	0 (0%)
		Total LTCF environment (n = 69)	10 (14.5%)
	LTCF dwelling medical tubes	Foley catheter-balloons from LTCF residents (n = 30)	7 (23.3%)
		Nasogastric tubes from LTCF residents (n = 15)	9 (60%)
		Tracheostomy tubes from LTCF residents (n = 18)	7 (38.9%)
		Total tubes from LTCF residents (n = 63)	23 (36.5%)
		Total LTCF samples (n = 132)	33 (25%)
	Hospital environment	Moist samples (n = 20)	6 (30%)
		Arid samples (n = 12)	0 (0)%
		Outpatient floor (n = 18)	0 (0%)
		Inpatient floor (n = 7)	2 (28.6%)
		Ward (used) (n = 7)	4 (57.1%)
		Total hospital samples (n = 32)	6 (18.8%)
		Total Changhua city samples (n = 164)	39 (23.8%)
Chiayi city	LTCF environment	Mild area (n = 26)	3 (11.5%)
		Severe area (n = 24)	8 (33.3%)
		Moist samples (n = 38)	7 (18.4%)
		Arid samples (n = 12)	4 (33.3%)
		Total LTCF samples (n = 50)	11 (22%)
	Hospital environment	Outpatient building 1F (n = 7)	1 (14.3%)
		Inpatient building 1F (n = 6)	3 (50%)
		Total building 1F (n = 13)	4 (30.8%)
		Ward (vacancy) (n = 9)	1 (11.1%)
		Ward (used) (n = 10)	3 (30%)
		Total wards (n = 19)	4 (21.1%)
		Moist samples (n = 16)	5 (31.3%)
		Arid samples (n = 16)	3 (18.8%)
		Total hospital samples (n = 32)	8 (25%)
		Total Chiayi city samples (n = 82)	19 (23.2%)
		Total Changhua city and Chiayi city samples (n = 246)	58 (23.6%)

2.2. SCCmec PCR Typing for Predicting the Source of the MRSA Strains

We purified 60 MRSA isolates from 246 samples. Their distribution in terms of sampling location and source, as well as different types of *SCCmec* PCR typing, are shown in Table 2. The majority of the 60 isolated MRSA strains belonged to *SCCmec* IV (48.3%, 29/60) and *SCCmec* III (41.7%, 25/60). Approximately 40% (24/60) of MRSA strains carried

PVL toxin genes. In addition, 51.7% (31/60) of all strains were related to hospital-associated MRSA (HA-MRSA), 30% (18/60) were community-associated MRSA (CA-MRSA) and 18.3% (11/60) were livestock-associated MRSA (LA-MRSA). The *SCCmec* III group was detected in both hospital environments (50%) and LTCF samples (54%) in Changhua; however, in Chiayi, this group was present at a higher percentage in hospital samples (37.5%) compared with that found in LTCF samples (9.1%). For *SCCmec* IV detection, the percentage in LTCF samples was much higher than in hospital samples for both Changhua (40% vs. 16.7%, respectively) and Chiayi (90.9% vs. 50%, respectively).

Table 2. *SCCmec* PCR typing results of the 60 MRSA isolates.

Sampling Locations	Sampling Sources	SCCmec I	SCCmec II	SCCmec III	SCCmec IV	SCCmec V	PVL	HA-MRSA (I, II, III)	CA-MRSA (IV+PVL, V+PVL)	LA-MRSA (IV, V)
Changhua City	LTCF environment ($n = 12$)	2 (16.7%)	0 (0%)	3 (25%)	7 (58.3%)	0 (0%)	2 (16.7%)	5 (41.7%)	2 (16.7%)	5 (41.7%)
	Tubes from LTCF residents ($n = 23$)	1 (4.3%)	0 (0%)	15 (65.2%)	7 (30.4%)	0 (0%)	9 (39.1%)	16 (69.6%)	6 (26.1%)	1 (4.3%)
	Total LTCF isolates ($n = 35$)	3 (8.6%)	0 (0%)	18 (51.4%)	14 (40%)	0 (0%)	11 (31.4%)	21 (60%)	8 (22.9%)	6 (17.1%)
	Hospital environment ($n = 6$)	0 (0%)	2 (33.3%)	3 (50%)	1 (16.7%)	0 (0%)	0 (0%)	5 (83.3%)	0 (0%)	1 (16.7%)
	Total Changhua city isolates ($n = 41$)	3 (7.3%)	2 (4.9%)	21 (51.2%)	15 (36.6%)	0 (0%)	11 (26.8%)	26 (63.4%)	8 (19.5%)	7 (17.1%)
Chiayi City	LTCF environment ($n = 11$)	0 (0%)	0 (0%)	1 (9.1%)	10 (90.9%)	0 (0%)	7 (63.6%)	1 (9.1%)	7 (63.6%)	3 (27.3%)
	Hospital environment ($n = 8$)	1 (12.5%)	0 (0%)	3 (37.5%)	4 (50%)	0 (0%)	6 (75%)	4 (50%)	3 (37.5%)	1 (12.5%)
	Total Chiayi city isolates ($n = 19$)	1 (5.3%)	0 (0%)	4 (21.1%)	14 (73.7%)	0 (0%)	13 (68.4%)	5 (26.3%)	10 (52.6%)	4 (21.1%)
Total Changhua City and Chiayi city isolates ($n = 60$)		4 (6.7%)	2 (3.3%)	25 (41.7%)	29 (48.3%)	0 (0%)	24 (40%)	31 (51.7%)	18 (30%)	11 (18.3%)

For MRSA, 31.4% of LTCF samples in Changhua but none of the hospital samples contained the PVL gene, whereas in Chiayi, the percentage of LTCF samples with PVL (64.6%) was less than that of hospital samples (75%). The detection percentages of HA-MRSA, CA-MRSA, and LA-MRSA in Changhua were 63.4%, 19.5%, and 17.1% ($n = 41$), respectively; isolates from the hospital environment accounted for 83.3% ($n = 6$) of HA-MRSA, 0% of CA-MRSA ($n = 6$), and 16.7% of LA-MRSA ($n = 6$). Samples from LTCF resident tubes contained higher amounts of HA-MRSA strains (69.6%, $n = 23$, vs. 41.7%, $n = 12$, respectively) and CA-MRSA (26.1%, $n = 23$, vs. 16.7%, $n = 12$, respectively) than those from the LTCF environment, although isolates from LTCF environments were mostly related to LA-associated MRSA (41.7%, $n = 12$) than to isolates from tube samples of LTCF residents (4.3%, $n = 23$). For Chiayi-isolated MRSA strains, 26.3% ($n = 19$) were HA-MRSA, 52.6% were CA-MRSA, and 21.1% were related to LA-MRSA. Furthermore, 50% ($n = 8$) of MRSA prevalence was HA-MRSA from the hospital environment, although, for the LTCF environment, this amount was lower (9.1%, $n = 11$); however, the detection rates of CA- and LA-associated MRSA isolates in LTCF environment samples (63.3% and 27.3%; $n = 11$, respectively) were higher than those collected from the hospital environment (37.5% and 12.5%; $n = 8$, respectively).

2.3. The Detection of Toxin Genes by PCR

All isolated MRSA strains carried the exfoliative toxin *eta* gene (100%, 60/60) (Table 3). A lower number of enterotoxin genes were present, including *entA*, *entB*, and *entC* (3.3%, 16.7%, and 13.3%, respectively), but no samples carried the *entD*, *entE*, or *tsst-1* genes. In Changhua samples, the *entA* (16.7%, $n = 6$) and *eta* (100%, $n = 6$) genes were detected in isolated MRSA strains from the hospital environment, whereas other toxin genes were not found in all other isolates from this area. However, for MRSA strains from LTCF environment, the only genes detected were *entC* and *eta* (8.3% and 100%; $n = 12$, respectively).

Enterotoxin genes *entB* (34.8%), *entC* (26.1%), and *eta* (100%) were found in MRSA isolates from medical tubes of LTCF residents. In Chiayi, isolates from the LTCF environment only carried the *eta* gene, whereas MRSA isolates from the hospital environment carried the *entA*, *entB*, *entC*, *etb*, and *eta* genes (12.5%, 25%, 12.5%, 25%, and 100%, $n = 8$, respectively).

Table 3. PCR detection of toxin genes from the 60 MRSA strains.

Sampling Locations	Sampling Sources	entA	entB	entC	entD	entE	Eta	etb	tsst-1
Changhua city	LTCF environment ($n = 12$)	0 (0%)	0 (0%)	1 (8.3%)	0 (0%)	0 (0%)	12 (100%)	0 (0%)	0 (0%)
	Tubes from LTCF residents ($n = 23$)	0 (0%)	8 (34.8%)	6 (26.1%)	0 (0%)	0 (0%)	23 (100%)	0 (0%)	0 (0%)
	Total LTCF isolates ($n = 35$)	0 (0%)	8 (22.9%)	7 (20%)	0 (0%)	0 (0%)	35 (100%)	0 (0%)	0 (0%)
	Hospital environment ($n = 6$)	1 (16.7%)	0 (0%)	0 (0%)	0 (0%)	0 (0%)	6 (100%)	0 (0%)	0 (0%)
	Total Changhua City isolates ($n = 41$)	1 (2.4%)	8 (19.5%)	7 (17.1%)	0 (0%)	0 (0%)	41 (100%)	0 (0%)	0 (0%)
Chiayi city	LTCF environment ($n = 11$)	0 (0%)	0 (0%)	0 (0%)	0 (0%)	0 (0%)	11 (100%)	0 (0%)	0 (0%)
	Hospital environment ($n = 8$)	1 (12.5%)	2 (25%)	1 (12.5%)	0 (0%)	0 (0%)	8 (100%)	2 (25%)	0 (0%)
	Total Chiayi City isolates ($n = 19$)	1 (5.3%)	2 (10.5%)	1 (5.3%)	0 (0%)	0 (0%)	19 (100%)	2 (10.5%)	0 (0%)
Total Changhua city and Chiayi city isolates ($n = 60$)		2 (3.3%)	10 (16.7%)	8 (13.3%)	0 (0%)	0 (0%)	60 (100%)	2 (3.3%)	0 (0%)

2.4. Antimicrobial Susceptibility of the MRSA Strains

Eight types of antibiotics were used to analyze the antibiotic resistance capability of the 60 isolated MRSA strains. Overall, the resistance was ranked in order of highest to lowest as erythromycin, gentamicin, ciprofloxacin, clindamycin, tetracycline, sulfamethoxazole-trimethoprim, rifampicin, and chloramphenicol (Table 4). MRSA isolates from Changhua city had higher antimicrobial resistance compared to the Chiayi city. In addition, the Changhua hospital environment's isolates had a higher percentage of resistance against most of the antibiotics, except chloramphenicol and rifampicin, compared to Changhua LTCF environment's isolates. However, a higher percentage of isolates from Changhua LTCF resident tube samples were capable of resisting gentamicin. All the isolates from the Chiayi city LTCF environment were resistant to ciprofloxacin and erythromycin (100%, $n = 11$), and only one isolate was resistant to tetracycline and gentamicin. In the case of the Chiayi hospital environment, although the percentages of isolates able to resist the ciprofloxacin and erythromycin (50% and 62.5%, $n = 8$) were observed, this value was significantly higher in Chiayi LTCF environment samples.

For MDR profiling (Table 5), six MRSA isolates (83%) from the Changhua hospital environment had the highest degree of MDR. In the Changhua LTCF environment, the degree of MDR reached 50% ($n = 12$). In addition, for tube samples, 65.2% ($n = 23$) of isolates were found to be MDR. For Chiayi, only 37.5% ($n = 8$) of the total isolates from the hospital environment were MDR, whereas in the LTCF environment, only one isolate was MDR (9.1%).

Table 4. Antimicrobial susceptibility results of the 60 MRSA strains.

Sampling Locations	Sampling Sources	C	CIP	DA	E	G	RA	S/T	T	MDR
Changhua city	LTCF environment (n = 12)	0 (0%)	5 (41.7%)	2 (16.7%)	7 (58.3%)	10 (83.3%)	3 (25%)	5 (41.7%)	5 (41.7%)	6 (50%)
	tubes from LTCF residents (n = 23)	3 (13.3%)	8 (34.8%)	10 (43.5%)	17 (73.9%)	18 (78.3%)	1 (4.3%)	4 (17.4%)	4 (17.4%)	15 (65.2%)
	LTCF isolates (n = 35)	3 (8.6%)	13 (37.1%)	12 (34.3%)	24 (68.6%)	28 (80%)	4 (11.4%)	9 (25.7%)	9 (25.7%)	21 (60%)
	Hospital environment (n = 6)	0 (0%)	5 (83.3%)	5 (83.3%)	6 (100%)	6 (100%)	0 (0%)	5 (83.3%)	5 (83.3%)	5 (83.3%)
	Total Changhua city isolates (n = 41)	3 (7.3%)	18 (43.9%)	17 (41.5%)	30 (73.2%)	34 (82.9%)	4 (9.8%)	14 (34.1%)	14 (34.1%)	26 (63.4%)
Chiayi city	LTCF environment (n = 11)	0 (0%)	11 (100%)	0 (0%)	11 (100%)	1 (9.1%)	0 (0%)	0 (0%)	1 (9.1%)	1 (9.1%)
	Hospital environment (n = 8)	0 (0%)	4 (50%)	2 (25%)	5 (62.5%)	1 (12.5%)	1 (12.5%)	1 (12.5%)	2 (25%)	3 (37.5%)
	Total Chiayi city isolates (n = 19)	0 (0%)	15 (78.9%)	2 (10.5%)	16 (84.2%)	2 (10.5%)	1 (5.3%)	1 (5.3%)	3 (15.8%)	4 (21.1%)
Total Changhua city and Chiayi city isolates (n = 60)		3 (5%)	33 (55%)	19 (31.7%)	46 (76.7%)	36 (60%)	5 (8.3%)	15 (25%)	17 (28.3%)	30 (50%)

C: chloramphenicol; CIP: ciprofloxacin; DA: clindamycin; E: erythromycin; G: gentamicin; RA: rifampicin; S/T: sulfamethoxazole-trimethoprim; T: tetracycline; MDR: multidrug resistance.

Table 5. MDR pattern profile results of 30 MRSA strains.

Sampling Locations	Changhua City			Chiayi City		Total MDR Strains
Sampling Sources	LTCF Environment	Tubes from LTCF Residents	Hospital Environment	LTCF Environment	Hospital Environment	
CIP-DA-E-G-S/T-T (6 drugs)	2		5			7
C-DA-E-G-S/T (5 drugs)		2				
CIP-E-G-RA-S/T (5 drugs)	1					4
CIP-E-G-RA-T (5 drugs)		1				
CIP-E-G-S/T (4 drugs)				1		
CIP-E-G-T (4 drugs)		1				
CIP-G-S/T-T (4 drugs)		1				5
DA-E-G-RA (4 drugs)					1	
G-RA-S/T-T (4 drugs)	1					
C-DA-E (3 drugs)		1				
CIP-E-G (3 drugs)		2				
CIP-ST-T (3 drugs)					1	
DA-E-G (3 drugs)		7				14
DA-E-T (3 drugs)					1	
E-G-T (3 drugs)	1					
G-RA-S/T (3 drugs)	1					
Total strains	6	15	5	1	3	30

C: chloramphenicol; CIP: ciprofloxacin; DA: clindamycin; E: erythromycin; G: gentamicin; RA: rifampicin; S/T: sulfamethoxazole-trimethoprim; T: tetracycline; MDR: multidrug resistance.

2.5. Genetic Diversity Analysis by ERIC-PCR

The combination of ERIC-PCR analysis with strain information for the 60 MRSA isolates is shown in Figure 1. The MRSA isolates in this study could be divided into three clusters by ERIC-PCR analysis: cluster 1 (24 isolates), cluster 2 (35 isolates), and cluster 3 (one isolate). We further divided cluster 1 into two sub-clusters (Cluster 1-1 and Cluster 1-2). Cluster 1-1 contained more MRSA strains than Cluster 1-2, and maximum number of this cluster's isolates were isolated from Chiayi city samples predominantly consist of SCCmec type IV + PVL genes, classified as community associated, non-MDR MRSA clones, and only carried the *eta* toxin gene. The MRSA isolates that belonged to Cluster 1-2 (6 isolates) were related to HA-MRSA and contained SCCmec element III and the *eta* toxin gene. These isolates were MDR strains from Changhua city's LTCF resident samples. Cluster 2 included three sub-clusters: 2-1-1, 2-1-2, and 2-2. The MRSA isolates of sub-cluster 2-1-1 presented a similar genetic profile as cluster 1-2, with the exception of the *entB* gene, which was present only in cluster 2-1-1.

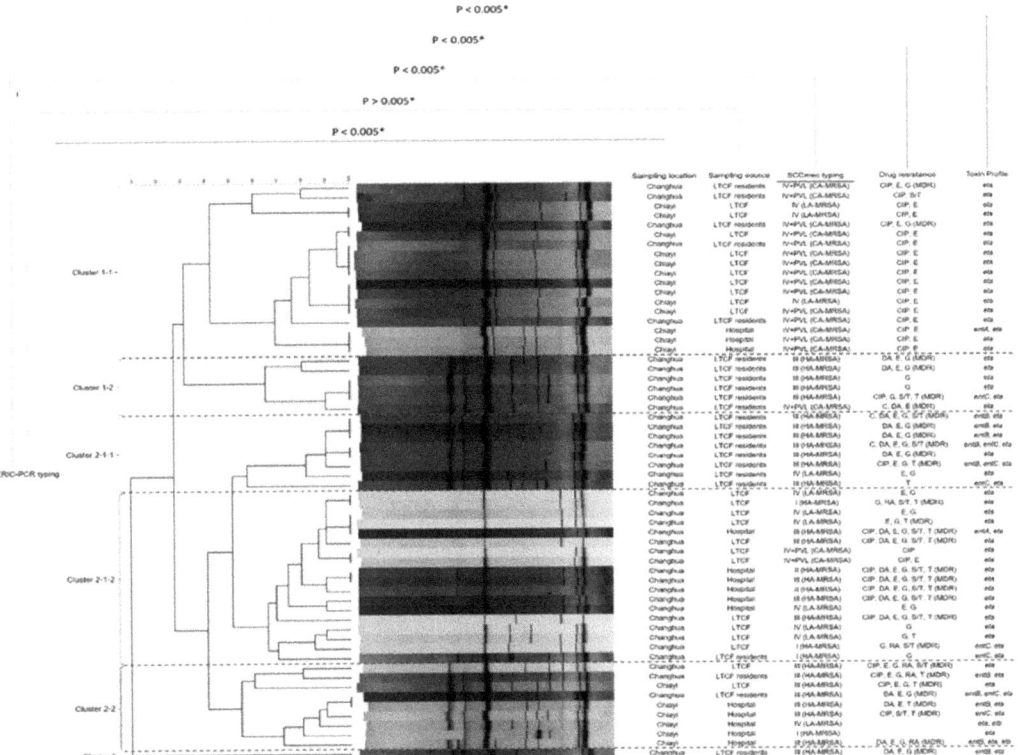

Figure 1. Genetical diversity of MRSA strains by ERIC-PCR combined with MDR pattern, SCCmec typing and toxin profile.

Furthermore, all isolates from clusters 2-1-1 and 1-2 were isolated from the dwelling medical tubes of Changhua LTFC residents. Eighteen MRSA isolates belonging to Cluster 2-1-2 showed high MDR properties combined with the *eta* gene and all were isolated from the hospital and LTCF environments of Changhua. The MRSA isolates of Cluster 2-2 were isolated from a range of samples, and the HA-MRSA isolates that contained SCCmec III elements and carried more than one toxin gene (*entB*, *entC*, *eta*, etc.) were predominant in this cluster. Cluster 3, considered as the outgroup, contained only one MRSA isolate isolated from a Changhua LTCF resident's tube sample.

The chi-square test was used to evaluate the discriminatory power of ERIC-PCR associated with the factors of all isolates, for example, sampling location, sampling source, SCCmec typing, drug resistance, and toxin gene profile. This showed that only the sampling source (P > 0.05) had no significant association with ERIC-PCR analysis while all the remaining parameters had a significant association with cluster classification of ERIC-PCR.

3. Discussion

MRSA is one of the most predominant multidrug-resistant pathogens worldwide, and Asia is among the regions with the highest incidence in the world [27–29]. The estimated percentage of MRSA in hospital samples varies from 28% to >70% in Asia [30]. Studies regarding hospital environmental MRSA showed that the average prevalence was 2.2% and 11.8% in Ireland and Canada, respectively [31,32]. Several studies have focused on the isolation of MRSA from hospital curtains with MRSA detection percentages ranging from 15.5% to 31.6% [26,29,33]. In our case, MRSA prevalence in hospital environment samples was 18.8% in Changhua city and 25% in Chiayi city. The differences in MRSA prevalence in hospital and LTCF environments may be due to the sample type and local hygiene conditions. A UK study showed that MRSA detection rates were 40% and 17% in LTCF environmental samples in 2011 and 2013, respectively [34]. This study also implied that the lower frequency in 2013 might be due to improved infrastructure in the new LTCF. This agreed with our results that showed a lower MRSA detection percentage in Chiayi LTCF, which had a better hygiene environment compared to that of Changhua LTCF. Liu et al. demonstrated a disparity in MRSA detection rates between six LTCFs and concluded that improved infrastructure and a good hygiene environment constitute a powerful approach for reducing MRSA prevalence [27]. Our results implied that MRSA strains were present with high occurrence in moist environments, which agreed with other investigations, as moist samples act as prominent hotspots of MRSA distribution [7,8]. Here, the highest detection rate of MRSA was in nasogastric tubes, which are frequently used in LTCF residents.

The predominant SCCmec types were SCCmec III and IV, which agrees with studies of LTCFs in Taiwan [27,29]. However, the predominant SCCmec types in the two hospital environments of this study were different. The dominant type was SCCmec III in Chunghua hospital but was SCCmec IV in Chiayi hospital. HA-MRSA (31 isolates) was the dominant classification in this study, where HA-MRSA typically belongs to SCCmec I, II, and III [30]. Clinical studies in Taiwan also indicated that most of the HA-MRSA strains from hospitals belonged to SCCmec III [30,35,36]. Between 17.1% and 21.1% of LA-MRSA strains were isolated from hospitals and CTCFs, respectively, and all LA-MRSA isolated here belonged to SCCmec IV+PVL. This type is the same as our previous LA-MRSA study in the river basin of Chiayi [37]. Huang and Che's study also concluded that more than 80% of Asian-specific LA-MRSA strains in Taiwan carried SCCmec IV and PVL genes, which strengthens our results [38].

The eta and etb enterotoxin-associated genes and tsst-1 are frequently prevalent virulence genes that vary between countries [30,33,39]. All the MRSA strains isolated in this study carry the eta gene; eta is reported to be the most privileged virulence factor-encoded gene, although this is contradicted in some reports [33,40–42]. Additionally, in contrast to other studies, we did not detect any entD, entE, and tsst-1-positive strains [33,42]. This showed that the distribution of toxin profiles of MRSA was highly diverse and implied geographic differences in these distributions. The MRSA isolates carrying the entB or entC genes all belonged to SSCmec III, except for one CA-MRSA isolate that carried two toxin genes, whereas all other isolates carried the eta gene only. This result is similar to the marginal differences identified in the distribution of toxin genes with SCCmec types reported by Fooladi et al. [33].

Antibiotic susceptibility testing revealed that MRSA isolates were more resistant to ciprofloxacin, erythromycin, and gentamicin than to other antibiotics, and 50% of these were related to MDR. MRSA from the hospital environment had more MDR ability compared with that from the LTCF environment. Furthermore, the prevalence of MDR MRSA was higher in Changhua city than in Chiayi city, and these were mainly HA-MRSA strains, followed by CA-MRSA from hospital environmental samples and LTCF resident samples, which agreed with a previous report [43]. Twenty-six of a total of 30 MDR MRSA isolates were identified in Changhua city and, among them, seven isolates were resistant to six antibiotics; this is an urgent and concerning issue and implies a cross-contamination problem.

ERIC-PCR is one of the most effective DNA-based molecular typing methods used to categorize MRSA isolates associated with epidemiological modeling and helps to track their spreading route [44]. In our ERIC-PCR fingerprinting, most of the MRSA isolates carrying the *SCCmec* IV + PVL genes (CA-MRSA) were from Chiayi LTCF environment samples and belonged to Cluster 1-1. Sub-clusters 1-1 and 2-1-1 were all from the Changhua LTFC resident samples, indicating that there were two main types of MRSA distributed in these LTCF residents.

In contrast, isolates in sub-cluster 2-1-1 from Changhua hospital and LTCFs generally consisted of *SCCmec* III (HA-MRSA) with MDR isolates. This finding implied that a genetically similar type of MRSA had spread between LTCFs and hospitals. ERIC-PCR aided the discrimination of resistance patterns among *SCCmec* types reported in our previous study [37]. ERIC-PCR is a popular tool for determining the genetic relatedness of different multidrug-resistant pathogenic bacteria from environmental samples, and previous analyses are consistent with our results [45,46]. This conclusion is further supported by the chi-square statistical hypothesis, where the individual significance score was < 0.05 with ERIC-PCR results. A similar analysis, adopted by Akindolire et. al. to distinguish the genetic diversity of isolated MRSA strains from their samples, strongly supported our ERIC-PCR results [47]. Therefore, using the ERIC-PCR figure combined with more detailed information, including toxin profiles, sampling location, other typing methods, and drug-resistant profiles, is a favorable approach to provide a complete understanding of pathogen transmission, microbial contamination, and surveillance spot information.

4. Materials and Methods

4.1. Sampling Information and Collection Method

Samples were taken from the hospital and LTCF environment of two cities in Taiwan (Changhua and Chiayi). For Changhua, the collected samples were from Hanming Christian Hospital (24.061271° N, 120.535643° E) and affiliated nursing homes (Auspicious Long-Term Care Center) (24.080745° N, 120.545247° E). Similarly, for Chiayi city, we collected samples from Chiayi Christian Hospital (23.499264° N, 120.450161° E) and affiliated nursing homes (Pau-Kang Long Term Care Center) (23.506819° N, 120.450287° E). A total of 246 samples were collected from LTCFs and hospital environments of both cities, including from medical tubes of LTCF residents, which are further categorized according to their type details, are described in Supplemental Table S1. Sterile cotton swabs were used to collect bacterial samples from the surface of each sampling point. Swabs were soaked in 5 mL of sterile phosphate buffer saline (PBS) in a centrifuge tube for storage and transported, at low temperature, to the laboratory for analysis.

4.2. Isolation Method of MRSA

To isolate MRSA from collected samples a two-step selective culture process was used. For the growth of MRSA colonies, we used CHROMagar™ MRSA (TPM ready-to-use media) and Baird-Parker agar (TPM ready-to-use media). The colonies that were grown on the respective cultured agar plate after the incubation period (30 °C for 24 h), were transferred into a sterile test tube containing brain heart infusion broth for pure culture [48]. Species identification, molecular characterization, and drug resistance analysis of isolated colony pure were performed using 300 µL broth from the enrichment culture.

4.3. PCR Identification of MRSA Strains

An aliquot of 300–600 µL of well-grown bacterial culture was centrifuged for 5 min at 10,000 rpm for DNA extraction. Genomic DNA was extracted using a commercial bacterial DNA extraction kit (MagPurix Bacterial DNA Extraction Kit, ZP02006, Taiwan, China). A reference bacterial genomic DNA (MRSA ATCC 29213) was used as a positive control (extracted by the same method and kit) [37]. After gDNA extraction, the PCR reaction mixture was prepared using 300 µg of gDNA with primers and master mix (Fast-RunTM Taq Master Mix with Dye). The total PCR reaction volume was 25 µL, and PCR reaction conditions are described in Supplemental Table S2. ERIC-PCR was used for PCR-based typing, and BioNumerics software was used to analyze kinship typing [37,49]. The *nuc* and *mecA* genes were used for the identification of MRSA strain types [50]. *SCCmec* and Panton–Valentine leukocidine (PVL) were used to confirm the classification of *mec* elements [51]. Some enterotoxins, toxic shock syndrome toxin-1 (*TSST-1*), and exfoliative toxins (ETs) genes were targeted for detection within the *S. aureus*. Finally, all PCR products were assessed by electrophoresis (110 V, 30 min, 1.5% agarose gel) to check the respective gene-specific amplicons.

4.4. Antibiotic Susceptibility Test

The following antibiotics—chloramphenicol (30 µg), ciprofloxacin (5 µg), clindamycin (2 µg), erythromycin (15 µg), gentamicin (10 µg), tetracycline (5 µg), rifampicin (30 µg) and sulfamethoxazole-trimethoprim (23.75/1.75 µg)—were used to test the antibiotic resistance of the MRSA isolates using the disc diffusion method as per the guidelines of the Clinical and Laboratory Standards Institute (CLSI, I-M45-P, 2006). These tests were conducted on Mueller–Hinton agar plates (TPM Ready-to-use media) [37].

5. Conclusions

This study showed that MRSA occurs at relatively higher rates in moist samples, especially in LTCF resident dwelling tubes. The eta gene was commonly found in all MRSA isolates. The hospital environmental MRSA isolates from Chiayi city carried the highest amount of enterotoxin genes, such as *entA*, *entB*, and *entC*, compared with those from Changhua city. Additionally, the MRSA isolates from the hospital environment and LTCF resident dwelling tubes exhibited high percentages of multidrug resistance to the following antibiotics: ciprofloxacin, clindamycin, erythromycin, sulfamethoxazole-trimethoprim, and tetracycline. The multidrug resistance problem of healthcare-associated MRSA is more severe in Changhua city than in Chiayi city. The *SCCmec* III containing HA-MRSA was identified as rank one and PVL + *SCCmec* IV element carrying CA-MRSA was rank two group of MRSA strain among 60 isolated *S. aureus* clones. ERIC-PCR was an effective tool for epidemiological characterization of MRSA isolates. The presence of genetically similar and multidrug-resistant MRSA in hospitals and their affiliated LTCFs is a threat to public health and needs to be closely monitored and controlled.

Supplementary Materials: The following are available online at https://www.mdpi.com/article/10.3390/antibiotics10060748/s1, Table S1: Details of samples location, source, types and number, Table S2: MRSA strain identification (ERIC-PCR), *SCCmec* typing and enterotoxin gene detection condition of PCR with primers information.

Author Contributions: Conceptualization, B.-M.H., J.-S.C., I.-C.L., G.-J.H. and H.-C.T.; Methodology, I.-C.L., S.K., G.-J.H., H.-C.T. and J.-S.C.; Software, H.-C.T. and J.-S.C.; Validation, G.-J.H., J.-S.C. and S.-W.H.; Formal Analysis, B.-M.H., J.-S.C. and G.-J.H.; Investigation, J.-S.C., S.-W.H., H.-C.T., B.H. and S.K.; Resources, I.-C.L. and G.-J.H.; Data Curation, J.-S.C., H.-C.T. and B.H.; Writing—Original Draft Preparation, S.K., B.-M.H., I.-C.L., G.-J.H. and H.-C.T.; Writing—Review and Editing, J.-S.C., B.-M.H., H.-C.T. and S.K.; Visualization, H.-C.T.; Supervision, S.-W.H., B.-M.H., B.H., and J.-S.C.; Project Administration, J.-S.C., B.-M.H., I.-C.L. and G.-J.H.; Funding Acquisition, B.-M.H., I.-C.L., G.-J.H. and H.-C.T. All authors have read and agreed to the published version of the manuscript.

Funding: This research was funded by the Ministry of Science and Technology of Taiwan (MOST 108-2116-M-194 -005 and 108-2811-M-194 -507), the Buddhist Tzu Chi Hospital (TCRD109-68; TCRD110-44) and Asia University Hospital (grant no. 10951003). This research was also supported by the Ditmanson Medical Foundation, Chia - Yi Christian Hospital (RCN011), and the Center for Innovative Research on Aging Society (CIRAS) through The Featured Areas Research Center Program, within the framework of the Higher Education Sprout Project by the Ministry of Education (MOEs) in Taiwan.

Institutional Review Board Statement: The study was conducted according to the guidelines of the Declaration of Helsinki and approved by the Institutional Review Board of Changhua Christian Hospital, Taiwan and Ditmanson Chia - Yi Christian Hospital (CCH IRB No. 190311, CYCH-IRB 2019031 and date of approval: 11 June 2019 and 14 May 2019).

Informed Consent Statement: Informed consent was obtained from all subjects involved in the study.

Data Availability Statement: The data presented in this study are available on request from the corresponding author.

Conflicts of Interest: The authors declare that they have no conflict of interest.

References

1. Bonomo, R. Multiple Antibiotic–Resistant Bacteria in Long-Term-Care Facilities: An Emerging Problem in the Practice of Infectious Diseases. *Clin. Infect. Dis.* **2001**, *31*, 1414–1422. [CrossRef]
2. Pai, H.-H. Multidrug resistant bacteria isolated from cockroaches in long-term care facilities and nursing homes. *Acta Trop.* **2013**, *125*, 18–22. [CrossRef]
3. Otto, M. MRSA virulence and spread. *Cell. Microbiol.* **2012**, *14*, 1513–1521. [CrossRef] [PubMed]
4. Lindsay, J. Hospital-associated MRSA and antibiotic resistance—What have we learned from genomics? *Int. J. Med. Microbiol.* **2013**, *303*. [CrossRef] [PubMed]
5. Ge, B.; Mukherjee, S.; Hsu, C.-H.; Davis, J.; Tran, T.; Yang, Q.; Abbott, J.; Ayers, S.; Young, S.; Crarey, E.; et al. MRSA and multidrug-resistant *Staphylococcus aureus* in U.S. retail meats, 2010–2011. *Food Microbiol.* **2017**, *62*, 289–297. [CrossRef] [PubMed]
6. Boyce, J. Methicillin-Resistant *Staphylococcus aureus* in Hospitals and Long-Term Care Facilities: Microbiology, Epidemiology, and Preventive Measures. *Infect. Control. Hosp. Epidemiol.* **1993**, *13*, 725–737. [CrossRef]
7. Pantosti, A.; Sanchini, A.; Monaco, M. Mechanisms of antibiotic resistance in *Staphylococcus aureus*. *Futur. Microbiol.* **2007**, *2*, 323–334. [CrossRef]
8. Kaito, C.; Saito, Y.; Nagano, G.; Ikuo, M.; Omae, Y.; Hanada, Y.; Han, X.; Kuwahara-Arai, K.; Hishinuma, T.; Baba, T.; et al. Transcription and Translation Products of the Cytolysin Gene psm-mec on the Mobile Genetic Element SCCmec Regulate *Staphylococcus* aureus Virulence. *PLoS Pathog.* **2011**, *7*, e1001267. [CrossRef] [PubMed]
9. Kim, C.; Mwangi, M.; Chung, M.; Milheiriço, C.; De Lencastre, H.; Tomasz, A. The Mechanism of Heterogeneous Beta-Lactam Resistance in MRSA: Key Role of the Stringent Stress Response. *PLoS ONE* **2014**, *9*. [CrossRef]
10. Valsesia, G.; Rossi, M.; Bertschy, S.; Pfyffer, G.E. Emergence of SCCmecType IV and SCCmecType V Methicillin-Resistant *Staphylococcus aureus* Containing the Panton-Valentine Leukocidin Genes in a Large Academic Teaching Hospital in Central Switzerland: External Invaders or Persisting Circulators? *J. Clin. Microbiol.* **2010**, *48*, 720–727. [CrossRef]
11. Jiménez, J.; Ocampo Rios, A.; Vanegas, J.; Rodriguez, E.; Mediavilla, J.; Chen, L.; Muskus, C.; Vélez, L.; Rojas, C.; Restrepo, A.; et al. CC8 MRSA Strains Harboring SCCmec Type IVc are Predominant in Colombian Hospitals. *PLoS ONE* **2012**, *7*, e38576. [CrossRef]
12. Otto, M. Community-associated MRSA: What makes them special? *Int. J. Med. Microbiol.* **2013**, *303*. [CrossRef] [PubMed]
13. Chuang, Y.-Y.; Huang, Y.-C. Molecular epidemiology of community-associated meticillin-resistant Staphylococcus aureus in Asia. *Lancet Infect. Dis.* **2013**, *13*. [CrossRef]
14. Chuang, Y.-Y.; Huang, Y.-C. Livestock-associated meticillin-resistant *Staphylococcus aureus* in Asia: An emerging issue? *Int. J. Antimicrob. Agents* **2014**, *45*. [CrossRef] [PubMed]
15. Goudarzi, M.; Seyedjavadi, S.S.; Nasiri, M.J.; Goudarzi, H.; Nia, R.S.; Dabiri, H. Molecular characteristics of methicillin-resistant *Staphylococcus aureus* (MRSA) strains isolated from patients with bacteremia based on MLST, SCCmec, spa, and agr locus types analysis. *Microb. Pathog.* **2017**, *104*, 328–335. [CrossRef]
16. Bush, K. Bench-to-bedside review: The role of β-lactamases in antibiotic-resistant Gram-negative infections. *Crit. Care* **2010**, *14*, 224. [CrossRef] [PubMed]
17. Palmer, A.; Kishony, R. Understanding, predicting and manipulating the genotypic evolution of antibiotic resistance. *Nat. Rev. Genet.* **2013**, *14*. [CrossRef]
18. Wellington, E.M.; Boxall, A.; Cross, P.; Feil, E.; Gaze, W.H.; Hawkey, P.; Johnson-Rollings, A.; Jones, D.; Lee, N.; Otten, W.; et al. The role of the natural environment in the emergence of antibiotic resistance in Gram-negative bacteria. *Lancet Infect. Dis.* **2013**, *13*, 155–165. [CrossRef]

19. Vernel-Pauillac, F.; Nandi, S.; Nicholas, R.A.; Goarant, C. Genotyping as a Tool for Antibiotic Resistance Surveillance of Neisseria gonorrhoeae in New Caledonia: Evidence of a Novel Genotype Associated with Reduced Penicillin Susceptibility. *Antimicrob. Agents Chemother.* **2008**, *52*, 3293–3300. [CrossRef]
20. Köser, C.; Ellington, M.; Cartwright, E.; Gillespie, S.; Brown, N.; Farrington, M.; Holden, M.; Dougan, G.; Bentley, D.; Parkhill, J.; et al. Routine Use of Microbial Whole Genome Sequencing in Diagnostic and Public Health Microbiology. *PLoS Pathog.* **2012**, *8*, e1002824. [CrossRef]
21. Ranjbar, R.; Tabatabaee, A.; Behzadi, P.; Kheiri, R. Enterobacterial Repetitive Intergenic Consensus Polymerase Chain Reaction (ERIC-PCR) Genotyping of Escherichia coli Strains Isolated from Different Animal Stool Specimens. *Iran. J. Pathol.* **2017**, *1212*, 25–34. [CrossRef]
22. Leclercq, R.; Cantón, R.; Brown, D.F.J.; Giske, C.G.; Heisig, P.; MacGowan, A.; Mouton, J.; Nordmann, P.; Rodloff, A.; Rossolini, G.; et al. EUCAST expert rules in antimicrobial susceptibility testing. *Clin. Microbiol. Infect.* **2011**, *24*. [CrossRef]
23. Hsueh, P.-R.; Chen, W.-H.; Luh, K.-T. Relationships between antimicrobial use and antimicrobial resistance in Gram-negative bacteria causing nosocomial infections from 1991–2003 at a university hospital in Taiwan. *Int. J. Antimicrob. Agents* **2006**, *26*, 463–472. [CrossRef]
24. March, A.; Aschbacher, R.; Dhanji, H.; Livermore, D.; Böttcher, A.; Sleghel, F.; Maggi, S.; Noale, M.; Larcher, C.; Woodford, N. Colonization of residents and staff of a long-term-care facility and adjacent acute-care hospital geriatric unit by multiresistant bacteria. *Clin. Microbiol. Infect.* **2009**, *16*, 934–944. [CrossRef] [PubMed]
25. Wu, C.-L.; Ku, S.-C.; Yang, K.-Y.; Fang, W.-F.; Tu, C.-Y.; Chen, C.-W.; Hsu, K.-H.; Fan, W.-C.; Lin, M.-C.; Chen, W.; et al. Antimicrobial drug-resistant microbes associated with hospitalized community-acquired and healthcare-associated pneumonia: A multi-center study in Taiwan. *J. Formos. Med. Assoc.* **2013**, *112*, 31–40. [CrossRef] [PubMed]
26. Lee, C.-M.; Lai, C.-C.; Chiang, H.; Lu, M.-C.; Wang, L.-F.; Tsai, T.-L.; Kang, M.-Y.; Jan, Y.-N.; Lo, Y.-T.; Ko, W.-C.; et al. Presence of multidrug-resistant organisms in the residents and environments of long-term care facilities in Taiwan. *J. Microbiol. Immunol. Infect.* **2017**, *50*. [CrossRef] [PubMed]
27. Liu, C.-Y.; Lai, C.-C.; Chiang, H.; Lu, M.-C.; Wang, L.-F.; Tsai, T.-L.; Kang, M.-Y.; Jan, Y.-N.; Lo, Y.-T.; Ko, W.-C.; et al. Predominance of methicillin-resistant *Staphylococcus aureus* in the residents and environments of long-term care facilities in Taiwan. *J. Microbiol. Immunol. Infect.* **2018**, *52*. [CrossRef] [PubMed]
28. Phoon, H.Y.; Hussin, H.; Hussain, B.M.; Lim, S.Y.; Woon, J.J.; Er, Y.X.; Thong, K.L. Distribution, genetic diversity and antimicrobial resistance of clinically important bacteria from the environment of a tertiary hospital in Malaysia. *J. Glob. Antimicrob. Resist.* **2018**, *14*. [CrossRef] [PubMed]
29. Tsai, H.-C.; Huang, T.-Y.; Chen, J.-S.; Chen, W.-J.; Lin, C.-Y.; Hsu, B.-M. Acinetobacter baumannii and methicillin-resistant *Staphylococcus aureus* in long-term care facilities in eastern Taiwan. *Tzu. Chi. Med. J.* **2019**, *31*. [CrossRef]
30. Chen, C.-J.; Huang, Y.-C. New epidemiology of *Staphylococcus aureus* infection in Asia. *Clin. Microbiol. Infect.* **2014**, *20*. [CrossRef]
31. Faires, M.; Pearl, D.; Ciccotelli, W.; Straus, K.; Zinken, G.; Berke, O.; Reid-Smith, R.; Weese, J. A prospective study to examine the epidemiology of methicillin-resistant *Staphylococcus aureus* and *Clostridium difficile* contamination in the general environment of three community hospitals in southern Ontario, Canada. *BMC Infect. Dis.* **2012**, *12*, 290. [CrossRef] [PubMed]
32. Kearney, A.; Kinnevey, P.; Shore, A.; Earls, M.; Poovelikunnel, T.T.; Brennan, G.; Humphreys, H.; Coleman, D.C. The oral cavity revealed as a significant reservoir of Staphylococcus aureus in an acute hospital by extensive patient, healthcare worker and environmental sampling. *J. Hosp. Infect.* **2020**, *105*, 389–396. [CrossRef]
33. Fooladi, A.A.I.; Ashrafi, E.; Tazandareh, S.G.; Koosha, R.Z.; Rad, H.S.; Amin, M.; Soori, M.; Larki, R.A.; Choopani, A.; Hosseini, H.M. The distribution of pathogenic and toxigenic genes among MRSA and MSSA clinical isolates. *Microb. Pathog.* **2015**, *81*. [CrossRef]
34. Ludden, C.; Brennan, G.; Morris, D.; Austin, B.; O'Connell, B.; Cormican, M. Characterization of methicillin-resistant *Staphylococcus aureus* from residents and the environment in a long-term care facility. *Epidemiol. Infect.* **2015**, *143*. [CrossRef] [PubMed]
35. Tsao, S.-M.; Wang, W.-Y.; Ko, W.-C.; Lu, C.-T.; Liu, C.-Y.; Liao, C.-H.; Chen, Y.-S.; Liu, Y.-C.; Jang, T.-N.; et al. Trend in vancomycin susceptibility and correlation with molecular characteristics of methicillin-resistant *Staphylococcus aureus* causing invasive infections in Taiwan: Results from the Tigecycline in vitro Surveillance in Taiwan (TIST) study, 2006–2010. *Diagn. Microbiol. Infect. Dis.* **2014**, *80*. [CrossRef]
36. Jean, S.-S.; Ko, W.-C.; Hsueh, P.-R. Susceptibility of clinical isolates of meticillin-resistant *Staphylococcus aureus* and phenotypic non-extended-spectrum β-lactamase-producing Klebsiella pneumoniae to ceftaroline in Taiwan: Results from Antimicrobial Testing Leadership and Surveillance (ATLAS) in 2012–2018 and Surveillance of Multicentre Antimicrobial Resistance in Taiwan (SMART) in 2018–2019. *Int. J. Antimicrob. Agents* **2020**, *56*, 106016. [CrossRef]
37. Tsai, H.-C.; Tao, C.-W.; Hsu, B.-M.; Yang, Y.-Y.; Tseng, Y.-C.; Huang, T.-Y.; Huang, S.-W.; Kuo, Y.-J.; Chen, J.-S. Multidrug-resistance in methicillin-resistant *Staphylococcus aureus* (MRSA) isolated from a subtropical river contaminated by nearby livestock industries. *Ecotoxicol. Environ. Saf.* **2020**, *200*, 110724. [CrossRef]
38. De Sousa, M.A.; Crisóstomo, M.; Sanches, I.S.; Wu, J.; Fuzhong, J.; Tomasz, A.; de Lencastre, H. Frequent Recovery of a Single Clonal Type of Multidrug-Resistant *Staphylococcus aureus* from Patients in Two Hospitals in Taiwan and China. *J. Clin. Microbiol.* **2003**, *41*, 159–163. [CrossRef] [PubMed]
39. Dulon, M.; Haamann, F.; Peters, C.; Schablon, A.; Nienhaus, A. MRSA prevalence in European healthcare settings: A review. *BMC Infect. Dis.* **2011**, *11*, 138. [CrossRef]

40. Mellmann, A.; Weniger, T.; Berssenbrügge, C.; Keckevoet, U.; Friedrich, A.; Harmsen, D.; Grundmann, H. Characterization of Clonal Relatedness among the Natural Population of *Staphylococcus aureus* Strains by Using spa Sequence Typing and the BURP (Based upon Repeat Patterns) Algorithm. *J. Clin. Microbiol.* **2008**, *46*, 2805–2808. [CrossRef]
41. Nubel, U.; Roumagnac, P.; Feldkamp, M.; Song, J.-H.; Ko, K.S.; Huang, Y.-C.; Coombs, G.; Ip, M.; Westh, H.; Skov, R.; et al. Frequent emergence and limited geographic dispersal of methicillin-resistant *Staphylococcus aureus*. *Proc. Natl. Acad. Sci. USA* **2008**, *105*, 14130–14135. [CrossRef]
42. Liu, M.; Liu, J.; Guo, Y.; Zhang, Z. Characterization of Virulence Factors and Genetic Background of *Staphylococcus aureus* Isolated from Peking University People's Hospital Between 2005 and 2009. *Curr. Microbiol.* **2010**, *61*, 435–443. [CrossRef] [PubMed]
43. Lee, T.-M.; Yang, M.-C.; Yang, T.-F.; Lee, P.-L.; Chien, H.-I.; Hsueh, J.-C.; Chang, S.-H.; Hsu, C.-H.; Chien, S.-T. Molecular Characterization of Community- and Healthcare-Associated Methicillin-Resistant *Staphylococcus aureus* Isolates in Southern Taiwan. *Microb. Drug Resist.* **2015**, *21*. [CrossRef] [PubMed]
44. Candan, E.; Idil, N.; Bilkay, I.S. Usefulness of REP and ERIC-PCR combination for tracking the spread of *Staphylococcus aureus* strains. *Minerva Biotecnol.* **2013**, *25*, 245–250.
45. Tsai, H.-C.; Chou, M.-Y.; Wu, C.-C.; Wan, M.-T.; Kuo, Y.-J.; Chen, J.-S.; Huang, T.-Y.; Hsu, B.-M. Seasonal Distribution and Genotyping of Antibiotic Resistant Strains of Listeria Innocua Isolated from A River Basin Categorized by ERIC-PCR. *Int. J. Environ. Res. Public Health* **2018**, *15*, 1559. [CrossRef] [PubMed]
46. Codjoe, F.; Brown, C.; Smith, T.; Miller, K.; Donkor, E. Genetic relatedness in carbapenem-resistant isolates from clinical specimens in Ghana using ERIC-PCR technique. *PLoS ONE* **2019**, *14*, e0222168. [CrossRef] [PubMed]
47. Akindolire, A.; Kumar, A.; Ateba, N. Genetic characterization of antibiotic-resistant *Staphylococcus aureus* from milk in the North-West Province, South Africa. *Saudi J. Biol. Sci.* **2015**, *25*. [CrossRef]
48. Onyango, L.A.; Dunstan, R.H.; Gottfries, J.; Von Eiff, C.; Roberts, T.K. Effect of Low Temperature on Growth and Ultra-Structure of *Staphylococcus* spp. *PLoS ONE* **2012**, *7*, e29031. [CrossRef]
49. Azis, N.M.; Pung, H.P.; Rachman, A.R.A.; Nordin, S.A.; Sarchio, S.N.E.; Suhaili, Z.; Desa, M.N.M. A persistent antimicrobial resistance pattern and limited methicil-lin-resistance-associated genotype in a short-term *Staphylococcus aureus* carriage isolated from a student population. *J. Infect. Public Health* **2017**, *10*, 156–164. [CrossRef]
50. Papadopoulos, P.; Papadopoulos, T.; Angelidis, A.S.; Boukouvala, E.; Zdragas, A.; Papa, A.; Hadjichristodoulou, C.; Sergelidis, D. Prevalence of *Staphylococcus aureus* and of methicillin-resistant *S. aureus* (MRSA) along the production chain of dairy products in north-western Greece. *Food Microbiol.* **2018**, *69*, 43–50. [CrossRef]
51. Halaji, M.; Karimi, A.; Shoaei, P.; Nahaei, M.; Khorvash, F.; Ataei, B.; Yaran, M.; Havaei, S.A. Distribution of SCCmec Elements and Presence of Panton-Valentine Leukocidin in Methicillin-Resistant *Staphylococcus epidermidis* Isolated from Clinical Samples in a University Hospital of Isfahan City, Iran. *J. Clin. Diagn. Res.* **2017**, *11*, DC27. [CrossRef] [PubMed]

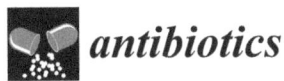

Article

Clinical and Economic Impact of Community-Onset Urinary Tract Infections Caused by ESBL-Producing *Klebsiella pneumoniae* Requiring Hospitalization in Spain: An Observational Cohort Study

Dawid Rozenkiewicz [1,2,3], Erika Esteve-Palau [1,2,3], Mar Arenas-Miras [1,2,3,4], Santiago Grau [3,4,5], Xavier Duran [6], Luisa Sorlí [1,2,3,4], María Milagro Montero [1,2,3,4] and Juan P. Horcajada [1,2,3,4,*]

1. Service of Infectious Diseases, Hospital del Mar, 08003 Barcelona, Spain; dawid.rozenkiewicz01@estudiant.upf.edu (D.R.); erika.esteve@pssjd.org (E.E.-P.); marenas@psmar.cat (M.A.-M.); lsorli@psmar.cat (L.S.); mmontero@psmar.cat (M.M.M.)
2. CEXS, Universitat Pompeu Fabra, Universitat Autònoma de Barcelona, 08003 Barcelona, Spain
3. Infectious Pathology and Antimicrobials Research Group (IPAR), Institut Hospital del Mar d'Investigacions Mèdiques (IMIM), 08003 Barcelona, Spain; sgrau@psmar.cat
4. REIPI, Instituto de Salud Carlos III (ISCIII), 28029 Madrid, Spain
5. Pharmacy Service, Hospital del Mar, 08003 Barcelona, Spain
6. Institut Hospital del Mar d'Investigacions Mèdiques (IMIM), 08003 Barcelona, Spain; xduran@imim.es
* Correspondence: jhorcajada@psmar.cat

Abstract: *Objective*: To analyze the clinical and economic impact of community-onset urinary tract infections (UTIs) caused by extended-spectrum beta-lactamase (ESBL)-producing *Klebsiella pneumoniae* requiring hospitalization. *Methods*: A retrospective cohort study that included all adults with a UTI caused by *K. pneumoniae* that were admitted to a tertiary care hospital in Barcelona, Spain, between 2011 and 2015. Demographic, clinical, and economic data were analyzed. *Results*: One hundred and seventy-three episodes of UTIs caused by *K. pneumoniae* were studied; 112 were non-ESBL-producing and 61 were ESBL-producing. Multivariate analysis identified ESBL production, acute confusional state associated with UTI, shock, and the time taken to obtain adequate treatment as risk factors for clinical failure during the first seven days. An economic analysis showed differences between ESBL-producing and non-ESBL-producing *K. pneumoniae* for the total cost of hospitalization per episode (mean EUR 6718 vs EUR 3688, respectively). Multivariate analysis of the higher costs of UTI episodes found statistically significant differences for ESBL production and the time taken to obtain adequate treatment. *Conclusion*: UTIs caused by ESBL-producing *K. pneumoniae* requiring hospitalization and the time taken to obtain adequate antimicrobial therapy are associated with worse clinical and economic outcomes.

Keywords: ESBL-producing *Klebsiella pneumoniae*; urinary tract infection; clinical impact; economic impact

1. Introduction

Extended-spectrum beta-lactamases (ESBLs) are enzymes produced by Gram-negative bacilli that inactivate oxyimino beta-lactam antibiotics (cephalosporins and aztreonam), but not cephamycins (cefoxitin) or carbapenems. They are generally plasmid-mediated and are derived from other enzymes with a narrower spectrum of hydrolysis. Al-though many species of Gram-negative bacilli can produce ESBLs, *Escherichia coli* and *Klebsiella pneumoniae* are the major ESBL producers. According to the WHO, ESBL-producing *Enterobacterales* must be regarded as critical priority pathogens due to their resistance to antibiotics [1]. ESBL-producing bacteria are a major cause of both community-based and healthcare-associated infections and are globally disseminated, although their incidence varies in different parts of the world [2]. An increase in community-acquired ESBL-producing

E. coli and *K. pneumoniae* has been recently reported [3]. *K. pneumoniae* is associated with pneumonia, urinary tract infections (UTIs), intra-abdominal infections and sepsis [4]. Data on the incidence of UTIs in Spain place *K. pneumoniae* as the second cause of UTIs of community and nosocomial origin [5].

ESBL-producing *K. pneumoniae* has been considered almost exclusively as a nosocomial pathogen due to its epidemiological behavior, although recent data show that it is also an important agent involved in processes of community origin [6]. Data from a multicenter study conducted in 11 hospitals in Spain from 2011 to 2016 showed an overall increase in ESBL-producing *K. pneumoniae*, compared to a similar study covering the 2002–2010 period, reaching a frequency of more than 18% in 2016. In that study, ESBLs were more prevalent in *K. pneumoniae* (16.3%) and *E. coli* (9.5%) isolates of nosocomial origin, followed by community-acquired *K. pneumoniae* (9.5%) [7].

Infections produced by ESBL-producing microorganisms pose important therapeutic challenges. The fact that ESBL-producing bacteria are resistant to all penicillins and cephalosporins, including third- and fourth-generation ones, means that infections due to these bacteria have limited therapeutic options [8]. As a result, infections caused by ESBL-producing bacteria can lead to increased mortality, an increased length of hospital stay, and higher hospital costs compared with infections caused by non-ESBL-producing bacteria of the same species [9,10]. The same phenomenon tends to be significantly stronger among patients with ESBL-producing *K. pneumoniae* infections compared with those with ESBL-producing *E. coli* infections [11].

A study was recently carried out to assess the clinical impact and consumption of health resources among patients with community-onset UTIs due to ESBL-producing *E. coli* admitted to our hospital. In that study, the presence of ESBL among *E. coli* strains was associated with higher clinical failure rates in the first seven days, as well as higher economic costs [12].

Bearing in mind that UTIs place an economic burden on both society and the healthcare system, that *K. pneumoniae* is a frequent cause of UTIs, and that ESBL-producing *Enterobacterales* cannot be considered a homogeneous group, the objective of this study was to analyze the clinical and economic impact of ESBL-producing *K. pneumoniae* as a cause of UTI in patients requiring admission to our hospital.

2. Results

One hundred and seventy-three UTI episodes met the criteria for inclusion during the study period and were included; 112 were due to non-ESBL-producing *K. pneumoniae* and 61 were due to ESBL-producing *K. pneumoniae*. The baseline characteristics of patients, broken down into those with and without ESBL infections, are shown in Table 1.

The bivariate analysis showed a significantly higher prevalence of men, AHA-UTIs, and previous antibiotic use (especially quinolones and cephalosporins) in the ESBL group. The clinical characteristics and procedures carried out on the studied patients, comparing ESBL and non-ESBL infections, are shown in Table 2. Among the admissions caused by ESBL-producing *K. pneumoniae*, there was a significantly higher clinical prevalence of cystitis; more frequent clinical failure at seven days; a longer time taken to obtain adequate treatment; longer hospitalization; and a more frequent use of infectious disease specialist consultants, pharmacy intervention, and home hospitalization. Among non-ESBL-producing *K. pneumoniae* infections, there was a more frequent use of adequate empirical antibiotics and a higher number of positive blood cultures, cases of pyelonephritis, and cases of sepsis.

Table 1. Univariate analysis of patient characteristics.

	Non-ESBL	ESBL	p-Value *
Total	112	61	
Sex, male	29 (25.9%)	28 (45.9%)	0.011
Age (in years)	72.8 ± 18.8	75.8 ± 12.1	0.200
AHA-UTI	34 (30.1%)	38 (63.3%)	<0.001
Diabetes mellitus	50 (44.6%)	30 (49.2%)	0.633
Dementia	28 (25%)	13 (21.3%)	0.709
Immunosuppressive treatment	40 (35.7%)	25 (41%)	0.515
McCabe Index	2.38 ± 0.67	2.4 ± 0.64	0.105
Charlson Comorbidity Index	6.02 ± 2.7	6.54 ± 2.12	0.198
Urinary catheterization	8 (7%)	10 (16.4%)	0.070
Other urinary catheters	9 (8%)	3 (4.9%)	0.543
Previous urological manipulation	16 (14.3%)	11 (18%)	0.519
Urological pathology	36 (32.1%)	22 (36.1%)	0.617
Kidney transplant	7 (6.3%)	2 (3.3%)	0.496
History of recurrent UTIs	39 (34.8%)	25 (41%)	0.510
History of pyelonephritis	16 (14.3%)	7 (11.5%)	0.648
Urinary incontinence	14 (12.5%)	14 (23%)	0.860
Previous antibiotic	38 (33.9%)	39 (63.9%)	<0.001
Amoxicillin/clavulanic acid	20 (17.9%)	10 (16.4%)	0.808
Trimethoprim/sulfamethoxazole	1 (0.9%)	2 (3.3%)	0.284
Quinolones	7 (6.3%)	10 (16.4%)	0.032
Fosfomycin	4 (3.6%)	3 (4.9%)	0.698
Cephalosporin	2 (1.8%)	6 (9.8%)	0.024
Carbapenems	1 (0.9%)	4 (6.6%)	0.053
Aminoglycosides	0 (0%)	1 (1.6%)	0.353
Linezolid	2 (1.8%)	1 (1.6%)	1.000
Others	1 (0.9%)	2 (3.3%)	0.284

* Student's t-test, or Mann–Whitney U was used for comparing quantitative variables. The Chi-square test was used for comparing qualitative variables. ESBL: extended spectrum betalactamases; AHA-UTI: ambulatory Health Care-Associated Urinary Tract Infection. HCA-UTI: Health Care-Associated Urinary Tract Infection. CA-UTI: Community-Acquired Urinary Tract Infection.

Table 2. Univariate analysis of clinical data.

	Non-ESBL	ESBL	p-Value *
Cystitis	17 (15.2%)	23 (37.7%)	0.001
Pyelonephritis	39 (34.8%)	12 (19.7%)	0.038
Confusion syndrome associated with UTIs	34 (30.4%)	21 (34.4%)	0.611
Prostatitis	6 (5.4%)	2 (3.3%)	0.714
Sepsis	40 (35.7%)	12 (19.7%)	0.037
Shock	6 (5.4%)	0 (0%)	0.091
Positive blood culture	45 (40.2%)	13 (21.3%)	0.012
Infectious diseases intervention	32 (28.6%)	43 (70.5%)	<0.001
Pharmacy intervention	9 (8%)	13 (21.3%)	0.017
Appropriate empirical treatment	104 (92.9%)	23 (37.7%)	<0.001
Time to adequate treatment (days)	0.54 ± 1.4	1.59 ± 2.1	<0.001
Duration of hospital treatment (days)	4.57 ± 2.64	4.06 ± 4.1	0.956
Clinical response at seven days	82 (73.2%)	31 (50.8%)	0.004
Days of hospitalization	8.43 ± 6.42	11.62 ± 7.1	0.003
Readmission for the same UTI	24 (21.4%)	17 (27.9%)	0.355
Emergency consultation [a]	25 (22.3%)	18 (29.5%)	0.358
Home hospitalization	5 (4.5%)	10 (16.4%)	0.011
ICU admission	6 (5.4%)	0 (0%)	0.091
Mortality within 30 days	12 (10.7%)	3 (4.9%)	0.263

[a] Re-consultation in the emergency room within 30 days after discharge; * Student's t-test or Mann–Whitney U was used for comparing quantitative variables. The Chi-square test was used for comparing qualitative variables. ESBL: extended spectrum betalactamases; ICU: intensive care unit.

In the non-ESBL-producing group, the most commonly used empiric antibiotics were cephalosporins (32.1%), amoxicillin/clavulanate (30.4%), and carbapenems (11.6%); adequate coverage was achieved in 92.9% of cases. In the ESBL-producing group, the most commonly used empiric treatments were amoxicillin/clavulanate (26.2%), cephalosporins (19.7%), and carbapenems (18%), and adequate coverage was achieved in only 37.7% of cases. The antibiotics most commonly used as directed therapy in the non-ESBL-producing group were ciprofloxacin (45.5%) and amoxicillin/clavulanate (19.6%), and, in the ESBL-producing group, ertapenem (45.6%) and imipenem (29.5%).

Table 3 shows the multivariate analysis of factors associated with clinical failure at seven days. ESBL production, the acute confusional state associated with a UTI, shock, and the time taken to obtain adequate therapy were factors independently associated with clinical failure at seven days.

An analysis of economic data can be found in Table 4. The analysis showed a mean difference of EUR 3.030 between the two groups for the total cost of hospitalization in favor of the ESBL-producing group. The costs associated with medication, nursing, and antibiotics accounted for this difference.

Table 5 shows the multivariate analysis of costs. The presence of ESBL, shock at admission, time taken to obtain adequate treatment, and the length of hospitalization were variables independently associated with higher hospitalization costs.

We performed a post-hoc power calculation to compare the median of the cost of hospitalization between non-ESBL and ESBL groups. The power of the study for comparing the costs was 1.0.

Table 3. Univariate and multivariate analysis of factors associated with clinical failure at seven days.

	OR (95%CI)	p-Value *	Adjusted OR	p-Value **
Sex, male	1.230 (0.626,2.415)	0.548	1.182 (0.501,2.785)	0.702
Age > 77	1.155 (0.886,1.505)	0.286	1.129 (0.856,1.487)	0.388
Infectious diseases intervention	1.676 (0.891,3.154)	0.109		
Pharmacy intervention	1.683 (0.681,4.161)	0.259		
Previous antibiotic	1.314 (0.700,2.465)	0.396	1.763 (0.756,4.114)	0.189
Immunosuppressive treatment	2.001 (1.052,3.805)	0.034		
Urinary catheterization	0.505 (0.159,1.609)	0.248		
Other catheters	0.157 (0.020,1.248)	0.080		
Previous urological manipulation	0.280 (0.092,0.851)	0.025		
Urological pathology	0.543 (0.270,1.089)	0.086		
History of recurrent UTIs	1.092 (0.572,2.084)	0.790		
Diabetes	0.679 (0.360,1.280)	0.231		
Urological neoplasms	0.176 (0.051,0.609)	0.006		
McCabe–Jackson Index > 2	0.899 (0.684,1.181)	0.446	1.108 (0.848,1.447)	0.451
Charlson Comobilidity Index > 5.8	1.062 (0.862,1.308)	0.571	1.695 (0.921,3.120)	0.090
Bacteremia	1.936 (1.006,3.724)	0.048	2.412 (0.351,16.538)	0.370
Cystitis	1.018 (0.485,2.138)	0.962	1.656 (0.562,4.877)	0.360
Pyelonephritis	0.410 (0.192,0.875)	0.021	0.782 (0.246,2.487)	0.678
Prostatitis	0 (0,0)	0.999		
Confusion syndrome associated with UTIs	2.215 (1.142,4.296)	0.019	5.155 (1.670,15.906)	0.004
Sepsis	2.275 (1.163,4.451)	0.016	3.758 (0.519,27.208)	0.190
Shock	3.964 (0.705,22.306)	0.118	7.239 (1.008,51.983)	0.049
ESBL	2.645 (1.376,5.084)	0.004	2.622 (1.086,6.328)	0.032
Time to adequate treatment	1.359 (1.092,1.692)	0.006	1.364 (1.059,1.755)	0.016
Appropriate empirical treatment	0.217 (0.106,0.443)	<0.001		
Duration of hospital treatment	1.285 (1.161,1.422)	<0.001		
CA-UTI	0.997 (0.528,1.881)	0.993		

* Univariate analysis: Student's t-test or Mann–Whitney U used for comparing quantitative variables. The Chi-square test was used for comparing qualitative variables. ** Multivariate analysis: binary logistic regression through the forward stepwise approach; ESBL: extended spectrum betalactamases; CA-UTI: Community-Acquired Urinary Tract Infection; OR: odds ratio.

Table 4. Univariate analysis of the economic impact of ESBL and non-ESBL-producing *K. pneumoniae* in Euros.

	Non-ESBL med[P$_{25}$,P$_{75}$]	ESBL med[P$_{25}$,P$_{75}$]	*p*-Value *
Cost of hospitalization	3688 [1783,4141]	6718 [3322,9611]	<0.001
Cost of pharmacy	457 [174,577]	888 [325,1158]	0.001
Cost of antibiotics	47 [7,31]	380 [87,544]	<0.001
Cost of nursery	1809 [880,2294]	4581 [2375,6630]	<0.001
Cost of laboratory	165 [39,201]	171 [81,192]	0.852
Cost of radiology	94 [0,111]	62 [1,72]	0.205
Cost of inter consultations	60 [0,33]	65 [0,71]	0.818
Cost of Emergency Room visits	341 [0,760]	463 [0,663]	0.218

* Student's *t*-test or Mann–Whitney U. ESBL: extended spectrum betalactamases; med: median; P$_{25}$:1st quartile; P$_{75}$:3rd quartile

Table 5. Univariate and multivariate analysis of the cost of the UTI episode.

	DM (95%CI)	*p*−Value *	Adjusted DM	*p*−Value **
ESBL	3446 (2330,4561)	<0.001	2569 (993,4144)	0.002
Sex, male	417 (−1126,1960)	0.594	−285 (−1578,1008)	0.663
Age > 77	−117 (−727,373)	0.526	−101 (−1578,1008)	0.602
Infectious diseases intervention	2718 (1582,3854)	<0.001		
Pharmacy intervention	2977 (814,5140)	0.007		
Previous antibiotic	957 (−592,2508)	0.224		
Immunosuppressive treatment	2304 (703,3904)	0.005		
Previous urological manipulation	−1202 (−3073,668)	0.206		
Urological pathology	−1353 (−2706,−1)	0.050		
History of recurrent UTIs	647 (−1013,2308)	0.442		
Urological neoplasms	−1648 (−3347,51)	0.057	−413 (−1953,1127)	0.596
McCabe–Jackson Index > 2	39 (−421,501)	0.865		
Charlson Comorbidity Index > 5.8	0.56 (−714,715)	0.999		
Bacteriemia	2031 (114,3949)	0.038	1617 (−762,3996)	0.181
Cystitis	1847 (115,3579)	0.037		
Pyelonephritis	401 (−1371,2173)	0.655		
Prostatitis	−1653 (−4984,1677)	0.328		
Sepsis	1772 (−144,3690)	0.070	−479 (−2944,1985)	0.701
Shock	8750 (4680,12820)	<0.001	6812 (3925,9699)	<0.001
Others	−413 (−2001,1174)	0.608		
Time to adequate treatment	612 (117,1107)	0.016	546 (82,1010)	0.021
Appropriate empirical treatment	−3552 (−4928,−2177)	<0.001	157 (−1635,1950)	0.862
Duration of hospital treatment	494 (298,629)	<0.001	266 (140,392)	<0.001
CA-UTI	−827 (−2371,717)	0.291	788 (−1101,1391)	0.818

* Univariate analysis: Student's *t*-test or Mann–Whitney U were used for comparing quantitative variables. The Chi-square test was used for comparing qualitative variables. ** Multivariate analysis: binary logistic regression through the forward stepwise approach; ESBLE: extended spectrum betalactamases; DM: difference between the median of the group that presents the variable and the median of the group that does not present it. The positivity of the value indicates an increase in the cost in the presence of the variable and the negativity decrease in the cost. CA-UTI: Community-Acquired Urinary Tract Infection.

3. Discussion

The present study showed that the clinical outcomes were worse and the hospital costs were higher for community-onset UTIs caused by ESBL-producing *K. pneumoniae* requiring hospitalization compared to the UTIs caused by non-ESBL-producing *K. pneumoniae*. These findings confirm that ESBL *Enterobacterales* are, as the WHO states, critical priority pathogens, adding more support for this argument. [1].

There are several risk factors for the acquisition of a UTI caused by ESBL-producing microorganisms, including healthcare contact, previous antibiotic use, recurrent UTIs, a urinary catheter, old age, and male gender [13]. Our study identified a higher prevalence of ambulatory healthcare-associated infections, previous antibiotic use, and male gender in the ESBL-producing group. Ambulatory healthcare-associated UTIs have previously been identified as more frequently caused by antibiotic-resistant microorganisms than community-acquired UTIs and have important clinical consequences [13]. Higher male gender prevalence could be attributed to the fact that UTIs in males tend to have more hospitalization criteria. These findings are similar to those from a recent study from Denmark [14].

There was a significant difference in the clinical response (22.4%) between the two groups, with lower response rates in the ESBL-producing group, similar to previous studies performed with *E. coli* [11]. A recent study was also carried out to assess the clinical impact and consumption of health resources among patients with community-onset UTIs due to ESBL-producing *E. coli* admitted to hospital. In that study, the presence of ESBL among *E. coli* strains was associated with higher clinical failure rates in the first seven days, as well as higher economic costs. Similar to the present study, in that study ESBL production was significantly related to clinical failure, and mean differences in the cost of hospitalization were EUR 2,368 [12]. Other variables associated with a worse clinical response were clinical presentation with a confusional state and shock. The time taken to obtain adequate antimicrobial therapy was also an independent factor associated with a worse clinical response. Previous studies have shown that patients who received adequate empirical treatment were more likely to have a better clinical course [15]. Hospital stay was significantly longer in ESBL-UTI patients. This is another important clinical consequence that could probably be avoided or reduced by improving initial or early antimicrobial management. Our data confirm that inadequate antimicrobial therapy is associated with a worse prognosis for patients with *K. pneumoniae* UTIs requiring hospital admission without differences in mortality. These findings are similar to those from a recent study from Denmark [16]. Infectious diseases specialist consultations or pharmacy interventions were more frequent in ESBL episodes. However, in the multivariate analysis of the clinical response at day 7, these interventions were not statistically significant, probably because they have an influence on the directed antimicrobial therapy, and not on the empirical therapy.

Interestingly, we observed that among patients with ESBL-producing *K. pneumoniae* infections, there was a higher prevalence of cystitis, whereas among patients with non-ESBL-producing *K. pneumoniae* UTIs clinical symptoms of pyelonephritis, positive blood cultures, sepsis, and ICU admission were more prevalent. These data seem to indicate a lower virulence in ESBL strains, a phenomenon that has already been reported in other studies involving *E. coli*, in which the acquisition of quinolone resistance was associated with a loss of virulence factors [17]. The relationship between resistance and bacterial virulence has also been studied in recent years. For instance, the acquisition by *E.coli* of the OXA-10, OXA-24 or SFO-1 family of beta-lactamases is known to be associated with a loss of virulence due to alterations in the formation of peptidoglycan, probably caused by residual enzymatic activity in the β-lactamases, similar to that of penicillin-binding proteins [18]. In the case of *K. pneumoniae*, there are studies describing the role of mechanisms such as the deletion of ompK36 and ompK36 porins in the loss of virulence and the acquisition of resistance [19]. Our cohort was comprised of community-acquired and ambulatory healthcare-associated UTIs, which are environments in which the selective pressure of antibiotics is not as high as in the nosocomial setting. It is likely that the loss of virulence in these environments due to the acquisition of resistance is better tolerated by microorganisms.

With respect to the economic impact, we showed that the total hospitalization costs associated with patients with ESBL-producing *K. pneumoniae* UTIs admitted to hospital were almost double those of patients with non-ESBL-producing *K. pneumoniae* UTIs. The cost of medication and the nursing costs accounted for the difference in total cost. The difference in medication cost was mainly due to the use of more expensive antibiotics such as carbapenems. The time taken to obtain adequate treatment was also identified as a variable related to the increased total cost of hospitalization and was probably an indirect effect of a worse clinical response, as seen in previous studies [9,12].

The main limitation of our study was its retrospective design. However, this design permitted the study of a higher number of patients in less time.

4. Materials and Methods

A retrospective cohort study was conducted from January 2011 to January 2016 at the Hospital del Mar, a tertiary university hospital with 420 beds serving a population of 340,000 people in the city of Barcelona (Spain). The study included all adults (older than 17 years) admitted to the Hospital del Mar during the study period with urinary tract infections and a urine culture that tested positive for *K. pneumoniae*. The only UTI origins considered were strictly community-acquired (CA) and ambulatory healthcare-associated (AHA). Hospital-acquired UTIs were excluded. In cases of multiple episodes requiring admission, only the first episode was studied. UTIs caused by microorganisms other than *K. pneumoniae*, cultures showing mixed flora, and patients with asymptomatic bacteriuria were excluded.

4.1. Variables

Patient data were collected retrospectively from hospital electronic medical records. The following variables were collected: demographic and epidemiological factors (age, gender, underlying diseases, use of immunosuppressive therapy, prior antibiotic treatment), clinical and microbiological data (UTI symptoms, sepsis, shock, empirical and definitive antibiotic treatment, time to obtain adequate treatment, clinical response at seven days, infectious diseases and/or pharmacy services interventions, ICU admission, emergency room visits after discharge, hospital readmissions, convalescent or subacute hospitalization after discharge, mortality at 30 days), and risk factors for ESBL-producing *K. pneumoniae* (urinary catheter, urological manipulation, urologic conditions, type of acquisition: community-acquired (CA) versus ambulatory healthcare-associated (AHA). The Charlson Index was used to classify comorbidities [20] and the McCabe–Jackson index was used to classify their severity [21]. The main variable used to analyze the clinical impact was clinical response seven days after admission. The variables selected to study the use of clinical resources were: duration of hospitalization, cost of hospitalization, use and cost of antibiotic treatment, emergency room visits, use of home hospitalization and the need for re-admission after 30 days. The costs of hospitalization were obtained from the hospital database and were broken down into cost of medication, cost of antibiotics, cost of nursing, laboratory costs, radiology costs, pharmacy costs, specialist consultations and emergency visits.

4.2. Definitions

A diagnosis of symptomatic UTI was established if the patient presented with one of the following signs or symptoms: a fever of >38 °C, urinary urgency, polyuria, dysuria or suprapubic pain, and a positive urine culture (more than 10^5 CFU of uropathogen per mL of urine). Five UTI syndromes were considered:

1. Cystitis: the presence of dysuria, urinary frequency, urgency and occasionally hematuria in patients without fever (axillary temperature < 38 °C).
2. Pyelonephritis: the presence of fever (axillary temperature > 38 °C) and spontaneous lumbar pain or pain on costovertebral percussion, with or without increased urinary frequency, dysuria or urine retention.
3. Acute prostatitis: a sudden febrile episode in men accompanied by lower back and perineal pain with polyuria or dysuria, and/or urinary retention.
4. The confusional state associated with UTIs was defined as an episode of confusion attributed to an underlying UTI after excluding other infectious foci and other causes.
5. Urinary sepsis: a systemic inflammatory response syndrome with a positive urine culture or blood culture for an uropathogen with no other apparent source of infection [22].

A CA-UTI was defined as a UTI detected within the first 48 h of hospital admission that did not meet the criteria for an AHA-UTI. An AHA-UTI was defined as a UTI detected within the first 48 h of hospital admission and met one of the following criteria [14]:

1. The patient had received specialized treatment at home by qualified healthcare workers within 30 days prior to hospital admission.
2. The patient had attended a day hospital, hemodialysis clinic or had received intravenous chemotherapy within 30 days prior to hospital admission.
3. Hospitalization for more than 48 h during the 90 days preceding the current admission.
4. Resident in a long-term care facility or nursing home.
5. The patient had undergone an invasive urinary procedure within 30 days of the episode or had a long-term indwelling urethral catheter.

A community-onset UTI was defined as any CA-UTI or AHA-UTI.

Previous antibiotic therapy was defined as the use of antibiotics in the three months prior to the diagnosis of a UTI. Empirical therapy was administered before the in vitro susceptibility of the uropathogen that caused the episode was known. Empirical therapy was considered inadequate if the microorganism causing the UTI was not fully susceptible to the antibiotic used.

The response to treatment at seven days was considered satisfactory if the patient was asymptomatic or there was a significant improvement in the signs and symptoms of infection; the treatment response was unsatisfactory if there was persistence or progression of signs and symptoms of infection, if a change in pharmacological agent was required after three days of treatment, or if an infection-related death occurred.

4.3. Statistical Analysis

Data from patients with and without ESBL-producing *K. pneumoniae* were compared. Quantitative variables were compared using the Student's *t*-test or the Mann–Whitney U test if the distribution of the data was not normal. Qualitative variables were compared using the Chi-square test. Bivariate and multivariate analyses were performed to elucidate the variables independently related to clinical failure at seven days and to higher hospital costs. The clinical response was analyzed by binary logistic regression. Multivariate median regression models were conducted through the forward stepwise approach. This was performed in terms of statistical signification of coefficients of variables ($p < 0.1$), but also to ensure clinical consistency of variables included in the model.

With respect to hospital costs, the normality of the variables was assessed by histogram inspection, testing for normality with a QQ-plot, and applying the Shapiro–Wilk W–test. Once non-normality was established ($p < 0.001$), hospital costs were analyzed by median regression. Associations with *p*-values < 0.05 were regarded as statistically significant. Statistical analyses were performed using the SPSS v.22 and STATA v.15.1 packages.

5. Conclusions

In conclusion, our study shows that the production of ESBL by *K. pneumoniae* causing community-onset UTIs and the time taken to obtain adequate antimicrobial therapy are independent factors for a worse clinical response and higher healthcare costs. It is important to identify risk factors in order to categorize these patients earlier so that they benefit from the appropriate empirical treatment that leads to a better clinical response and reduced hospitalization costs. Rapid diagnostic tests are also important in this scenario.

More studies of infections caused by multidrug-resistant bacteria in the community should be performed in order to prevent acquisition and optimize the management of infections in an attempt to reduce their clinical and economic burden.

Author Contributions: Conceptualization: J.P.H.; methodology: J.P.H., E.E.-P., D.R.; validation, J.P.H., E.E.-P., L.S., M.M.M., S.G.; formal analysis: X.D., J.P.H.; investigation: D.R., E.E.-P.; data curation: D.R., X.D.; writing—original draft preparation: D.R., J.P.H.; writing—review and editing: M.A.-M., J.P.H., L.S., M.M.M., S.G.; supervision: J.P.H. All authors have read and agreed to the published version of the manuscript.

Funding: This research did not receive any specific grant from funding agencies in the public, commercial, or not-for-profit sectors.

Institutional Review Board Statement: The study was conducted in accordance with the Declaration of Helsinki and the protocol was approved by the Ethics for Clinical Research (Nr. 2016/6572/I)) of the IMIM-Parc de Salut MAR, Barcelona, Spain. The study followed legal regulations on the confidentiality of data (Spanish Organic Law 15/1999 of 13 December on the Protection of Personal Data [LOPD]).

Informed Consent Statement: Informed consent was waived due to the retrospective observational nature of the study.

Data Availability Statement: Not applicable.

Conflicts of Interest: J.P.H. has received honoraria for speaker activities and advisory boards from MSD, Pfizer, Angelini, Menarini. All the other authors declare no conflict of interest.

References

1. WHO Publishes List of Bacteria for Which New Antibiotics Are Urgently Needed. Available online: https://www.who.int/news/item/27-02-2017-who-publishes-list-of-bacteria-for-which-new-antibiotics-are-urgently-needed (accessed on 9 May 2021).
2. Paterson, D.L.; Bonomo, R.A. Extended-spectrum beta-lactamases: A clinical update. *Clin. Microbiol. Rev.* 2005, *18*, 657–686. [CrossRef]
3. Richelsen, R.; Smit, J.; Anru, P.L.; Schønheyder, H.C.; Nielsen, H. Incidence of community-onset extended-spectrum β-lactamase-producing Escherichia coli and Klebsiella pneumoniae infections: An 11-year population-based study in Denmark. *Infect. Dis.* 2020, *52*, 547–556. [CrossRef]
4. Podschun, R.; Ullmann, U. Klebsiella spp. as nosocomial pathogens: Epidemiology, taxonomy, typing methods, and pathogenicity factors. *Clin. Microbiol. Rev.* 1998, *11*, 589–603. [CrossRef]
5. Cantón, R.; Loza, E.; Aznar, J.; Castillo, F.J.; Cercenado, E.; Fraile-Ribot, P.A.; Gonzalez-Romo, F.; Lopez-Hontangas, J.L.; Rodriguez-Lozano, J.; Suarez-Barrenechea, A.I.; et al. Monitoring the antimicrobial susceptibility of Gram-negative organisms involved in intraabdominal and urinary tract infections recovered during the SMART study (Spain, 2016 and 2017). *Rev. Esp. Quimioter.* 2019, *32*, 145–155. [PubMed]
6. Boix-Palop, L.; Xercavins, M.; Badia, C.; Obradors, M.; Riera, M.; Freixas, N.; Perez, J.; Rodriguez-Carballeira, M.; Garau, J.; Calbo, E. Emerging extended-spectrum β-lactamase-producing Klebsiella pneumoniae causing community-onset urinary tract infections: A case–control–control study. *Int. J. Antimicrob. Agents* 2017, *50*, 197–202. [CrossRef] [PubMed]
7. Cantón, R.; Loza, E.; Aznar, J.; Barrón-Adúriz, R.; Calvo, J.; Castillo, F.J.; Cercenado, E.; Cisterna, R.; González-Romo, F.; López-Hontangas, J.L.; et al. Antimicrobial susceptibility trends and evolution of isolates with extended spectrum β-lactamases among Gram-negative organisms recovered during the SMART study in Spain (2011–2015). *Rev. Esp. Quimioter.* 2018, *31*, 136–145.
8. Paterson, D.L. Recommendation for treatment of severe infections caused by Enterobacteriaceae producing extended-spectrum-lactamases (ESBLs). *Clin. Microbiol. Infect.* 2000, *6*, 460–463. [CrossRef] [PubMed]
9. MacVane, S.H.; Tuttle, L.O.; Nicolau, D.P. Impact of extended-spectrum B-lactamase-producing organisms on clinical and economic outcomes in patients with urinary tract infection. *J. Hosp. Med.* 2014, *4*, 232–238. [CrossRef]
10. Lautenbach, E.; Patel, J.B.; Bilker, W.B.; Edelstein, P.H.; Fishman, N.O. Extended-spectrum beta-lactamase-producing Escherichia coli and Klebsiella pneumoniae: Risk factors for infection and impact of resistance on outcomes. *Clin. Infect. Dis.* 2001, *32*, 1162–1171. [CrossRef]
11. Scheuerman, O.; Schechner, V.; Carmeli, Y.; Gutiérrez-Gutiérrez, B.; Calbo, E.; Almirante, B.; Viale, P.; Oliver, A.; Ruiz-Garbajosa, P.; Gasch, O.; et al. Comparison of Predictors and Mortality Between Bloodstream Infections Caused by ESBL-Producing Escherichia coli and ESBL-Producing Klebsiella pneumoniae. *Infect. Control Hosp. Epidemiol.* 2018, *39*, 660–667. [CrossRef] [PubMed]
12. Esteve Palau, E.; Solande, G.; Sánchez, F.; Sorlí, L.; Montero, M.; Güerri, R.; Villar, J.; Grau, S.; Horcajada, J.P. Clinical and economic impact of urinary tract infections caused by ESBL-producing Escherichia coli requiring hospitalization: A matched cohort study. *J. Infect.* 2015, *71*, 667–674. [CrossRef] [PubMed]
13. Horcajada, J.P.; Shaw, E.; Padilla, B.; Pintado, V.; Calbo, E.; Benito, N.; Gamallo, R.; Gozalo, M.; Rodriguez-Bano, J.; ITUBRAS group; et al. Healthcare-associated, community-acquired and hospital-acquired bacteraemic urinary tract infections in hospitalized patients: A prospective multicentre cohort study in the era of antimicrobial resistance. *Clin. Microbiol. Infect.* 2013, *19*, 962–968. [CrossRef]

14. Richelsen, R.; Smit, J.; Laxsen Anru, P.; Schønheyder, H.C.; Nielsen, H. Risk factors of community-onset extended-spectrum β-lactamase *Escherichia coli* and *Klebsiella pneumoniae* bacteraemia: An 11-year population-based case-control-control study in Denmark. *Clin. Microbiol. Infect.* **2020**, S1198–S1743.
15. Lee, S.Y.; Kotapati, S.; Kuti, J.L.; Nightingale, C.H.; Nicolau, D.P. Impact of extended-spectrum beta-lactamase-producing Escherichia coli and Klebsiella species on clinical outcomes and hospital costs: A matched cohort study. *Infect. Control Hosp. Epidemiol.* **2006**, *27*, 1226–1232. [CrossRef] [PubMed]
16. Richelsen, R.; Smit, J.; Schønheyder, H.C.; Laxsen Anru, P.; Gutiérrez-Gutiérrez, B.; Rodríguez-Baño, J.; Nielsen, H. Outcome of community-onset ESBL-producing Escherichia coli and Klebsiella pneumoniae bacteraemia and urinary tract infection: A population-based cohort study in Denmark. *J. Antimicrob. Chemother.* **2020**, *75*, 3656–3664. [CrossRef] [PubMed]
17. Horcajada, J.P.; Soto, S.; Gajewski, A.; Smithson, A.; de Anta, M.T.J.; Mensa, J.; Vila, J.; Johnson, J.R. Quinolone-Resistant Uropathogenic Escherichia coli Strains from Phylogenetic Group B2 Have Fewer Virulence Factors than Their Susceptible Counterparts. *J. Clin. Microbiol.* **2005**, *43*, 2962–2964. [CrossRef]
18. Fernández, A.; Pérez, A.; Ayala, J.A.; Mallo, S.; Rumbo-Feal, S.; Tomas, M.; Poza, M.; Bou, G. Expression of OXA-type and SFO-1 beta-lactamases induces changes in peptidoglycan composition and affects bacterial fitness. *Antimicrob. Agents Chemother.* **2012**, *56*, 1877–1884. [CrossRef]
19. Tsai, Y.K.; Fung, C.P.; Lin, J.C.; Chen, J.; Chang, F.; Chen, T.; Siu, L.K. Klebsiella pneumoniae Outer Membrane Porins OmpK35 and OmpK36 Play Roles in both Antimicrobial Resistance and Virulence. *Antimicrob. Agents Chemother.* **2011**, *55*, 1485–1493. [CrossRef] [PubMed]
20. Charlson, M.E.; Pompei, P.; Ales, K.L.; MacKenzie, C.R. A new method of classifying prognostic comorbidity in longitudinal studies: Development and validation. *J. Chronic Dis.* **1987**, *40*, 373–383. [CrossRef]
21. McCabe, W.R. Gram-negative bacteremia. *Adv. Intern Med.* **1974**, *19*, 135–158. [PubMed]
22. Levy, M.M.; Fink, M.P.; Marshall, J.C.; Abraham, E.; Angus, D.; Cook, D.; Cohen, J.; Opal, S.M.; Vincent, J.; Ramsay, G. 2001 SCCM/ESICM/ACCP/ATS/SIS International Sepsis Definitions Conference. *Crit. Care Med.* **2003**, *31*, 1250–1256. [CrossRef] [PubMed]

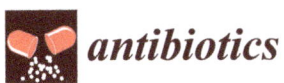

Article

Heterogeneity of Antibiotics Multidrug-Resistance Profile of Uropathogens in Romanian Population

Răzvan-Cosmin Petca [1,2,†], Silvius Negoiță [1,3,†], Cristian Mareș [1,2,*], Aida Petca [1,4,*], Răzvan-Ionuț Popescu [1,2] and Călin Bogdan Chibelean [5,6]

[1] "Carol Davila" University of Medicine and Pharmacy, 8 Eroii Sanitari Blvd., 050474 Bucharest, Romania; drpetca@gmail.com (R.-C.P.); silvius.negoita@umfcd.ro (S.N.); dr.razvanp@gmail.com (R.-I.P.)
[2] Department of Urology, "Prof. Dr. Th. Burghele" Clinical Hospital, 20 Panduri Str., 050659 Bucharest, Romania
[3] Department of Anesthesiology and Critical Care, Elias University Hospital, 17 Marasti Blvd., 011461 Bucharest, Romania
[4] Department of Obstetrics and Gynecology, Elias University Hospital, 17 Marasti Blvd., 011461 Bucharest, Romania
[5] George Emil Palade University of Medicine, Pharmacy, Science, and Technology of Targu-Mures, 38 Gheorghe Marinescu Str., 540139 Targu-Mures, Romania; calin.chibelean@umfst.ro
[6] Department of Urology, Mureș County Hospital, 1st Gheorghe Marinescu Str., 540136 Targu-Mures, Romania
* Correspondence: dr.marescristian@gmail.com (C.M.); aida.petca@umfcd.ro (A.P.); Tel.: +40-745-383-552 (C.M.); +40-745-787-448 (A.P.)
† These authors contributed equally to this work.

Abstract: Urinary tract infections (UTIs) are a leading cause of morbidity for both males and females. The overconsumption of antibiotics in general medicine, veterinary, or agriculture has led to a spike in drug-resistant microorganisms; obtaining standardized results is imposed by standard definitions for various categories of drug-resistant bacteria—such as multiple-drug resistant (MDR), extensive drug-resistant (XDR), and pan drug-resistant (PDR). This retrospective study conducted in three university teaching hospitals in Romania has analyzed urine probes from 15,231 patients, of which 698 (4.58%) presented multidrug-resistant strains. *Escherichia coli* was the leading uropathogen 283 (40.54%), presenting the highest resistance to quinolones (R = 72.08%) and penicillin (R = 66.78%) with the most important patterns of resistance for penicillin, sulfonamides, and quinolones (12.01%) and aminoglycosides, aztreonam, cephalosporins, and quinolones (9.89%). *Klebsiella* spp. followed—260 (37.24%) with the highest resistance to amoxicillin-clavulanate (R = 94.61%) and cephalosporins (R = 94.23%); the leading patterns were observed for aminoglycosides, aminopenicillins + β-lactams inhibitor, sulfonamides, and cephalosporins (12.69%) and aminoglycosides, aztreonam, cephalosporins, quinolones (9.23%). The insufficient research of MDR strains on the Romanian population is promoting these findings as an important tool for any clinician treating MDR-UTIs.

Keywords: urinary tract infections; UTIs; MDR; *Escherichia coli*; *Klebsiella*; uropathogens; AMR; antibiotic resistance

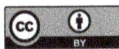

1. Introduction

Urinary tract infections (UTIs) represent a common disorder treated by urologists and general medical practitioners, accounting for an important percentage of the yearly healthcare costs [1]. Most UTIs are treated on ambulatory patients [2]. However, the increasing resistance to the first-line antibiotic treatment [3–5] and the rising quota of this condition [6] have urged the research of new lines of therapy. In practice, we must combine updated data on uropathogens' resistance profiles and sensibility rates of antimicrobial agents used in the treatment of UTIs.

Several factors are linked to promoting the increasing spread of bacterial resistance to antibiotics in community settings. The most important vector of increasing resistance is represented by the overuse of antimicrobials in general medicine, veterinary, or agriculture, which enables the selection and spread of drug-resistant strains [7]. Other risk factors are host-related; an extensive review of the literature [8] aiming to detect the risk factors associated with multidrug-resistance (MDR) UTIs has highlighted 12 possible factors:

- Probable factors: urinary catheterization, previous hospitalization, previous antibiotic treatment, nursing home resident;
- Possible risk factor: age, previous UTI, male gender;
- Unlikely risk factors: diabetes, recent travel, ethnicity, immunocompromised, female gender.

International assemblies of heads of departments from international specialized forums such as the European Center for Disease Prevention and Control (Stockholm, Sweden), Office of Infectious Diseases, Department of Health and Human Services from Center for Disease Prevention and Control (Atlanta, GA, USA), and Division of Epidemiology, Tel Aviv Sourasky Medical Center (Tel Aviv, Israel) [9] proposed standard definitions for various categories of drug-resistant bacteria. These are classified as [9]:

- "multiple drug-resistant" (MDR)—nonsusceptible to one or more antibiotic agent in three or more antimicrobial categories,
- "extensive" or "extremely" drug-resistant (XDR)—nonsusceptible to one or more antibiotic agents in all but two or less antimicrobial classes, and
- "pan drug-resistant"(PDR)—nonsusceptible to all antimicrobial agents listed.

They admitted that a better understanding of highly resistant bacterial strains and obtaining comparability data would be facilitated if these definitions were applied worldwide.

The European Association of Urology (EAU) via EAU Guidelines on Urological Infections from 2020 [10] recommends empirical treatment of uncomplicated urological infections using sulfonamides (TMP-SMX), phosphonic acids (fosfomycin), or nitrofurantoin. Fluoroquinolones (ciprofloxacin and levofloxacin) may be used only as an alternative therapy while also considering locoregional resistance rates. Carbapenems (imipenem and meropenem) should be used only as reserved therapy or in special conditions such as urosepsis.

This study aimed to determine the resistance profiles of the most frequent multidrug-resistant uropathogen strains involved in UTIs on a Romanian male and female cohort. The preliminary data [11] have shown *Escherichia coli* as the most frequent bacteria (42.9%) implicated in UTIs, followed by *Klebsiella* spp. (21.17%), *Enterococcus* spp. (18.66%), *Proteus* spp. (7.75%), *Staphylococcus* spp. (4.91%), and *Pseudomonas aeruginosa* (4.58%). The limited number of MDR strains studied in previous research, the necessity of determining specific resistance patterns for each bacteria against common antibiotic classes in treating UTIs, and comparing the results with the international findings were the decisive factors in initiating the study.

2. Results

A total number of 698 cases of MDR-UTIs were registered in all three centers during research, as follows: 262 patients (37.53%) at "Prof. Dr. Th Burghele" Clinical Hospital (BCH), 278 cases (39.82%) at Elias University Hospital (EUH), and 158 samples (22.63%) at Mures County Hospital (MCH). A detailed report on MDR-UTIs uropathogen distributions for each center is presented in Table 1 and Figure 1.

Table 1. MDR isolated uropathogens.

Isolated Bacteria	BCH		EUH		MCH		Total	
	n	%	n	%	n	%	n	%
Gram negative	226	86.25	266	95.68	152	96.20	644	92.26
Escherichia coli	75	28.62	109	39.20	99	62.65	283	40.54
Klebsiella spp.	114	43.51	111	39.92	35	22.15	260	37.24
Pseudomonas aeruginosa	20	7.63	29	10.43	11	6.96	60	8.59
Proteus spp.	17	6.48	17	6.11	7	4.43	41	5.87
Gram positive	36	13.74	12	4.31	6	3.79	54	7.73
Enterococcus spp.	13	4.96	11	3.95	6	3.79	30	4.29
Staphylococcus spp.	23	8.77	1	0.35	-	-	24	3.43

n—number, %—percentage, BCH—Burghele Clinical Hospital, EUH—Elias University Hospital, and MCH—Mures County Hospital.

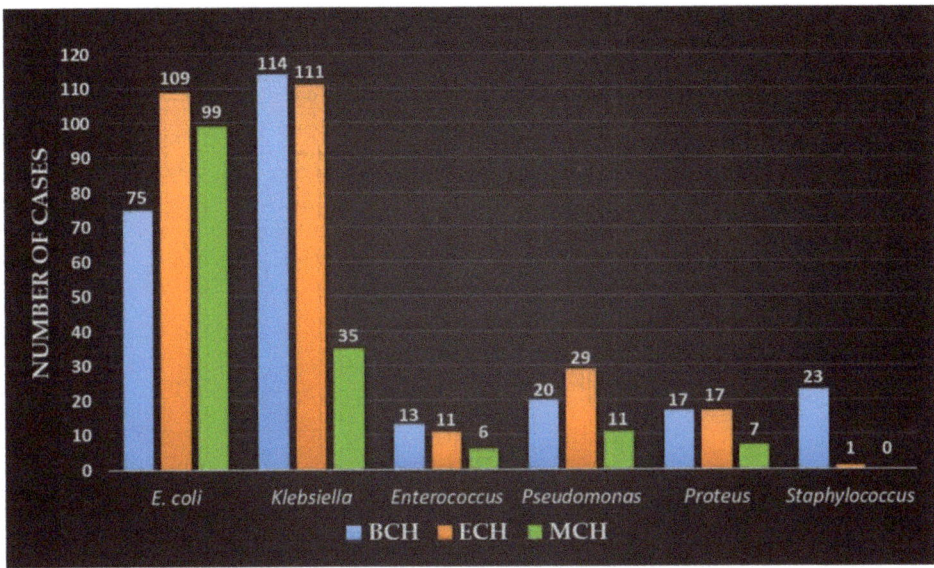

Figure 1. Distribution of the MDR uropathogens in the study centers.

Except for BCH center, where *Klebsiella* spp. (43.51%) surpassed *E. coli* (28.62%) in prevalence, the rest of the Gram-negative uropathogens respected the distribution in all subjects. Overall, *Enterococcus* spp. was the most incriminated Gram-positive bacterial strain, except for the BCH center, where *Staphylococcus* spp. surpassed it in prevalence; in the EUH center, a single strain of MDR-*Staphylococcus* spp. was detected; as for the MCH center, none of these pathogens were registered.

In terms of age-group distribution, both males and females showed an increased prevalence at the lower pole of the distribution axis with 6.45% females and 6.68% males in their 18–29 years. We noted a progressive increase in MDR-UTIs with every decade of life. This highlights the correlation between age and incidence of UTIs; a high quota was observed in seniors between 60–69, representing 24.73% in females and 30.07% in males, with a peak of incidence in patients over 70 years old—48.28% in the overall population. Detailed data on age-group distribution is displayed in Table 2.

Table 2. Female and male age group distribution of the MDR uropathogens.

Age Groups (Years)	Females		Males		Total	
	n	%	n	%	n	%
18–29	18	6.45	28	6.68	46	6.59
30–39	14	5.01	9	2.14	23	3.29
40–49	16	5.73	15	3.57	31	4.44
50–59	33	11.82	33	7.87	66	9.45
60–69	69	24.73	126	30.07	195	27.93
≥70	129	46.23	208	49.64	337	48.28

n—number and %—percentage.

E. coli, the most frequent microbial strain, showed the highest resistance rate (R) to quinolones-levofloxacin—72.08%, followed by penicillin-ampicillin—66.78%, cephalosporins-ceftazidime—60.07%, and aminopenicillins + β lactamase-amoxicillin-clavulanate—56.89%. A good sensitivity (S) was observed for fosfomycin—83.74%, followed by amikacin—66.78% and nitrofurantoin—39%.

Detailed information of each Gram-negative bacterial strains, including resistance and sensitivity profiles and overall statistics, are included in Figure 2 and Table 3.

Klebsiella ranked as the second-most common uropathogen in the study. It showed an outstanding resistance to all antibiotic classes, led by amoxicillin-clavulanate—94.61%, followed by ceftazidime—94.23%, levofloxacin—63.84%, and amikacin—53.07%. No good sensitivity was observed for either of the tested antibiotics. None of them showed resistance below 10%. The lowest resistance was obtained for fosfomycin—15.75%, nitrofurantoin—21.92%, and carbapenems—imipenem and meropenem—21.15% and 23.46%, respectively.

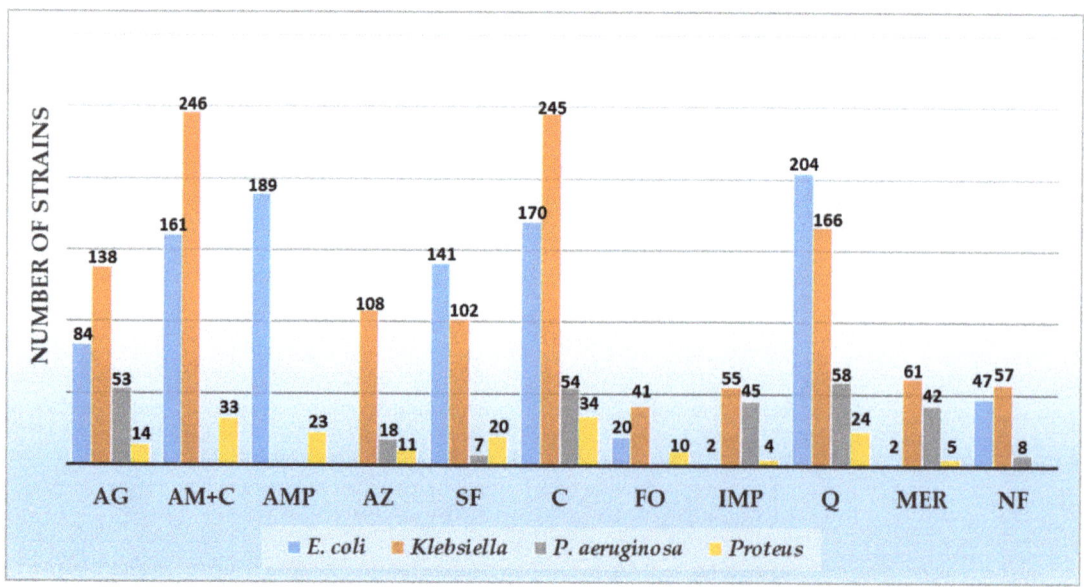

Figure 2. Gram-negative uropathogen resistance profiles (AG—aminoglycosides, AM + C—amoxicillin + clavulanic ac., AMP—ampicillin, AZ—aztreonam, SF—sulfonamides, C—cephalosporins, FO—Fosfomycin, IMP—imipenem, Q—quinolones, MER—meropenem, and NF—nitrofurantoin).

Table 3. Gram-negative uropathogen resistance profiles.

Antibiotics	Gram-Negative Organisms Isolated														
	Escherichia coli			*Klebsiella* spp.			*Pseudomonas aeruginosa*			*Proteus* spp.			Total		
	R	S	NA	R	S	NA	R	S	NA	R	S	NA	R	S	NA
	n (%)	*n* (%)	*n* (%)	*n* (%)	*n* (%)	*n* (%)	*n* (%)	*n* (%)	*n* (%)	*n* (%)	*n* (%)	*n* (%)	*n* (%)	*n* %	*n* %
Amikacin	84 (29.68)	189 (66.78)	10 (3.53)	138 (53.07)	120 (46.15)	2 (0.76)	53 (88.33)	6 (10.0)	1 (1.66)	14 (34.14)	27 (65.85)	-	289 (44.87)	342 (53.1)	13 (2.01)
Amoxicillin-Clavulanic ac.	161 (56.89)	114 (40.28)	8 (2.82)	246 (94.61)	11 (4.23)	3 (1.15)	-	-	-	33 (80.48)	7 (17.07)	1 (2.43)	440 (75.34)	132 (22.6)	12 (2.05)
Ampicillin	189 (66.78)	6 (2.12)	88 (31.09)	-	-	-	-	-	-	23 (56.09)	2 (4.87)	16 (39.02)	212 (65.43)	8 (2.46)	104 (32.09)
Aztreonam	-	-	-	108 (41.53)	3 (1.15)	149 (57.3)	18 (30.0)	2 (3.33)	40 (66.66)	11 (26.82)	6 (14.63)	24 (58.53)	137 (37.95)	11 (3.04)	213 (59.0)
Trimethoprim/Sulfamethoxazole	141 (49.82)	58 (20.49)	84 (29.68)	102 (39.23)	35 (13.46)	123 (47.3)	7 (11.66)	1 (1.66)	52 (86.66)	20 (48.78)	4 (9.75)	17 (41.46)	270 (41.92)	98 (15.21)	276 (42.85)
Ceftazidime	170 (60.07)	101 (35.68)	12 (4.24)	245 (94.23)	14 (5.38)	1 (0.38)	54 (90.0)	6 (10.0)	0	34 (82.92)	6 (14.63)	1 (2.43)	503 (78.10)	127 (19.72)	14 (2.17)
Fosfomycin	20 (7.06)	237 (83.74)	26 (9.18)	41 (15.76)	60 (23.07)	159 (61.15)	-	-	-	10 (24.39)	6 (14.63)	25 (60.97)	71 (12.15)	303 (51.88)	210 (35.95)
Imipenem	2 (0.7)	81 (28.62)	200 (70.67)	55 (21.15)	136 (52.3)	69 (26.53)	45 (75.0)	6 (10.0)	9 (15.0)	4 (9.75)	12 (29.26)	25 (60.97)	106 (16.45)	235 (36.49)	303 (47.04)
Levofloxacin	204 (72.08)	47 (16.6)	32 (11.30)	166 (63.84)	68 (26.15)	26 (10.0)	58 (96.66)	1 (1.66)	1 (1.66)	24 (58.53)	10 (24.39)	7 (17.07)	452 (70.18)	126 (19.56)	66 (10.24)
Meropenem	2 (0.7)	86 (30.38)	195 (68.90)	61 (23.46)	145 (55.76)	54 (20.76)	42 (70.0)	10 (16.66)	8 (13.33)	5 (12.19)	27 (65.85)	9 (21.95)	110 (17.08)	268 (41.61)	266 (41.3)
Nitrofurantoin	47 (16.6)	111 (39.22)	125 (44.16)	57 (21.92)	38 (14.61)	165 (63.46)	8 (13.33)	5 (8.33)	47 (78.33)	-	-	-	112 (18.57)	154 (25.53)	337 (55.88)

n—number, %—percentage; R—resistant, S—sensitive, and NA—not available.

The third-most frequent uropathogen, *P. aeruginosa*, shows almost complete resistance in MDR strains to quinolones-levofloxacin—96.66%; alarmingly, a high resistance is also observed for cephalosporins-ceftazidime—88.33%, followed by aminoglycosides-amikacin—88.33%. Surprisingly, the resistance to carbapenems in MDR *P. aeruginosa* is the highest in all pathogens for this antimicrobial class, accounting for imipenem—75% and meropenem—70%.

Proteus spp. is considered a nosocomial uropathogen, consistently discovered in patients presenting complicated UTIs. *Protea* (a group of pathogens including *Proteus, Providentia,* and *Morganella* spp.) are naturally resistant to colistin and nitrofurantoin and have raised resistance to carbapenems [12]. Our study discovered lower resistance rates than other Gram-negative bacteria, showing the highest resistance profile to ceftazidime—82.92%, followed by amoxicillin-clavulanate—80.48%, levofloxacin—58.53%, and ampicillin—56.09%. Relatively preserved sensitivity was observed for amikacin and meropenem—both 65.85%.

Both Gram-positive bacteria in this study make up for less than 10% of the total strains: *Staphylococcus* spp.—3.43% and *Enterococcus* spp.—4.29%; in both cases, the highest resistance was observed for quinolones (*Staphylococcus* spp.—91.66% and *Enterococcus* spp.—63.33%) and penicillin (*Staphylococcus* spp.—83.33% and *Enterococcus* spp.—70.0%).

The most frequent association of antimicrobial classes involved in common MDR strains was represented by amoxicillin-clavulanate, aztreonam, cephalosporins, and quinolones in 56 isolates (8.02%), followed by aminoglycosides, amoxicillin + clavulanate, sulfonamides, and cephalosporins in 5.01%; penicillin, sulfonamides, and quinolones in 4.87%; and aminoglycosides, amoxicillin + clavulanate, aztreonam, cephalosporins, carbapenems, and quinolones in 4.01%. Detailed outcomes of the 10th-most common MDR strain resistance patterns can be found in Table 4.

Table 4. Most common MDR profiles.

Antibiotics	n (%)
Amoxicillin + Clavulanate, Aztreonam, Cephalosporins, Quinolones	56 (8.02)
Aminoglycosides, Amoxicillin + Clavulanate, Sulfonamides, Cephalosporins	35 (5.01)
Penicillin, Sulfonamides, Quinolones	34 (4.87)
Aminoglycosides, Amoxicillin + Clavulanate, Aztreonam, Cephalosporins, Carbapenems, Quinolones	28 (4.01)
Amoxicillin + Clavulanate, Aztreonam, Cephalosporins, Quinolones, Nitrofurantoin	21 (3.0)
Aminoglycosides, Amoxicillin + Clavulanate, Aztreonam, Cephalosporins, Quinolones	19 (2.72)
Aminoglycosides, Penicillin, Cephalosporins	17 (2.43)
Aminoglycosides, Sulfonamides, Cephalosporins	14 (2.0)
Penicillin, Cephalosporins, Quinolones	12 (1.71)
Aminoglycosides, Cephalosporins, Carbapenems, Quinolones	11 (1.57)

n—number and %—percentage.

The resistance profile for *E. coli* and *Klebsiella* presented similarities, as well as noticeable differences, in the results. For *E. coli*, a high resistance to various combinations can be observed, such as penicillin, sulfonamides, and quinolones ($n = 34$ strains); aminoglycosides, aztreonam, cephalosporins, and quinolones ($n = 28$ strains); and aminoglycosides, aminopenicillins + β-lactams inhibitor, aztreonam, cephalosporins, and quinolones ($n = 9$ strains)—Figure 3.

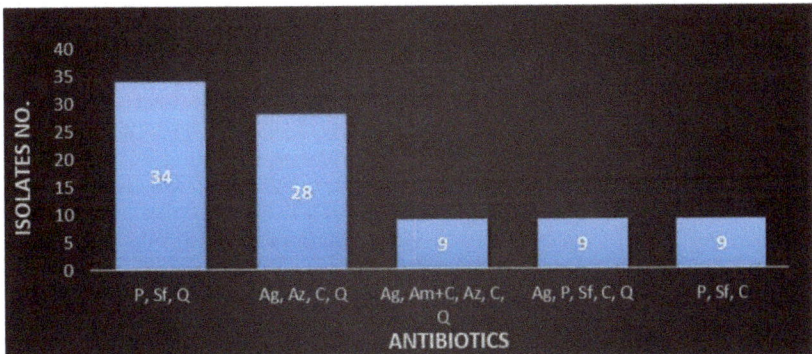

Figure 3. *Escherichia coli* resistance profiles of MDR strains (Ag—aminoglycosides, Am + C—aminopenicillins + β-lactams inhibitor, Az—aztreonam, C—cephalosporins, P—penicillin, Q—quinolones, and Sf—sulfonamides).

Klebsiella spp. revealed resistance to aminoglycosides, aminopenicillins + β-lactams inhibitor, sulfonamides, and cephalosporins (n = 33 strains), followed by aminoglycosides, aztreonam, cephalosporins, and quinolones (n = 24 strains) and aminoglycosides, aminopenicillins + β-lactams inhibitor, aztreonam, cephalosporins, carbapenems, and quinolones (n = 18 strains)—Figure 4. *E. coli* proved resistant mostly to penicillin and quinolones, while *Klebsiella* spp. to aminoglycosides, the aminopenicillins+ β-lactams inhibitor, or even carbapenems.

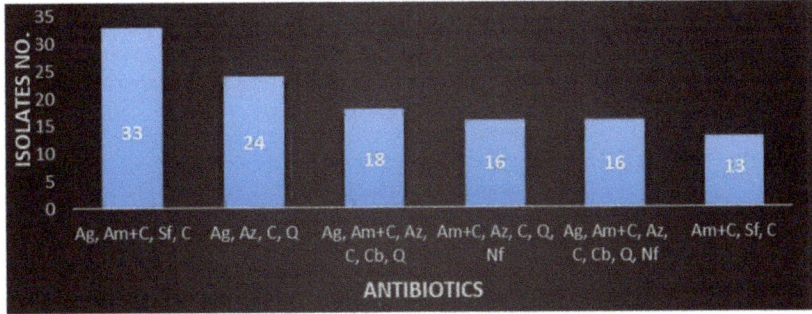

Figure 4. *Klebsiella* spp. resistance profiles of MDR strains (Ag—aminoglycosides, Am + C—aminopenicillins + β-lactams inhibitor, Az—aztreonam, C—cephalosporins, Cb—carbapenems, Nf—nitrofurantoin, Q—quinolones, and Sf—sulfonamides).

E. coli proved resistant mostly to penicillin and quinolones, while *Klebsiella* spp. to aminoglycosides, the aminopenicillins+ β -lactams inhibitor, or even carbapenems.

3. Discussion

Infections located in the urinary tract are a common cause of urological treatment among the general population. Moreover, acquiring a bacterial strain that shows resistance to multiple antimicrobial agents in use overlaps the primary morbidity of UTIs alone, leading to an excessively dangerous disease that in the absence of prompt and adequate treatment, can cause lots of problems. Due to overuse of antibiotics in various fields, such as general medicine, veterinary, or agriculture, an alarming increase of MDR strains among uropathogens was detected; taking into account the lack of locoregional data on MDR-UTIs incidence and resistance patterns, results from a six-month multicenter "cross-sectional" retrospective study are provided.

3.1. MDR Uropathogens in Relation with Patients Age

Throughout the entire cohort of patients, one could see a general trend of progressive growth in MDR-UTIs with every decade of life. This highlights the correlation between age and incidence of UTIs, just like Rowe et al. [13] summarized in a literature review. A high quota was observed in seniors between 60–69 years old, representing 24.73% in females and 30.07% in males, with a peak of incidence in patients over 70 years old—48.28% in the overall population. It has been shown that multiple risk factors are associated with the prevalence of UTIs in the elderly male population, such as prostate enlargement, urolithiasis, urinary tract neoplasia, renal failure, or urethral strictures [14,15].

In the elderly female population, various risk factors are associated with UTIs. The studies performed by Hu et al. [16], Brown et al. [17], and a literature review from Mody et al. [18] demonstrated that a history of UTIs during early lifetime, diabetes, functional disability, urinary retention, presence of urinary catheters, history of urogynecology surgery (all of them eventually combined with estrogen deficiency) are common risk factors-related with this age category. As an exception, a spike of incidence is underlined at the lower pole of the distribution axis; the increased number of positive MDR urine cultures in these patients is linked to the most active sexual period in both sexes, at the end of puberty, as Foxman B. [19] and Chu et al. [20] previously showed in their papers. It has been proven that high frequency of sexual intercourse, use of male condoms, contraceptive diaphragms, spermicides, and abusing some of the antimicrobials are key factors of acquiring UTIs at a younger age [21].

3.2. Comparison of MDR Escherichia coli Patterns with Other Studies

For the most common uropathogen in the tested cohort, high resistance rates to the most common antimicrobial agents were observed; similar results for MDR *E. coli* strains, with amoxicillin R = 55.6% and nitrofurantoin R = 7.9%, were obtained by Baral et al. [22] in 2012, while the results for ceftazidime and amikacin were R = 100% and R = 6.2%, respectively. Dehbanipour et al. [23] performed a study in Iran in 2016 that showed an alarming resistance in MDR *E. coli* to amikacin (R = 89.1%) higher than our findings and with an even higher difference compared to nitrofurantoin (R = 85.9%). The same paper admitted increasing resistance to carbapenems (meropenem), while we observed a still very low resistance in this group—R = 0.7%—both to imipenem and meropenem.

In terms of MDR patterns, *E. coli* showed the highest one to penicillin and quinolones; the last one appeared in almost all MDR *E. coli* patterns. Linhares et al. [24] developed a similar study in 2015 in Aveiro, Portugal analyzing 4376 MDR uropathogens strains, searching for resistance patterns in MDR microorganisms; the report highlighted the highest resistance to the combination of penicillin, sulfonamides, and quinolones with 12.6%, followed by cephalosporins, nitrofurans, and penicillin with 7.8%; cephalosporins, penicillin, and sulfonamides in 6.6%; and cephalosporins, penicillin, quinolones, and sulfonamides with 6.0%. Contrary to the Portuguese research, the current findings suggest an increasing resistance for aminopenicillins and aminoglycosides in the tested MDR strains. A recent study from Iasi, Romania, conducted in early 2020 [25], obtained similar locoregional results, highlighting an increasing resistance to carbapenems. Surprisingly, the tested strains showed good sensitivity to fosfomycin (S = 83.74%); similar findings were reported by Sultan et al. in 2014 [26]. His study analyzed the resistance rates among uropathogens, especially MDR strains, highlighting 100% sensitivity to this drug from ESBL and non-ESBL *Enterobacteriaceae, Staphylococcus aureus,* and *Enterococcus fecalis*.

3.3. Comparison of MDR Klebsiella Patterns with Other Studies

Klebsiella spp. is the Gram-negative bacteria ranked as the second-most frequent uropathogen in MDR-UTIs but the first in terms of resistance, as previously shown. Mishra et al. [27] published in 2013 extensive research on 996 MDR uropathogen strains sampled from hospitalized patients that were tested for common antibiotics in three different time phases. High rates of resistance were observed for *Klebsiella* spp. to multiple antibiotic classes. The Indian study highlighted higher resistance in 2013 compared to our results for amikacin (R = 65%, 76%, and 79%); trimethoprim-sulfamethoxazole (R = 66%, 69%, and 78%); and nitrofurantoin (R = 69%, 71%, and 76%), while, for amoxicillin-clavulanate (R = 54%, 67%, and 76%); ceftazidime (R = 64%, 69%, and 73%); and levofloxacin (R = 47%, 49%, and 53%), better sensitivity in all three phases was observed, contrary to our results.

One can see that, for both *E. coli* and *Klebsiella* spp., the two most common uropathogens in MDR strains, an alarmingly increased resistance for beta-lactams and fluoroquinolones has been reported by many researchers. Various mechanisms of resistance—such as enzymatic inactivation, target modification, reduced permeability reduction, or active efflux, are cited for the beta-lactams [28]. For fluoroquinolones, chromosomal mutations altering target enzymes DNA gyrase and topoisomerase IV or activating the efflux systems and pumping drugs out of the cytoplasm, concomitant with the loss of porin channels for drug entry [29], are key factors in the resistance patterns. Numerous studies have highlighted the increasing resistance to beta-lactams (penicillin, aminopenicillins, and cephalosporins) and—even if numbers are still low—a continuous growth for carbapenems [30] for all uropathogens (especially for *E. coli* and *Klebsiella* spp. [31–33]). The same can be stated in regard to quinolones [34,35].

Thus, a careful administration for both antimicrobial classes is recommended, always considering the locoregional studies on antimicrobial resistance patterns. The European Guidelines on Urological Infections [10] also suggest similar cautiousness.

3.4. How MDR Strains Modify Our Daily Practice in UTIs

According to the European Association of Urology [10], the primal evaluation of a patient suspecting an UTI imposes an empiric antibiotic treatment, taking into account locoregional patterns of resistance, followed by the collection of urine specimens for uroculture; the antibiogram will later conduct the definitive treatment of the specific UTI. In suspected cases of MDR microorganisms, a careful decision on recommending an antibiotic should be made.

A recent study from Germany conducted by Bischoff et al. [36] that was following the empiric antibiotic therapy in UTIs in patients with risk factors for resistant uropathogens noticed that, in patients with two or more risk factors, the lowest susceptibility was represented by quinolones-ciprofloxacin (S = 51.8%). A second-generation cephalosporin-cefuroxime (S = 53.7%) followed, then a third-generation cephalosporin-cefpodoxime (S = 60.7%), a wide broad-spectrum penicillin with a beta lactamase inhibitor-piperacillin/tazobactam (S = 75.0%), an aminoglycoside-gentamycin (S = 75.0%), another third-generation cephalosporin-ceftazidime (S = 76.8%), and the highest susceptibility was reported for carbapenems-imipenem (S = 91.1%). Another recent study from Italy published by Gasperini et al. [37] concerning MDR UTI bacteria in geriatric population also highlighted the increased uropathogen resistance for quinolones-levofloxacin (R = 80.0%) and ciprofloxacin (R = 55.3%); cephalosporins-cefepime, cefotaxime, and ceftazidime (R = 45.8%, 59.4%, and 51.6%, respectively); and aminopenicillin with beta lactamase inhibitor-amoxicillin/clavulanic acid (R = 50.0%) was noted. Favorable sensitivity patterns for aminoglycosides-amikacin (R = 9.4%) and carbapenems-meropenem (R = 8.5%) were also noted.

All this data endorses the presented results, as this study observed the highest resistance for quinolones, cephalosporins, and aminopenicillins; intermediate resistance was noted for amikacin; and confined sensitivity was observed for carbapenems, although not enough ubiquitous testing in all three centers was conducted for this drug class. Surprisingly, promising sensibility was noted for fosfomycin; this "old forgotten drug", as Bradley J Gardiner [38] referred to it in a study from early 2019 concerning the resistance patterns for nitrofurantoin and fosfomycin, could be an effective alternative for these patients, especially in uncomplicated UTIs.

Although fosfomycin is both a safe and effective drug in the management of the empiric treatment of a UTI, as MDR strains breed complicated features, its efficiency and usage must be limited to cystitis.

When a MDR uropathogen is suspected in complicated UTIs, the only viable treatment is represented by carbapenems.

3.5. Limitations

The impossibility of determining each bacterial species' genus in all involved centers is the major limitation of the study. It would have been helpful if the minimal inhibitory concentration of each drug was measured, providing a better understanding of the resistance dynamics in each of the tested strains. The clinical information of every patient was not available, especially in the ambulatory patients, to allow a correlation between resistance profiles and risk factors, plus medical history. One of the study's primary limitations was represented by the lack of assessment of the risk factors contributing to the emerging of multidrug resistance, resulting in the impossibility of suggesting specific recommendations. Considering that the study was performed only in tertiary-care hospitals where patients with more severe pathology are managed, this could represent a risk of selection bias.

All the aforementioned would have improved the accuracy of the recommendations that would eventually reduce acquiring MDR bacteria.

4. Materials and Methods

4.1. Study Design and Sample Population

This descriptive "cross-sectional" retrospective study was conducted at three different clinical hospitals in two University centers: "Prof Dr. Th Burghele" Clinical Hospital (BCH) and Elias University Hospital (EUH) from Bucharest, Romania and Mures County Hospital (MCH) from Targu Mures, Romania. The data collection was conducted for six months, between 1 September 2018 and 28 February 2019.

Urine probes from 15,231 patients were collected for bacterial analysis, out of which 3444 (22.61%) presented positive urine cultures with more than 10^5 CFU/mL and 698 (4.58%) showed criteria of MDR-UTIs. The representative diagram of patient dynamics is illustrated in Figure 5.

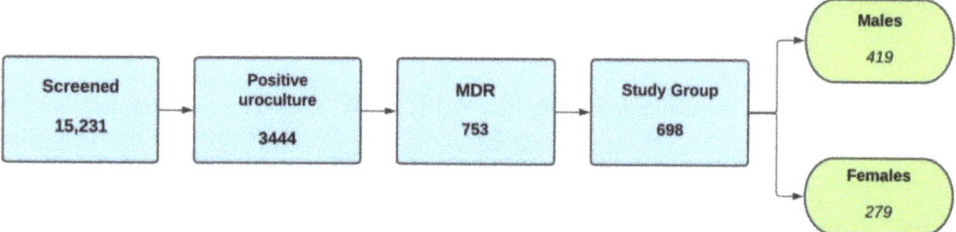

Figure 5. Diagram of the screened and enrolled patients in the study.

Information on age, sex, and social–demographic status were registered for each patient; both hospitalized and ambulatory treated patients were considered for this study; thus, an exhaustive medical history for the second group was not available.

4.2. Inclusion and Exclusion Criteria

The inclusion criteria:
1. Positive urine culture $\geq 10^5$ CFU/mL;
2. Single bacteria strain on urine culture;
3. Age $\geq$ 18 years;

4. Standards of MDR-UTIs (nonsusceptible uropathogen to one or more antibiotic agents in three or more antimicrobial categories).

The exclusion criteria:

1. Urine culture $< 10^5$ CFU/mL;
2. Two or more bacterial strains on uroculture;
3. No requirements of admission into the MDR group;
4. Presence of permanent urinary catheter (>1 month).

4.3. Sample Collection, Bacterial Culture, Identification of Uropathogens, and Antibiotic Susceptibility Test

The European and Romanian Association of Urology guidelines [10,39] on urological infections are followed to treat UTIs among patients from all clinics. In each case, a minimum 7–10 days were considered between the last antibiotic treatment and urine sampling for proper microbiological testing.

International Safety Standards [40] were followed for urine collecting techniques. After inoculation and incubation, microorganisms were identified based on specific Gram reactions, morphology, and biochemical characteristics. In all cases, the Clinical Laboratory Standard Institute (CLSI) [41] guidelines were followed for a comprehensive determination of sensitivity and resistance rates for each of the antibiotics tested to obtain the antibiogram.

Bacterial culture, the identification of uropathogens, and the antibiotic susceptibility test used were previously described in more detail [3,4,11].

4.4. Statistical Analysis

Data analysis was conducted using Microsoft Excel software (version 2020, Microsoft Corporation, Redmond, WA, USA); simple descriptive statistics were calculated. The relations of the variables were analyzed using frequency and percentage.

5. Conclusions

The current study acknowledged *E. coli* as the most common urinary pathogen among the MDR bacteria involved in UTIs among hospitalized and ambulatory patients. The incidence of MDR-UTIs increases with age distribution, peaking among the over 70 years old group of patients. In both the Gram-negative and Gram-positive groups, the highest resistance was noted for quinolones and β-lactams; alarmingly, the resistance to carbapenems rose, peaking with *P. aeruginosa*. Overall, the most common MDR resistance profiles were associated with aminopenicillins, quinolones, and cephalosporins. Together, *E. coli* and *Klebsiella* represented more than three-quarters of the identified MDR strains.

As MDR in urological infections are evolving, we strongly recommend the surveillance of resistance profiles and assessing the risk factors. A proper antibiotic administration policy should be implemented considering new MDR resistance data entailing the locoregional results.

Author Contributions: Conceptualization, R.-C.P., A.P. and C.B.C.; methodology, R.-C.P., S.N. and C.M.; validation, C.M. and R.-I.P.; formal analysis, C.M. and R.-I.P.; investigation, S.N., CM, R.-I.P. and C.B.C.; resources, S.N. and A.P.; data curation, R.-C.P. and A.P.; writing—original draft preparation, S.N., C.M., R.-I.P., and C.B.C.; writing—review and editing, R.-C.P. and A.P.; visualization, S.N. and C.B.C.; and supervision, R.-C.P. All authors have read and agreed to the published version of the manuscript.

Funding: This research received no external funding.

Institutional Review Board Statement: The study was conducted according to the guidelines of the Declaration of Helsinki. The ethics committee from every hospital approved the protocol: Burghele Clinical Hospital (no.2/2019), Mures County Hospital (no. 6522/2020), and Elias University Hospital (no. 2517/2020).

Informed Consent Statement: The data collected retrospectively did not contain any personal information. For each patient, written informed consent was obtained.

Data Availability Statement: Data supporting the reported results are available from the authors.

Acknowledgments: The results from BCH, regarding MDR, were partially presented in the paper "Antibiotic resistance profile of common uropathogens implicated in urinary tract infections in Romania" published by Petca R.C. et al. in Farmacia, 2019, 67, 994–1004, doi:10.31925/farmacia. 2019.6.9. The results from BCH, EUH, and MCH, not regarding MDR, were partially presented in the papers: "A clinical perspective on the antimicrobial resistance spectrum of uropathogens in a Romanian male population" published by Chibelean C.B. et al. in Microorganisms, 2020, 8, 848, doi:10.3390/microorganisms8060848 and "Spectrum and antibiotic resistance of uropathogens in Romanian females" published by Petca R.C. in Antibiotics, 2020, 9, 472, doi:10.3390/antibiotics9080472.

Conflicts of Interest: The authors declare no conflict of interest.

References

1. Simmering, J.E.; Tang, F.; Cavanaugh, J.E.; Polgreen, L.A.; Polgreen, P.M. The increase in hospitalizations for urinary tract infections and the associated costs in the United States, 1998–2011. *Open Forum Infect. Dis.* **2017**, *4*, ofw281. [CrossRef] [PubMed]
2. Gupta, K.; Hooton, T.M.; Stamm, W.E. Increasing antimicrobial resistance and the management of uncomplicated community-acquired urinary tract infections. *Ann. Intern. Med.* **2001**, *135*, 41–50. [CrossRef] [PubMed]
3. Chibelean, C.B.; Petca, R.-C.; Mareș, C.; Popescu, R.-I.; Enikő, B.; Mehedințu, C.; Petca, A. A clinical perspective on the antimicrobial resistance spectrum of uropathogens in a Romanian male population. *Microorganisms* **2020**, *8*, 848. [CrossRef] [PubMed]
4. Petca, R.-C.; Mareș, C.; Petca, A.; Negoiță, S.; Popescu, R.-I.; Boț, M.; Barabás, E.; Chibelean, C.B. Spectrum and Antibiotic Resistance of Uropathogens in Romanian Females. *Antibiotics* **2020**, *9*, 472. [CrossRef] [PubMed]
5. Sanchez, G.V.; Master, R.N.; Karlowsky, J.A.; Bordon, J.M. In vitro antimicrobial resistance of urinary Escherichia coli isolates among US outpatients from 2000 to 2010. *Antimicrob. Agents Chemother.* **2012**, *56*, 2181–2183. [CrossRef] [PubMed]
6. Medina, M.; Castillo-Pino, E. An introduction to the epidemiology and burden of urinary tract infections. *Ther. Adv. Urol.* **2019**, *11*, 1756287219832172. [CrossRef] [PubMed]
7. Furuya, E.; Lowy, F. Antimicrobial-resistant bacteria in the community setting. *Nat. Rev. Microbiol.* **2006**, *4*, 36–45. [CrossRef] [PubMed]
8. Tenney, J.; Hudson, N.; Alnifaidy, H.; Li, J.T.C.; Fung, K.H. Risk factors for aquiring multidrug-resistant organisms in urinary tract infections: A systematic literature review. *Saudi Pharm. J.* **2018**, *26*, 678–684. [CrossRef] [PubMed]
9. Magiorakos, A.P.; Srinivasan, A.; Carey, R.B.; Carmeli, Y.; Falagas, M.E.; Giske, C.G.; Harbarth, S.; Hindler, J.F.; Kahlmeter, G.; Olsson-Liljequist, B.; et al. Multidrug-resistant, extensively drug-resistant and pandrug-resistant bacteria: An international expert proposal for interim standard definitions for acquired resistance. *Clin. Microbiol. Infect.* **2012**, *18*, 268–281. [CrossRef] [PubMed]
10. Bonkat, G.; Bartoletti, R.; Bruyere, F.; Cai, T.; Geerlings, S.E.; Köves, B.; Schubert, S.; Wagenlehner, F. *EAU Guidelines on Urological Infections*; European Association of Urology: Arnhem, The Netherlands, 2018.
11. Petca, R.C.; Popescu, R.I.; Mares, C.; Petca, A.; Mehedintu, C.; Sandu, I.; Maru, N. Antibiotic resistance profile of common uropathogens implicated in urinary tract infections in Romania. *Farmacia* **2019**, *67*, 994–1004. [CrossRef]
12. Gajdács, M.; Urbán, E. Comparative epidemiology and resistance trends of Proteae in urinary tract infections of inpatients and outpatients: A 10-year retrospective study. *Antibiotics* **2019**, *8*, 91. [CrossRef]
13. Rowe, T.A.; Juthani-Mehta, M. Urinary tract infection in older adults. *Aging Health* **2013**, *9*, 519–528. [CrossRef]
14. Alpay, Y.; Aykin, N.; Korkmaz, P.; Gulduren, H.M.; Caglan, F.C. Urinary tract infections in the geriatric patients. *Pak. J. Med. Sci.* **2018**, *34*, 67–72. [CrossRef]
15. Rodriguez-Mañas, L. Urinary tract infections in the elderly: A review of disease characteristics and current treatment options. *Drugs Context* **2020**, *9*. [CrossRef]
16. Hu, K.K.; Boyko, E.J.; Scholes, D.; Normand, E.; Chen, C.L.; Grafton, J.; Fihn, S.D. Risk factors for urinary tract infections in postmenopausal women. *Arch. Intern. Med.* **2004**, *164*, 989–993. [CrossRef]
17. Brown, J.S.; Vittinghoff, E.; Kanaya, A.M.; Agarwal, S.K.; Hulley, S.; Foxman, B. Heart and Estrogen/Progestin Replacement Study Research Group. Urinary tract infections in postmenopausal women: Effect of hormone therapy and risk factors. *Obstet. Gynecol.* **2001**, *98*, 1045–1052. [CrossRef]
18. Mody, L.; Juthani-Mehta, M. Urinary tract infections in older women: A clinical review. *JAMA* **2014**, *311*, 844–854. [CrossRef]
19. Foxman, B. Epidemiology of urinary tract infections: Incidence, morbidity, and economic costs. *Am. J. Med.* **2002**, *113* (Suppl. 1A), 5S–13S. [CrossRef]
20. Chu, C.M.; Lowder, J.L. Diagnosis and treatment of urinary tract infections across age groups. *Am. J. Obstet. Gynecol.* **2018**, *219*, 40–51. [CrossRef]

21. Lema, V.M.; Lema, A.P.V. Sexual activity and the risk of acute uncomplicated urinary tract infection in premenopausal women: Implications for reproductive health programming. *Obstet. Gynecol. Int. J.* **2018**, *9*, 00303. [CrossRef]
22. Baral, P.; Neupane, S.; Marasini, B.P.; Ghimire, K.R.; Lekhak, B.; Shrestha, B. High prevalence of multidrug resistance in bacterial uropathogens from Kathmandu, Nepal. *BMC Res. Notes* **2012**, *5*, 38. [CrossRef] [PubMed]
23. Dehbanipour, R.; Rastaghi, S.; Sedighi, M.; Maleki, N.; Faghri, J. High prevalence of multidrug-resistance uropathogenic Escherichia coli strains, Isfahan, Iran. *J. Nat. Sci. Biol. Med.* **2016**, *7*, 22–26. [CrossRef] [PubMed]
24. Linhares, I.; Raposo, T.; Rodrigues, A.; Almeida, A. Incidence and diversity of antimicrobial multidrug resistance profiles of uropathogenic bacteria. *Biomed Res. Int.* **2015**, *2015*, 354084. [CrossRef] [PubMed]
25. Manciuc, C.; Mihai, I.F.; Filip-Ciubotaru, F.; Lacatusu, G.A. Resistance profile of multidrug-resistant urinary tract infections and their susceptibility to carbapenems. *Farmacia* **2020**, *68*, 715–721. [CrossRef]
26. Sultan, A.; Rizvi, M.; Khan, F.; Sami, H.; Shukla, I.; Khan, H.M. Increasing antimicrobial resistance among uropathogens: Is fosfomycin the answer? *Urol. Ann.* **2015**, *7*, 26–30. [CrossRef]
27. Mishra, M.P.; Debata, N.K.; Padhy, R.N. Surveillance of multidrug resistant uropathogenic bacteria in hospitalized patients in Indian. *Asian Pac. J. Trop. Biomed.* **2013**, *3*, 315–324. [CrossRef]
28. Padmini, N.; Ajilda, A.A.K.; Sivakumar, N.; Selvakumar, G. Extended spectrum β-lactamase producing Escherichia coli and Klebsiella pneumoniae: Critical tools for antibiotic resistance pattern. *J. Basic Microbiol.* **2017**, *57*, 460–470. [CrossRef]
29. Martínez-Martínez, L.; Pascual, A.; García, I.; Tran, J.; Jacoby, G. Interaction of plasmid and host quinolone resistance. *J. Antimicrob. Chemother.* **2003**, *51*, 1037–1039. [CrossRef]
30. Shahbazi, S.; Asadi Karam, M.R.; Habibi, M.; Talebi, A.; Bouzari, S. Distribution of extended-spectrum β-lactam, quinolone and carbapenem resistance genes, and genetic diversity among uropathogenic Escherichia coli isolates in Tehran, Iran. *J. Glob. Antimicrob. Resist.* **2018**, *14*, 118–125. [CrossRef]
31. Toner, L.; Papa, N.; Aliyu, S.H.; Dev, H.; Lawrentschuk, N.; Al-Hayek, S. Extended-spectrum beta-lactamase producing Enterobacteriaceae in hospital urinary tract infections: Incidence and antibiotic susceptibility profile over 9 years. *World J. Urol.* **2016**, *34*, 1031–1037. [CrossRef]
32. Sbiti, M.; Lahmadi, K.; Louzi, L. Profil épidémiologique des entérobactéries uropathogènes productrices de bêta lactamases à spectre élargi. *Pan. Afr. Med. J.* **2017**, *28*, 29. [CrossRef]
33. Grude, N.; Tveten, Y.; Kristiansen, B.E. Urinary tract infections in Norway: Bacterial aetiology and susceptibility. A retrospective study of clinical isolates. *Clin. Microbiol. Infect.* **2001**, *7*, 543–547. [CrossRef]
34. Corkill, J.E.; Anson, J.J.; Hart, C.A. High prevalence of the plasmid-mediated quinolone resistance determinant qnrA in multidrug-resistant Enterobacteriaceae from blood cultures in Liverpool, UK. *J. Antimicrob. Chemother.* **2005**, *56*, 1115–1117. [CrossRef]
35. Jacoby, G.A.; Walsh, K.E.; Mills, D.M.; Walker, V.J.; Oh, H.; Robicsek, A.; Hooper, D.C. qnrB, another plasmid-mediated gene for quinolone resistance. *Antimicrob. Agents Chemother.* **2006**, *50*, 1178–1182. [CrossRef]
36. Bischoff, S.; Walter, T.; Gerigk, M.; Ebert, M.; Vogelmann, R. Empiric antibiotic therapy in urinary tract infection in patients with risk factors for antibiotic resistance in a German emergency department. *BMC Infect. Dis.* **2018**, *18*, 56. [CrossRef]
37. Gasperini, B.; Cherubini, A.; Lucarelli, M.; Espinosa, E.; Prospero, E. Multidrug-resistant bacterial infections in geriatric hospitalized patients before and after the COVID-19 outbreak: Results from a retrospective observational study in two geriatric wards. *Antibiotics* **2021**, *10*, 95. [CrossRef]
38. Gardiner, B.J.; Stewardson, A.J.; Abbott, I.J.; Peleg, A.Y. Nitrofurantoin and fosfomycin for resistant urinary tract infections: Old drugs for emerging problems. *Aust. Prescr.* **2019**, *42*, 14–19. [CrossRef]
39. Benea, E.O.; Gavriliu, L.C.; Popescu, C.; Popescu, G.A. *Ghidul Angelescu. Terapie Antimicrobiana 2018*, 3rd ed.; Editura Bucuresti: Bucharest, Romania, 2018; pp. 181–192.
40. World Health Organization. *Guidelines for the Collection of Clinical Specimens during Field Investigation of Outbreaks*; World Health Organization: Geneva, Switzerland, 2000; pp. 1–51.
41. Clinical and Laboratory Standards Institute®(CLSI). M 100 Performance Standards for Antimicrobial Susceptibility Testing, 28th ed. Available online: https://clsi.org/standards/products/microbiology/documents/m100/ (accessed on 10 May 2020).

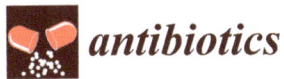

Article

Short-Course Versus Long-Course Colistin for Treatment of Carbapenem-Resistant *A. baumannii* in Cancer Patient

Wasan Katip [1,2,*], Suriyon Uitrakul [3] and Peninnah Oberdorfer [2,4]

1. Department of Pharmaceutical Care, Faculty of Pharmacy, Chiang Mai University, Chiang Mai 50200, Thailand
2. Epidemiology Research Group of Infectious Disease (ERGID), Chiang Mai University, Chiang Mai 50200, Thailand; aoberdor@med.cmu.ac.th
3. Department of Pharmaceutical Care, School of Pharmacy, Walailak University, Thai Buri 80160, Thailand; Suriyon.ui@wu.ac.th
4. Division of Infectious Diseases, Department of Pediatrics, Faculty of Medicine, Chiang Mai University, Chiang Mai 50200, Thailand
* Correspondence: wasankatip@gmail.com; Tel.: +66-53-944342-3

Abstract: Carbapenem-resistant *Acinetobacter baumannii* (CRAB) is one of the most commonly reported nosocomial infections in cancer patients and could be fatal because of suboptimal immune defenses in these patients. We aimed to compare clinical response, microbiological response, nephrotoxicity, and 30-day mortality between cancer patients who received short (<14 days) and long (≥14 days) courses of colistin for treatment of CRAB infection. A retrospective cohort study was conducted in cancer patients with CRAB infection who received short or long courses of colistin between 2015 to 2017 at Chiang Mai University Hospital (CMUH). A total of 128 patients met the inclusion criteria. The results of this study show that patients who received long course of colistin therapy had a higher rate of clinical response; adjusted odds ratio (OR) was 3.16 times in patients receiving long-course colistin therapy (95%CI, 1.37–7.28; *p* value = 0.007). Microbiological response in patients with long course was 4.65 times (adjusted OR) higher than short course therapy (95%CI, 1.72–12.54; *p* value = 0.002). Moreover, there was no significant difference in nephrotoxicity (adjusted OR, 0.91, 95%CI, 0.39–2.11; *p* value = 0.826) between the two durations of therapy. Thirty-day mortality in the long-course therapy group was 0.11 times (adjusted OR) compared to the short-course therapy group (95%CI, 0.03–0.38; *p* value = 0.001). Propensity score analyses also demonstrated similar results. In conclusion, cancer patients who received a long course of colistin therapy presented greater clinical and microbiological responses and lower 30-day mortality but similar nephrotoxicity as compared with those who a received short course. Therefore, a long course of colistin therapy should be considered for management of CRAB infection in cancer patients.

Keywords: cancer patients; duration of treatment; colistin; propensity score analysis; multidrug-resistant *Acinetobacter baumannii*

Citation: Katip, W.; Uitrakul, S.; Oberdorfer, P. Short-Course Versus Long-Course Colistin for Treatment of Carbapenem-Resistant *A. baumannii* in Cancer Patient. *Antibiotics* **2021**, *10*, 484. https://doi.org/10.3390/antibiotics10050484

Academic Editor: Pavel Bostik

Received: 9 March 2021
Accepted: 20 April 2021
Published: 22 April 2021

Publisher's Note: MDPI stays neutral with regard to jurisdictional claims in published maps and institutional affiliations.

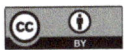

Copyright: © 2021 by the authors. Licensee MDPI, Basel, Switzerland. This article is an open access article distributed under the terms and conditions of the Creative Commons Attribution (CC BY) license (https://creativecommons.org/licenses/by/4.0/).

1. Introduction

Patients with cancer are at-risk of infections caused by antibiotic resistant Gram-negative bacteria. *Acinetobacter baumannii* is one of the most commonly reported nosocomial infections in cancer patients [1]. *A. baumannii* has been identified in patients with solid tumors, hematological malignancies, neutropenia, and those in the Intensive Care Unit (ICU) [2–4]. Infections caused by *A. baumannii* can be fatal in patients with suboptimal immune defenses, especially cancer patients [1,2]. Moreover, the prevalence and mortality rate of carbapenem-resistant *A. baumannii* (CRAB) has increased. The mortality rate of patients with cancer and multidrug-resistant (MDR) *A. baumannii* infection has reached 55% [5].

Colistin treatment for *Acinetobacter baumannii* infection is one of the most debated regimens [6]. Therefore, several alternative treatments are suggested, such as tigecycline, amikacin, and sulbactam. Tigecycline is one of the active antibiotics against CRAB and appears to be a potential alternative therapeutic option for the treatment of CRAB [6,7]. However, tigecycline provides low concentration in plasma, and this limits its use in blood stream infections [6]. Furthermore, tigecycline has been shown to be inferior to the comparator drugs and has shown higher mortality rate in VAP patients [7]. For amikacin and sulbactam, although they have shown anti-CRAB efficacy, their nephrotoxicity and high resistance rate among CRAB limits their use [6]. Therefore, as compared with the other drugs, colistin is still safe and effective for the treatment of CRAB infection [6].

Colistin is one of the most widely prescribed medicines for the treatment of carbapenem-resistant *A. baumannii* (CRAB). It has long been acknowledged that higher consumption of colistin resulted in higher risk of MDR bacteria, as well as higher treatment cost [6]. Theoretically, short-course treatment decreases ecological pressure and eliminates adverse effects without affecting the outcome [8]. Nonetheless, a subgroup of ventilator-associated pneumonia (VAP) patients who were infected with non-maturing Gram-negative microorganisms had higher recurrence of pulmonary infection with the short-course (8 days) treatment regimen than with the long-course regimen [9].

The duration of colistin treatment CRAB is typically ≥ 7 to 14 days [10–12]. However, CRAB is known as a significant and difficult-to-treat pathogen with complex resistance. This characteristic is a real challenge to all clinicians and leads to the use of colistin for longer than 2 weeks for established infections in many patients [12].

There was a randomized, open-label, clinical trial that studied 210 patients with life-threatening infections due to extensively drug-resistant (XDR) *A. baumannii*. The recruited patients were randomly assigned to either colistin alone or colistin plus rifampicin groups. The primary end point of the study was overall 30-day mortality. Treatment had to be administered for at least 10 days and up to a maximum of 21 days [12].

However, the optimal treatment duration for a specific group of CRAB-infected cancer patients still remains to be determined. Therefore, the primary objective of this study was to compare clinical outcome, microbiological response, and nephrotoxicity between cancer patients receiving a short course (<14 days) and long course (≥ 14 days) of colistin for treatment of CRAB. The secondary objective of this study was to compare 30-day mortality rates between patients who received short and long courses of antimicrobial therapy for CRAB pneumonia.

2. Results

One hundred and twenty-eight cancer patients with CRAB infection were recruited in the study; there were 84 patients in the short course and 44 patients in the long course of colistin therapy. For median duration of therapy, the short-course group had 7 days duration (interquartile range (IQR), 5–9 days) while the long-course group had 14 days duration (IQR, 14–15 days). Overall, the median age was 62 years, and 78 patients (61%) were female. The majority of infectious disease was pneumonia (72%). Patients in the short and long courses of colistin therapy were comparable in most baseline demographics and clinical characteristics, although the numbers of patient in both group were different (Table 1). The number of patients who received short and long courses of colistin therapy is shown in Figure 1.

When assessing the outcomes and toxicity of colistin therapy, Fisher's exact test showed that the clinical and microbiological response of CRAB infection was higher in the long-course therapy group than in the short-course. There was no significant difference in nephrotoxicity between both patient groups (54 cases (64.29%) in short-course group and 27 cases (61.36%) in long-course group, p value = 0.847). Moreover, the 30-day mortality of CRAB infection was higher in the short course than in the long course of colistin therapy group (32 (38.10%) and 5 (11.36%), respectively, p value = 0.002), as shown in Table 2.

Table 1. Demographic and clinical characteristics of patients in short and long courses of colistin therapy.

Characteristic	Short Course (*n* = 84)	Long Course (*n* = 44)	*p* Value
Sex (no. (%) of patients)			
Male	31 (36.90)	19 (43.18)	0.568
Female	53 (63.10)	25 (56.82)	
Age (years), mean ± SD	61.39 ± 13.44	63.41 ± 14.22	0.431
Type of malignancy, *n* (%)			
Solid tumor	73 (86.91)	38 (86.36)	1.000
- Lung cancer	17 (20.24)	10 (22.73)	
- Brain cancer	9 (10.71)	1 (2.27)	
- Liver, bile duct, and GI cancer	10 (11.90)	3 (6.82)	
- Urogenital cancer	7 (8.33)	6 (13.64)	
- Colon cancer	9 (10.71)	8 (18.18)	
- Bone cancer	6 (7.14)	1 (2.27)	
- Head and neck cancer	6 (7.14)	4 (3.70)	
- Gynecologic cancer	9 (10.71)	5 (11.36)	
Hematologic malignancies	11 (13.09)	6 (13.64)	1.000
- Lymphoma	6 (7.14)	4 (9.09)	
- Leukemia	5 (5.95)	2 (4.55)	
Comorbidities *, *n* (%)	44 (52.38)	23 (52.27)	1.000
- Hypertension	20 (23.81)	13 (29.55)	0.527
- Cardiovascular disease	17 (20.24)	10 (22.73)	0.821
- Diabetes mellitus	7 (8.33)	4 (9.09)	1.000
- Chronic kidney disease	7 (8.33)	1 (2.27)	0.262
- Chronic liver disease	5 (5.95)	0 (0.00)	0.164
- Chronic obstructive pulmonary disease	8 (9.52)	9 (20.45)	0.103
ICU status, *n* (%)	50 (59.52)	28 (63.64)	0.706
Septic shock, *n* (%)	51 (60.71)	27 (61.36)	1.000
Mechanical ventilation, *n* (%)	58 (69.05)	39 (88.64)	0.017
Charlson score, mean ± SD	4.14 ± 2.39	4.32 ± 2.32	0.691
Baseline SCr, mg/dl, median (IQR)	0.7 (0.5–1.2)	0.9 (0.5–1.6)	0.281

Table 1. Cont.

Characteristic	Short Course (n = 84)	Long Course (n = 44)	p Value
Baseline GFR, ml/min, median (IQR)	94.96 (29.65–114.68)	67.6 (29.83–110.21)	0.394
Baseline GFR < 50, mL/min, n (%)	27 (32.14)	17 (38.64)	0.557
Baseline GFR < 20, mL/min, n (%)	16 (19.05)	7 (15.91)	0.810
Total CMS dose, g, median (IQR)	1.68 (1.04–2.40)	3.22 (2.10–4.50)	0.001
Meropenem, n (%)	25 (29.76)	13 (29.55)	1.000
Concomitant nephrotoxic medications **, n (%)			
Aminoglycosides	3 (3.57)	3 (6.82)	0.413
Diuretics	59 (70.24)	37 (84.09)	0.131
Amphotericin B	4 (4.76)	7 (15.91)	0.046
Vasopressor	49 (58.33)	29 (65.91)	0.450
Vancomycin	38 (45.24)	30 (68.18)	0.016
Duration of IV colistin (day), mean ± SD	7.13 ± 2.99	15.82 ± 4.10	0.001
Length of hospital stay (day), median (IQR)	31.5 (20–52)	43.5 (35–57.5)	0.001
Source of CRAB infection, n (%)			0.065
Pneumonia	56 (66.67)	36 (81.82)	
Bacteremia	3 (3.57)	3 (6.82)	
UTI	17 (20.24)	2 (4.55)	
Other #	8 (9.52)	3 (6.82)	
Colistin MICs, median (min–max)	0.25 (0.094–1.5)	0.25 (0.064–1.5)	0.853

IV, intravenous; SCr, serum creatinine; GFR, glomerular filtration rate; SD, standard deviation; GI, gastrointestinal tract; UTI, urinary tract infection; IQR, interquartile range. * Patients with > 1 disease; ** Patients prescribed > 1 drug; # Other included intercostal drainage, surgical site infection.

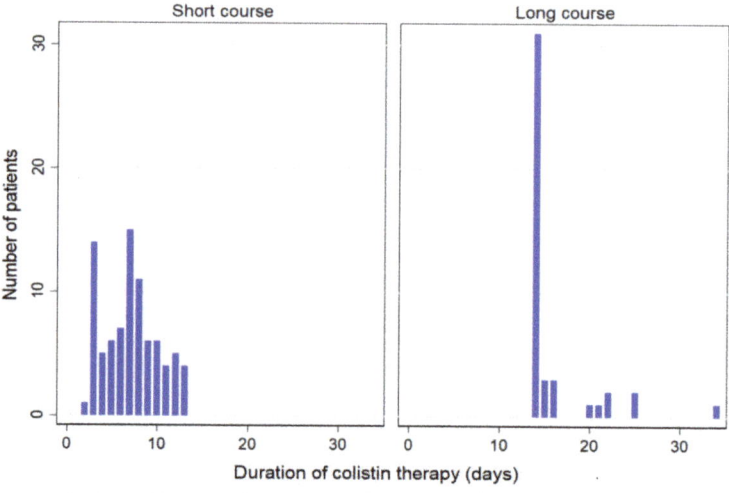

Figure 1. Number of patients who received short and long courses of colistin therapy.

Table 2. Overall outcomes and toxicity in short and long courses of colistin therapy.

Outcome	Short Course (n = 84)	Long Courses (n = 44)	p Value
Clinical response	39 (46.43)	31 (70.45)	0.015
Microbiological response	49 (58.33)	38 (86.36)	0.001
Nephrotoxicity (RIFLE criteria)	54 (64.29)	27 (61.36)	0.847
- Risk	17 (20.23)	10 (22.72)	
- Injury	17 (20.23)	4 (9.09)	
- Failure	20 (23.83)	13 (29.55)	
- Loss	-	-	
- ESRD	-	-	
30-day mortality	32 (38.10)	5 (11.36)	0.002

Univariate and Multiple Logistic Regression Analyses of the Outcomes

The results of univariate analysis indicate significant differences in clinical response, microbiologic response, and 30-day mortality rates between the short- and long-course groups. Table 3 shows similar nephrotoxicity rates in both groups. However, a significantly higher clinical response rate (odds ratio (OR), 3.16; 95% confidence interval (CI), 1.37–7.28; p value = 0.007), higher microbiological response rate (OR, 4.65; 95% CI, 1.72 to 12.54; p value = 0.002), and lower 30-day mortality rate (OR, 0.11; 95% CI, 0.03 to 0.38; p value = 0.001) were observed in patients who received long-course therapy as compared with short-course therapy based on multiple logistic regression analysis. However, the nephrotoxicity rates were not different (OR, 0.91; 95% CI, 0.39 to 2.11; p value = 0.826) (Table 3). Other predictors of clinical response were septic shock and Charlson score ≥ 4, and the predictor of microbiological response was septic shock. Age of 60 years or more could predict higher nephrotoxicity. Other independent risk factors for 30-day mortality were septic shock, Charlson score ≥ 4, and baseline Scr ≥ 1 mg/dl (Table 3).

The results of propensity score analysis using inverse probability weighting with variables associated with long-course therapy showed a significant difference in clinical response, microbiological response, and 30-day mortality rate (p value = 0.001, p value = 0.001 and p value = 0.001, respectively, Table 3). Factors that were used in the analysis were age, sex, vancomycin, amphotericin B, septic shock, Charlson score, comorbidities, stay in ICU during infection, mechanical ventilation during infection, baseline serum creatinine, source of CRAB infection, and type of malignancy.

Table 3. The outcomes of cancer patients receiving short-course and long-course colistin for CRAB infection (n = 128).

Outcome and Variable	Univariate Analysis			Logistic Regression Analysis			Propensity Score Analysis (IPW)		
	Crude OR	95%CI	p Value	Adjusted OR	95%CI for Adjusted OR	p Value	OR	95%CI	p Value
Clinical response									
Long course colistin therapy	2.75	1.26–5.98	0.011	3.16	1.37–7.28	0.007	1.30	1.11–1.52	0.001
Septic shock	0.35	0.16–0.74	0.006	0.30	0.13–0.68	0.004			
Charlson score ≥ 4	0.39	0.19–0.79	0.010	0.34	0.16–0.74	0.006			
Microbiological response									
Long course colistin therapy	4.52	1.73–11.86	0.002	4.65	1.72–12.54	0.002	1.32	1.14–1.52	0.001
Septic shock	0.38	0.17–0.87	0.022	0.37	0.15–0.88	0.024			

Table 3. Cont.

Outcome and Variable	Univariate Analysis			Logistic Regression Analysis			Propensity Score Analysis (IPW)		
	Crude OR	95%CI	p Value	Adjusted OR	95%CI for Adjusted OR	p Value	OR	95%CI	p Value
Nephrotoxicity									
Long course colistin therapy	0.88	0.42–1.87	0.745	0.91	0.39–2.11	0.826	1.02	0.85–1.22	0.861
Age ≥ 60 years	1.72	0.83–3.57	0.146	2.31	1.01–5.33	0.049			
30 days mortality									
Long course colistin therapy	0.21	0.07–0.58	0.003	0.11	0.03–0.38	0.001	0.73	0.65–0.83	0.001
Septic shock	6.26	2.29–17.50	0.001	6.20	1.67–23.10	0.007			
Charlson score ≥ 4	4.53	1.95–10.49	0.001	7.12	2.40–21.10	0.001			
Baseline Scr ≥ 1 mg/dl	2.39	1.10–5.22	0.028	2.85	1.02–7.97	0.046			

CI, confidence interval; ICU, intensive care unit; OR, odds ratio; IPW, inverse probability weighting.

3. Discussion

The results from this study point out that greater clinical and microbiological responses were achieved in cancer patients who received a long-course colistin therapy compared with a short-course. Additionally, no significant difference in nephrotoxicity rate between the two groups was detected. Furthermore, cancer patients who received long-course colistin therapy had lower 30-day mortality rate than the short-course. These findings were supported by logistic regression analysis and propensity score analysis using inverse probability weighting for both primary outcome (i.e., clinical response, microbiologic response, and nephrotoxicity) and secondary outcome (30-day mortality).

Guidelines of antimicrobial therapy are important tools that can help clinicians to make decisions about the duration of treatment. The optimization of antimicrobial duration might also be an important factor for management of CRAB infection in cancer patients. However, prior studies examining the impact of duration of antimicrobial therapy in cancer patients with CRAB infection remain limited. Most randomized controlled trials on duration of antibiotic therapy do not include difficult-to-treat patients or pathogens, such as immunocompromised patients, critically ill patients, specific infection foci, *P. aeruginosa* infection, and *A. baumannii* infection [13]. Therefore, the optimal duration of antimicrobial therapy for cancer patients with CRAB infection remains uncertain and needs to be investigated.

In some recent studies, the duration of antibiotic therapy for *Acinetobacter baumannii* infection was not well defined [10–14]. In previous studies, the definition typically used for short-course treatment was less than 10 days, while long-course treatment was typically defined as more than or equal to 10 days [15–17]. However, some studies defined treatment of longer than 7 or 8 days as a long-course duration [9,18]. In the clinical practice guidelines by the Infectious Diseases Society of America and the American Thoracic Society (IDSA/ATS), a 7-day course of antimicrobial therapy was strongly recommended for hospital-acquired and ventilator-associated pneumonia rather than a longer duration, even in non-fermentative Gram-negative bacilli infection including *P. aeruginosa* and *A. baumannii* [19]. Remarkably, *A. baumannii* might be one of the most debated pathogens for antibiotic treatment duration; many clinicians usually consider continuation of antibiotic therapy for up to 2 weeks in many patients with established infection [10–14]. However, using antibiotics for 14 days was classified as a long treatment duration in many studies and guidelines [9–12,14–19]. Based on the mentioned information, especially in immunocompromised patients, a 14-day duration was defined as long course therapy; this cut-off was longer than most studies but was set based on the principle of immunocompromised status of patients [9–12,14–19]. Nevertheless, with regard to the patient distribution, where approximately 70% of patients in the long-course group received 14 days of treatment, the effect on the 14-day patients could dominate the effect of other patients. This, therefore, should be considered because the results might be altered if another cut-off were used.

The difference in duration of treatment between 8 and 15 days was analyzed by subgroup in a randomized controlled trial that was conducted in 401 patients with VAP. There was no significant difference in 28-day mortality rate between the two groups with non-fermentative Gram-negative bacilli; the 8-day group had 23.4% and the 15-day group had 30.2% 28-day mortality rates (−6.8% difference; 90% CI: −17.5–4.1). Likewise, no significant difference was observed in clinical response. However, in the 8-day group, the rate of recurrent pulmonary infection was higher than in the other group: 40.6% and 25.4%, respectively (15.2% difference; 90% CI: 3.9–26.6) [9]. Therefore, longer antibiotic therapy might be necessary and should be considered in patients with VAP caused by non-fermentative Gram-negative bacilli (1.7% was *A. baumannii*) [9].

Multiple logistic regression and propensity score analysis showed that patients in this study who received a long course of colistin were more likely than those who received a short course to experience clinical response (61% and 26%, respectively; p value = 0.005) and microbiological response (61% and 34%, respectively; p value = 0.013). These data further support the notion that longer colistin therapy is highly useful in the treatment of MDR *A. baumannii* in cancer patients.

The results of this study were consistent with the retrospective study by Nelson et al. [20] that included 117 patients with a short course and 294 patients with a long course of antimicrobial therapy (median duration of 8.5 and 13.3 days, respectively) for uncomplicated Gram-negative bloodstream infection. The propensity score adjusted risk of treatment failure was higher in patients with a short course of antimicrobial agents compared with a long course (HR 2.60, 95% CI: 1.20–5.53, p value = 0.02). Moreover, the compromised immune status was found to be a risk factor for treatment failure (HR 4.30, 95% CI: 1.57–10.80, p value = 0.006). However, the abovementioned study was not conducted using a specific treatment for *A. baumannii* infection, so this result might not be applicable in this pathogen [20].

Another study by Hachem et al. [21] evaluated the efficacy of colistin in cancer patients, mostly patients with hematological malignancy treated for multidrug-resistant *Pseudomonas aeruginosa* infection; it was found that clinical cure rate was 61% and median treatment duration of colistin was 20 days (range from 5–58). However, the objective of this study was not to investigate duration of treatment, so the result found for duration in the Hachem et al. [21] study could not indicate a suitable duration of treatment.

Nazer et al. [22] described that microbiological clearance was observed in 51 patients (66.2%) on day 13 ± 9 (mean ± SD) after starting colistin therapy. They found that 35 out of 89 patients with cancer and CRAB infection (39.3%) met the RIFLE criteria for nephrotoxicity, with a mean of 9 ± 7 days from the initiation of colistin therapy. Duration of IV colistin was 15.8 ± 11 days (mean ± SD). However, the mentioned study was not designed to compare the courses of antibiotic therapy, so there was no control group for comparison [22].

Theoretically, in cases where a patient has good clinical response without clinical features of infection, the duration of antibiotic therapy should be shortened from the traditional 14–21 days (long course) to a period as short as 7 days (short course) because a short-course therapeutic approach can reduce ecological pressure and diminish side effects. However, cancer patients with CRAB in this recent study had lower clinical and microbiological responses when using a short-course treatment regimen. There were several reasons for the requirement of a long course (>14 days) of antibiotic therapy in CRAB-infected patients. First, one of the potential causes of delayed eradication of CRAB from the body might be attributed to chemotherapy administration, which diminishes neutrophil function [23]. Since neutrophils have several essential roles in host resistance to respiratory infection from many organisms as well as from *A. baumannii* [24], cancer patients infected with CRAB should considered for longer antibiotic therapy. Secondly, antibacterial therapy aims to reduce the number of bacteria, but in most cases, antibacterial efficacy relies on the immune system to eliminate bacteria completely. However, patients with malignancy can sometimes have neutropenia and lack of the defense mechanisms that are present in patients with intact immune systems. Therefore, a higher pharmacokinetic (PK)–pharmacodynamic (PD) target and longer antibiotic therapy may be required in immunosuppressed patients such as cancer patients. This hypothesis is supported by the neutropenic mouse thigh model, where it was found that neutropenia increased the required magnitude of PK/PD index by 50% to 100% (i.e., 1.5–2.0-fold) [25,26].

The poor outcomes reported in this study might be caused by underlying malignant diseases in patient population, but there were also other potential contributing factors. After adjusting the potential confounders, other predictors of clinical response were detected, including septic shock (OR, 0.3; 95% CI, 0.13 to 0.68; p value = 0.004) and Charlson score ≥ 4 (OR, 0.34; 95% CI, 0.16 to 0.74; p value = 0.006), and the predictor of microbiological response was septic shock (OR, 0.37; 95% CI, 0.15 to 0.88; p value = 0.024). The other independent risk factors for 30-day mortality were septic shock (OR, 6.20; 95% CI, 1.67 to 23.10; p value = 0.007), Charlson score ≥ 4 (OR, 7.12; 95% CI, 2.40 to 21.10; p value = 0.001), and baseline Scr ≥ 1 mg/dl (OR, 2.85; 95% CI, 1.02 to 7.97; p value = 0.046).

In the present study, 54 (64.29%) and 27 (61.36%) patients developed nephrotoxicity during short course and long course therapy (p value = 0.847), respectively. The incidence of nephrotoxicity observed in this study was within the range that has been reported in previous studies, ranging from 20% to 69% [27–29]. The other factor that was found correlated with nephrotoxicity was age equal or greater than 60 years (OR, 2.31; 95%CI, 1.01–5.33).

Regarding antimicrobial stewardship, reducing the length of antibiotic course might be effective in reducing antibiotic resistance through the abovementioned mechanism. However, this study observed higher rates of clinical and microbiological response, similar nephrotoxicity, and a lower rate of 30-day mortality in the long-course therapy than in short-course therapy. Therefore, in the specific group of cancer patients with CRAB infection, consideration of longer treatment was necessary.

This study differed from other previously reported studies since all patients here had underlying cancer. Eighty-six percent of the patients had solid tumor, and the rest had hematologic malignancy. Additionally, all patients in this study had CRAB infection without any other infections.

There were some limitations in this study. Firstly, the methodology of this study was retrospective, which could possibly have allowed unknown variables to affect the results. However, sensitivity analysis was used to adjust for the suspected confounding factors, and the obtained results still led to the same conclusion. Secondly, in a previous prospective study, the incidence of acute kidney injury (AKI) during therapy was strongly correlated with baseline renal function and plasma colistin concentration. Patients with a higher creatinine clearance (CL_{CR}) had higher rates of AKI than those with a lower CL_{CR} [30]. As this study did not measure plasma colistin concentration, there was a lack of pharmacokinetic information, which was considered one of limitations of this study. However, therapeutic drug monitoring, especially for colistin, is not routinely performed in clinical practice in Thailand. RIFLE criteria were therefore used to assess nephrotoxicity outcome. The baseline renal functions were not significantly different between short- and long-course treatment groups. Moreover, logistic regression analysis and propensity score analysis using inverse probability weighting with variables associated with long-course therapy were performed to adjust any variables that were different between short- and long-course treatment groups. Thirdly, this study did not describe the type of chemotherapy that patients might have been administered, so the results of this study should be carefully interpreted based on cancer patient status. Fourthly, this study did not explore patient blood counts, which might affect the outcomes.

4. Materials and Methods

This retrospective cohort study was conducted at Chiang Mai University Hospital (CMUH), Chiang Mai, Thailand, from January 2015 to August 2017. The methodology was approved by the ethics committee on human research of the Faculty of Medicine, Chiang Mai University, with a waiver of informed consent for retrospective data collection under the condition of anonymously stored data collected. Medical chart records and microbiology laboratory data of cancer patients with CRAB infection were reviewed. The criteria used to identify and classify infection were outlined by the Center for Disease Control and Prevention (CDC) [31]. The inclusion criteria were age equal or greater than 18 years, colistin treatment for more than 2 days for documented CRAB infection, and receipt of only one course of colistin treatment. The exclusion criteria were the presence of other types of Gram-negative infection, and treatment with hemodialysis or renal replacement therapy. The primary exposure was duration of antibiotic treatment, divided into short-course and long-course therapy. The first day of colistin therapy was defined as the day that CRAB cultures were obtained. Short-course antimicrobial therapy was defined as a total duration of colistin <14 days after the first day. Long-course therapy was defined as a total duration of colistin $\geq$14 days after the first day. The duration was the first day of intravenous colistin use until fully discontinuation.

The following information was collected: age, sex, type and site of malignancy, co-morbidities, dates of admission and discharge, medical history, ICU admission, the need for mechanical ventilation, Charlson score, previous nosocomial infection, clinical course, length of hospital stay, and hospital discharge diagnosis. Data on positive bacterial cultures, antibiotic susceptibilities, colistin minimum inhibitory concentration (MIC), source of CRAB infection, subsequent culture results, and the duration of colistin therapy were also collected. Side effects related to colistin, baseline serum creatinine, baseline GFR, total colistin dose, and the development of septic shock during the evolution of CRAB infection were recorded, as well as the concomitant nephrotoxic medications that could potentially cause nephrotoxicity, hospital discharge diagnosis, outcome, nephrotoxicity (base on RIFLE criteria), and 30-day mortality.

CRAB was defined as *A. baumannii* that was resistant to carbapenems but sensitive to colistin. Dosage of antibiotic regimens was based on the respective hospital guidelines: LD colistin 300 mg of colistin base activity (CBA) once at the start of treatment course and then 150 mg of CBA every 12 h. Colistin administration was adjusted according to renal function. Dose and interval were adjusted according to Cockcroft and Gault creatinine clearance estimates if patients had moderate-to-severe renal impairment (creatinine clearance rate, <50 mL/min). For example, a loading dose of 300 mg followed by maintenance dose of 150! mg CBA every 24 h was administered for creatinine clearance rate of 20–50 mL/min, or 150 mg CBA every 48 h was administered for creatinine clearance rate of <20 mL/min.

4.1. Outcome Assessment

Three primary outcomes in this study were clinical response, microbiological response, and nephrotoxicity after treatment. Clinical response of treatment was assessed by resolution or partial resolution of the present symptoms and signs of CARB infection at the end of colistin treatment. Patients who failed to achieve all criteria for clinical response were defined as clinical failures. Microbiological response was defined as obtaining two consecutive negative CARB cultures from the site of infection after the initial positive culture, whereas microbiological failure was defined as persistence of CARB in the subsequent specimen cultures. Renal toxicity was defined as detection of any stage of acute kidney injury outlined in the RIFLE classification [32]. The secondary outcome of the study was 30-day mortality, which was defined as death within 30 days after initial colistin treatment for CARB infection.

4.2. Antimicrobial Susceptibility Testing

A. baumannii was discovered using traditional cultures and biochemical methods at CMUH's Clinical Microbiology Division. The Clinical and Laboratory Standards Institute (CLSI) protocol [33] was used to assess antimicrobial susceptibility. Antibiotic susceptibility to *A. baumannii* was determined using the VITEK 2 method, and colistin susceptibility was determined using broth microdilution, with resistance identified as a colistin MIC breakpoint >2 mg/L. The Vitek 2 system (bioMerieux, Marcy I 'Etoile, France) is a fully automated system that uses a fluorogenic approach to identify organisms and a turbidimetric process to assess susceptibility. Antimicrobial susceptibility testing with VITEK 2 demonstrated high compliance with standard methods for evaluating antimicrobial MICs, with a time benefit of hours to days and increased reproducibility [34,35].

4.3. Statistical Analysis

Stata 14 software was used to analyze all of the results (Stata-Corp, College Station, TX, USA). The duration of colistin therapy was mainly compared between the two treatment groups.

General characteristics and basic information of patients were analyzed with descriptive statistics, including percentage, frequency, average, and standard deviation. Using Fisher's exact test, the average comparison case of sample basic data and the average of other statistical methods was the independent t test when data were distributed normally, and the Mann–Whitney U test when data were not normally distributed. The significance level was set as 0.05. Fisher's exact test was used to compare differences in rates of clinical response, microbiologic response, nephrotoxicity, and 30-day mortality between short-course and long-course colistin therapy.

Furthermore, factors that might affect the four outcomes, i.e., clinical response, microbiologic response, nephrotoxicity, and 30-day mortality, were adjusted using logistic regression. The evaluated factors included age, comorbidities, stay in an intensive care unit (ICU) during infection, course of colistin therapy, septic shock, Charlson score, baseline serum creatinine, type of malignancy, mechanical ventilation during infection, type of nephrotoxic medication, and source of CRAB infection. Firstly, univariate analysis was performed to evaluate the predictive effect of each factor. Next, any factors with a p value of < 0.25 from univariate test were included in a full multiple logistic model. Lastly, factors were removed from the model one at a time until all factors remaining in the model had 5% significance level, except that course of colistin therapy remained in the model, regardless of its p value.

For sensitivity analysis, a propensity score for courses of colistin therapy and estimated ORs with inverse probability weighting methods was developed using variables likely to influence the outcomes of both primary outcome (i.e., clinical response, microbiologic response and nephrotoxicity) and secondary outcome (30-day mortality).

5. Conclusions

The results of this study suggest that a long course of colistin was preferred in the treatment of CRAB infection in a cancer population, based on higher rates of clinical and microbiological response. Furthermore, cancer patients who received a long course of colistin had a lower 30-day mortality rate but the same nephrotoxicity rate. A long course of colistin therapy, therefore, should be considered for the management of CRAB infection in cancer patients.

Author Contributions: Conceptualization, W.K.; data curation, W.K.; formal analysis, W.K.; investigation, W.K.; methodology, W.K.; project administration, W.K.; software, W.K.; supervision, P.O.; validation, P.O.; writing—original draft, W.K.; writing—review and editing, W.K. and S.U. All authors have read and agreed to the published version of the manuscript.

Funding: This research received no external funding.

Institutional Review Board Statement: The study was conducted according to the guidelines of the Declaration of Helsinki and approved by the Ethics Committee of the Faculty of Medicine, Chiang Mai University (NONE-2560-04839).

Informed Consent Statement: Patient consent was waived due to retrospective data collection under the condition of anonymously stored data collected.

Data Availability Statement: The datasets used and analyzed during the current study are available from the corresponding author on reasonable request.

Acknowledgments: This research work was partially supported by Chiang Mai University.

Conflicts of Interest: The authors declare no conflict of interest.

References

1. Perez, F.; Adachi, J.; Bonomo, R.A. Antibiotic-resistant gram-negative bacterial infections in patients with cancer. *Clin. Infect. Dis.* **2014**, *59*, S335–S339. [CrossRef] [PubMed]
2. Turkoglu, M.; Mirza, E.; Tunçcan, Ö.G.; Erdem, G.U.; Dizbay, M.; Yağcı, M.; Aygencel, G.; Türköz Sucak, G. Acinetobacter baumannii infection in patients with hematologic malignancies in intensive care unit:risk factors and impact on mortality. *J. Crit. Care* **2011**, *26*, 460–467. [CrossRef]
3. Chiang, M.C.; Kuo, S.C.; Chen, S.J.; Yang, S.P.; Lee, Y.T.; Chen, T.L.; Fung, C.P. Clinical characteristics and outcomes of bacteremia due to different genomic species of *Acinetobacter baumannii* complex in patients with solid tumors. *Infection* **2012**, *40*, 19–26. [CrossRef] [PubMed]
4. El Far, M.Y.; El-Mahallawy, H.A.; Attia, A.S. Tracing the dissemination of the international clones of multidrug-resistant *Acinetobacter baumannii* among cancer patients in Egypt using the PCR-based open reading frame typing (POT) method. *J. Glob. Antimicrob. Resist.* **2019**, *19*, 210–215. [CrossRef] [PubMed]
5. Fukuta, Y.; Muder, R.R.; Agha, M.E.; Clarke, L.G.; Wagener, M.M.; Hensler, A.M.; Doi, Y. Risk factors for acquisition of multidrug-resistant *Acinetobacter baumannii* among cancer patients. *Am. J. Infect. Control* **2013**, *41*, 1249–1252. [CrossRef] [PubMed]
6. Isler, B.; Doi, Y.; Bonomo, R.A.; Paterson, D.L. New Treatment Options against Carbapenem-Resistant Acinetobacter baumannii Infections. *Antimicrob. Agents Chemother.* **2018**, *63*, e01110-18. [CrossRef]
7. Freire, A.T.; Melnyk, V.; Kim, M.J.; Datsenko, O.; Dzyublik, O.; Glumcher, F.; Chuang, Y.C.; Maroko, R.T.; Dukart, G.; Cooper, C.A.; et al. Comparison of tigecycline with imipenem/cilastatin for the treatment of hospital-acquired pneumonia. *Diagn. Microbiol. Infect. Dis.* **2010**, *68*, 140–151. [CrossRef]
8. Tamma, P.D.; Avdic, E.; Li, D.X.; Dzintars, K.; Cosgrove, S.E. Association of adverse events with antibiotic use in hospitalized patients. *JAMA Intern. Med.* **2017**, *177*, 1308–1315. [CrossRef]
9. Chastre, J.; Wolff, M.; Fagon, J.Y.; Chevret, S.; Thomas, F.; Wermert, D.; Clementi, E.; Gonzalez, J.; Jusserand, D.; Asfar, P.; et al. Comparison of 8 vs 15 days of antibiotic therapy for ventilator-associated pneumonia in adults: A randomized trial. *JAMA* **2003**, *290*, 2588–2598. [CrossRef]
10. Park, H.J.; Cho, J.H.; Kim, H.J.; Han, S.H.; Jeong, S.H.; Byun, M.K. Colistin monotherapy versus colistin/rifampicin combination therapy in pneumonia caused by colistin-resistant *Acinetobacter baumannii*: A randomised controlled trial. *J. Glob. Antimicrob. Resist.* **2019**, *17*, 66–71. [CrossRef]
11. Katip, W.; Uitrakul, S.; Oberdorfer, P. The effectiveness and nephrotoxicity of loading dose colistin combined with or without meropenem for the treatment of carbapenem-resistant *A. baumannii*. *Int. J. Infect. Dis.* **2020**, *97*, 391–395. [CrossRef]
12. Durante-Mangoni, E.; Signoriello, G.; Andini, R.; Mattei, A.; De Cristoforo, M.; Murino, P.; Bassetti, M.; Malacarne, P.; Petrosillo, N.; Galdieri, N.; et al. Colistin and rifampicin compared with colistin alone for the treatment of serious infections due to extensively drug-resistant *Acinetobacter baumannii*: A multicenter, randomized clinical trial. *Clin. Infect. Dis.* **2013**, *57*, 349–358. [CrossRef]
13. De Waele, J.J.; Martin-Loeches, I. Optimal duration of antibiotic treatment in Gram-negative infections. *Curr. Opin. Infect. Dis.* **2018**, *31*, 606–611. [CrossRef] [PubMed]
14. Katip, W.; Oberdorfer, P. Clinical Efficacy and Nephrotoxicity of Colistin Alone versus Colistin Plus Vancomycin in Critically Ill Patients Infected with Carbapenem-Resistant *Acinetobacter baumannii*: A Propensity Score-Matched Analysis. *Pharmaceutics* **2021**, *13*, 162. [CrossRef] [PubMed]
15. Tansarli, G.S.; Andreatos, N.; Pliakos, E.E.; Mylonakis, E. A Systematic Review and Meta-analysis of Antibiotic Treatment Duration for Bacteremia Due to *Enterobacteriaceae*. *Antimicrob. Agents Chemother.* **2019**, *63*, e02495-18. [CrossRef] [PubMed]
16. Sousa, A.; Pérez-Rodríguez, M.T.; Suárez, M.; Val, N.; Martínez-Lamas, L.; Nodar, A.; Longueira, R.; Crespo, M. Short-versus long-course therapy in gram-negative bacilli bloodstream infections. *Eur. J. Clin. Microbiol. Infect. Dis.* **2019**, *38*, 851–857. [CrossRef]
17. Lee, C.C.; Hsieh, C.C.; Yang, C.Y.; Hong, M.Y.; Lee, C.H.; Tang, H.J.; Ko, W.C. Short versus long duration antimicrobial treatment for community-onset bacteraemia: A propensity score matching study. *Int. J. Antimicrob. Agents* **2019**, *54*, 176–183. [CrossRef] [PubMed]
18. Pugh, R.; Grant, C.; Cooke, R.P.; Dempsey, G. Short-course versus prolonged-course antibiotic therapy for hospital-acquired pneumonia in critically ill adults. *Cochrane Database Syst. Rev.* **2015**, *2015*, CD007577. [CrossRef]

19. Kalil, A.C.; Metersky, M.L.; Klompas, M.; Muscedere, J.; Sweeney, D.A.; Palmer, L.B.; Napolitano, L.M.; O'Grady, N.P.; Bartlett, J.G.; Carratalà, J.; et al. Executive Summary: Management of Adults With Hospital-acquired and Ventilator-associated Pneumonia: 2016 Clinical Practice Guidelines by the Infectious Diseases Society of America and the American Thoracic Society. *Clin. Infect. Dis.* **2016**, *63*, 575–582. [CrossRef]
20. Nelson, A.N.; Justo, J.A.; Bookstaver, P.B.; Kohn, J.; Albrecht, H.; Al-Hasan, M.N. Optimal duration of antimicrobial therapy for uncomplicated Gram-negative bloodstream infections. *Infection* **2017**, *45*, 613–620. [CrossRef] [PubMed]
21. Hachem, R.Y.; Chemaly, R.F.; Ahmar, C.A.; Jiang, Y.; Boktour, M.R.; Rjaili, G.A.; Bodey, G.P.; Raad, I.I. Colistin is effective in treatment of infections caused by multidrug-resistant *Pseudomonas aeruginosa* in cancer patients. *Antimicrob. Agents Chemother.* **2007**, *51*, 1905–1911. [CrossRef] [PubMed]
22. Nazer, L.H.; Rihani, S.; Hawari, F.I.; Le, J. High-dose colistin for microbiologically documented serious respiratory infections associated with carbapenem-resistant *Acinetobacter baumannii* in critically ill cancer patients: A retrospective cohort study. *Infect. Dis.* **2015**, *47*, 755–760. [CrossRef] [PubMed]
23. Hong, C.-Y.; Peng, J.; Wei, Y.-S.; Peng, H.-P.; Yang, H.; Zhao, C.-X.; Liang, G.-J.; Wang, G.-Q. The impact of chemotherapy-associated neutrophil/ lymphocyte counts on prognosis of adjuvant chemotherapy in colorectal cancer. *BMC Cancer* **2013**, *13*, 177.
24. Van Faassen, H.; KuoLee, R.; Harris, G.; Zhao, X.; Conlan, J.W.; Chen, W. Neutrophils play an important role in host resistance to respiratory infection with *Acinetobacter baumannii* in mice. *Infect. Immun.* **2007**, *75*, 5597–5608. [CrossRef]
25. Andes, D.R.; Van Ogtrop, M.L.; Craig, W.A. Impact of neutrophils on the in vivo activity of fluoroquinolones. In Proceedings of the Program and abstracts of the 37th Meeting of the Infectious Diseases Society of America (Philadelphia), Arlington, VA, USA, 18–21 November 1999; Infectious Diseases Society of America: Arlington, VA, USA, 1999.
26. Theuretzbacher, U. Pharmacokinetic and pharmacodynamic issues for antimicrobial therapy in patients with cancer. *Clin. Infect. Dis.* **2012**, *54*, 1785–1792. [CrossRef]
27. Karaiskos, I.; Giamarellou, H. Multidrug-resistant and extensively drug-resistant Gram-negative pathogens: Current and emerging therapeutic approaches. *Expert Opin. Pharmacother.* **2014**, *15*, 1351–1370. [CrossRef]
28. Pogue, J.M.; Lee, J.; Marchaim, D.; Yee, V.; Zhao, J.J.; Chopra, T.; Lephart, P.; Kaye, K.S. Incidence of and risk factors for colistin-associated nephrotoxicity in a large academic health system. *Clin. Infect. Dis.* **2011**, *53*, 879–884. [CrossRef]
29. Hartzell, J.D.; Neff, R.; Ake, J.; Howard, R.; Olson, S.; Paolino, K.; Vishnepolsky, M.; Weintrob, A.; Wortmann, G. Nephrotoxicity associated with intravenous colistin (colistimethate sodium) treatment at a tertiary care medical center. *Clin. Infect. Dis.* **2009**, *48*, 1724–1728. [CrossRef]
30. Forrest, A.; Garonzik, S.M.; Thamlikitkul, V.; Giamarellos-Bourboulis, E.J.; Paterson, D.L.; Li, J.; Silveira, F.P.; Nation, R.L. Pharmacokinetic/Toxicodynamic Analysis of Colistin-Associated Acute Kidney Injury in Critically Ill Patients. *Antimicrob. Agents Chemother.* **2017**, *61*, e01367-17. [CrossRef]
31. Horan, T.C.; Andrus, M.; Dudeck, M.A. CDC/NHSN surveillance definition of health care-associated infection and criteria for specific types of infections in the acute care setting. *Am. J. Infect. Control* **2008**, *36*, 309–332. [CrossRef] [PubMed]
32. Kellum, J.A.; Bellomo, R.; Ronco, C. Definition and classification of acute kidney injury. *Nephron Clin. Pract.* **2008**, *109*, c182–c187. [CrossRef] [PubMed]
33. Clinical and Laboratory Standards Institute. *Performance Standards for Antimicrobial Susceptibility Testing: Twentieth Informational Supplement M100-S20*; CLSI: Wayne, PA, USA, 2010.
34. Choi, S.H.; Cho, E.B.; Chung, J.W.; Lee, M.K. Changes in the early mortality of adult patients with carbapenem-resistant *Acinetobacter baumannii* bacteremia during 11 years at an academic medical center. *J. Infect. Chemother.* **2019**, *25*, 6–11. [CrossRef] [PubMed]
35. Bitew, A.; Molalign, T.; Chanie, M. Species distribution and antibiotic susceptibility profile of bacterial uropathogens among patients complaining urinary tract infections. *BMC Infect. Dis.* **2017**, *17*, 654. [CrossRef] [PubMed]

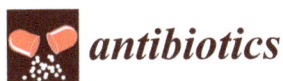

Article

Effect of N-Acetylcysteine Administration on 30-Day Mortality in Critically Ill Patients with Septic Shock Caused by Carbapenem-Resistant *Klebsiella pneumoniae* and *Acinetobacter baumannii*: A Retrospective Case-Control Study

Alessandra Oliva [1,2,*], Alessandro Bianchi [1], Alessandro Russo [1], Giancarlo Ceccarelli [1], Francesca Cancelli [1], Fulvio Aloj [2], Danilo Alunni Fegatelli [3], Claudio Maria Mastroianni [1] and Mario Venditti [1]

[1] Department of Public Health and Infectious Diseases, Sapienza University of Rome, 00185 Rome, Italy; alessandro.bianchi@uniroma1.it (A.B.); alessandro.russo1982@gmail.com (A.R.); giancarlo.ceccarelli@uniroma1.it (G.C.); francesca.cancelli@uniroma1.it (F.C.); claudio.mastroianni@uniroma1.it (C.M.M.); mario.venditti@uniroma1.it (M.V.)

[2] IRCCS Neuromed, Istituto Neurologico Mediterraneo, 86077 Pozzilli (IS), Italy; aloj@neuromed.it

[3] Department of Statistical Science, Sapienza University of Rome, 00185 Rome, Italy; danilo.alunnifegatelli@uniroma1.it

* Correspondence: alessandra.oliva@uniroma1.it

Abstract: Carbapenem-resistant *Klebsiella pneumoniae* (CR-Kp) and *Acinetobacter baumannii* (CR-Ab) represent important cause of severe infections in intensive care unit (ICU) patients. N-Acetylcysteine (NAC) is a mucolytic agent with antioxidant and anti-inflammatory properties, showing also in-vitro antibacterial activity. Aim was to evaluate the effect on 30-day mortality of the addition of intravenous NAC to antibiotics in ICU patients with CR-Kp or CR-Ab septic shock. A retrospective, observational case:control study (1:2) in patients with septic shock caused by CR-Kp or CR-Ab hospitalized in two different ICUs was conducted. Cases included patients receiving NAC plus antimicrobials, controls included patients not receiving NAC. Cases and controls were matched for age, SAPS II, causative agent and source of infection. No differences in age, sex, SAPS II score or time to initiate definitive therapy were observed between cases and controls. Pneumonia and bacteremia were the leading infections. Overall, mortality was 48.9% (33.3% vs. 56.7% in cases and controls, $p = 0.05$). Independent risk factors for mortality were not receiving NAC ($p = 0.002$) and CR-Ab ($p = 0.034$) whereas therapy with two in-vitro active antibiotics ($p = 0.014$) and time to initial definite therapy ($p = 0.026$) were protective. NAC plus antibiotics might reduce the 30-day mortality rate in ICU patients with CR-Kp and CR-Ab septic shock.

Keywords: carbapenem-resistant *Klebsiella pneumoniae*; carbapenem-resistant *Acinetobacter baumannii*; N-acetylcysteine; septic shock; critically ill patients

1. Introduction

Carbapenem-resistant *Klebsiella pneumoniae* (CR-Kp) and *Acinetobacter baumannii* (CR-Ab) represent nowadays an important cause of severe infections in intensive care unit (ICU) patients and mortality rates are significantly associated to septic shock [1–6]. Protective factors that influence the clinical outcome include early appropriate antibiotic treatment, adequate source control and number of in-vitro active antimicrobials, whereas septic shock caused by CR-Ab might exhibit a mortality rate up to 60% [6,7]. Therefore, in the context of increasing antimicrobial resistance and restricted therapeutic options typical of the contemporary era, there is a growing scientific interest on finding possible therapeutic adjuvants for sepsis and septic shock [8–11]. Since septic shock is characterized by excessive and unbalanced production of pro-inflammatory cytokines, reactive oxygen species and a marked alteration of circulation, compounds able to counteract these effects might find a rationale in the treatment of this condition [12–17].

N-Acetylcysteine (NAC) is a mucolytic agent with antioxidant and anti-inflammatory properties, commonly used for the treatment of acetaminophen overdose or respiratory conditions with high mucus production [18–20]. Beyond this, NAC showed also in-vitro activity against several bacteria including multi-drug resistant (MDR) ones and viruses and demonstrated a synergistic interaction with antibiotics or antivirals [21–30]. In addition, animal models showed improvement of organ damage and a reduction of microvascular dysfunction following NAC administration in endotoxin-induced shock [12,31], rendering this compound attractive for the clinical use as a therapeutic adjuvant in case of infections.

To date, clinical studies evaluating NAC in septic shock gave conflicting results; however, most of them were not recent [32–37]. On the other hand, a recent randomized clinical trial investigating the effect of different anti-oxidants as adjuvants in septic shock showed that NAC was able to improve antioxidant capacity [38].

Besides the common use of NAC in the clinical practice, currently in some Italian centers including the ICU of IRCCS Neuromed (Pozzilli, Italy), intravenous NAC is routinely administered in critically ill patients with respiratory conditions characterized by excessive and/or thick mucus production.

Therefore, based on these premises, the purpose of the study was to evaluate the effect on 30-day mortality of the addition of intravenous NAC to antibiotic therapy in ICU patients with septic shock caused by CR-Kp or CR-Ab.

2. Results

During the study period, there were 41 cases of patients who had septic shock caused by CR-Kp or CR-Ab treated with NAC. Eleven out of 41 (26.8%) were excluded from the study: central nervous system infections (four cases), no sufficient data (four cases) or no matched controls (three cases). Eventually, 90 patients were enrolled in the study (30 cases and 60 matched controls) (Figure 1).

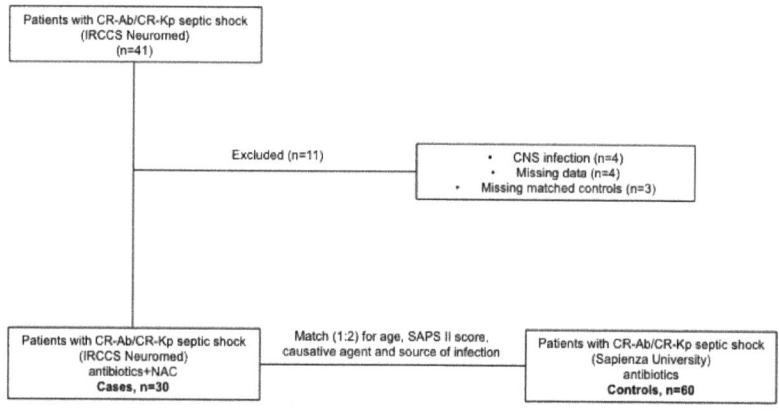

Figure 1. Flow-chart of the study.

Mean age was 58.1 and 59.2 years in case and control groups, respectively. 80% of cases and 68.3% of controls were male. SAPS II was 35.3 and 38.6 in cases and controls, respectively. Previous antibiotic therapy was recorded in 63.3% and 48.3% of cases and controls, respectively, whereas a previous CR-Kp or CR-Ab colonization was found in 43.3% and 28.3% of cases and controls, respectively. Length of ICU stay was statistically significant longer in cases than in controls (51.4 vs. 27.8 days, $p < 0.001$). Study population characteristics are shown in Table 1.

Table 1. Characteristics of patients with septic shock caused by carbapenem-resistant *Klebsiella pneumoniae* (CR-Kp) and *Acinetobacter baumannii* (CR-Ab).

	Cases ° n = 30	Controls ° n = 60	p-Value
Age, years (mean ± SD)	58.1 ± 17.7	59.2 ± 14.19	*
Male sex, n (%)	24 (80)	41 (68.3)	0.32
SAPS II	35.33 ± 17.7	38.57 ± 11.5	*
Lenght of ICU stay, days (mean ± SD)	51.4 ± 27.9	27.8 ± 20	<0.0001
Previous (90-d) hospitalization, n (%)	14 (46.6)	21 (35)	0.36
Previous (90-d) ICU admission, n (%)	4 (13.3)	6 (10)	0.72
Previous (90-d) surgery, n (%)	14 (43.3)	17 (28.3)	0.16
Previous (90-d) antibiotic therapy, n (%)	19 (63.3)	29 (48.3)	0.26
Previous colonization with CR-Kp or CR-Ab, n (%)	13 (43.3)	17 (28.3)	0.16
Comorbidities, n (%) - chronic liver disease - neoplasm - diabetes mellitus - cardiovascular diseases - chronic renal failure - COPD	 6 (20) 6 (20) 6 (20) 18 (60) 0 (0) 3 (10)	 7 (11.6) 2 (3.3) 15 (25) 19 (31.6) 2 (3.3) 11 (18.3)	 0.34 0.01 0.79 0.01 0.55 0.37
Causes of ICU admission, n (%) - respiratory failure - septic shock - stroke - post-surgery - trauma - cardiac arrest	 6 (20) 3 (10) 12 (40) 6 (20) 2 (6.6) 1 (3.3)	 20 (33.3) 14 (23.3) 4 (6.6) 7 (11.6) 9 (15) 6 (10)	 0.22 0.16 0.0002 0.34 0.32 0.41
Source of infection, n (%) - pneumonia - primary bacteremia	 20 (66.7) 10 (33.3)	 40 (66.7) 20 (33.3)	 *
Causative agent, n (%) - CR-Kp - CR-Ab	 18 (60) 12 (40)	 36 (60) 24 (40)	 *
Colistin-resistant strains, n (%)	8 (26.7)	29 (31.7)	0.54
Adequate source control, n (%)	10 (33.3)	31 (51.6)	0.12
Number of antibiotics used as definitive therapy, n (%) - no definite therapy - 1 antibiotic - 2 antibiotics - 3 antibiotics - 4 antibiotics	 1 (3.4) 0 (0) 12 (40) 13 (43.3) 4 (13.3)	 1 (1.7) 5 (8.3) 19 (31.6) 28 (46.7) 7 (11.7)	 0.99 0.16 0.48 0.82 0.99
Type of antimicrobial combinations, n (%) - Carbapenem-containing regimen - Colistin-containing regimen - Tigecycline-containing regimen - Aminoglycoside-containing regimen - Rifampin-containing regimen	 22 (73.3) 24 (80) 7 (23.3) 6 (20) 2 (6.7)	 44 (73.3) 33 (55) 33 (55) 8 (13.33) 13 (20)	 0.99 0.02 0.007 0.53 0.12
≥2 in-vitro active antibiotics within 24 h from septic shock, n (%)	5 (16.7)	14 (23.3)	0.58
≥2 in-vitro active antibiotics definitive, n (%)	6 (20)	16 (26.7)	0.60
Time to initial definitive therapy, days (mean ± SD)	2.7 ± 0.4	2.65 ± 0.2	0.86
NAC dosage, mg/die (mean± SD) Range	1520 ± 504 (1200–3000)	NA	
Length of antibiotic therapy, days (mean± SD)	15.1 ± 7.9	12.3 ± 8.3	0.12
Length of NAC therapy, days (mean± SD)	16.6 ± 7.1	NA	
Adverse effects of NAC therapy, n(%)	0 (0)	NA	
Outcome, n (%) - 7-day mortality - 14-day mortality - 30-day mortality	 4 (13.3) 6 (20) 10 (33.3)	 15 (25) 19 (31.7) 34 (56.7)	 0.18 0.32 0.051

°: Cases included patients receiving intravenous NAC in combination with antimicrobials, controls included patients not receiving NAC. Data collection for cases was blinded for the outcome. *: Cases and controls were matched for age, SAPS II, source of infection and causative agent. ICU: Intensive Care Unit. CR-Kp: Carbapenem-resistant *Klebsiella pneumoniae*; CR-Ab: Carbapenem-resistant *Acinetobacter baumannii*; COPD: Chronic Obstructive Pulmonary Disease. NA: not applicable.

In both groups pneumonia was the most frequent source of infection (66.7%), followed by primary bacteremia (33.3%). As for causative agent, 60% and 40% of patients had a septic shock caused by CR-Kp and CR-Ab, respectively. Colistin resistant strains represented 26.7% and 31.7% of isolates in case and control group, respectively, without statistical differences.

Combination therapy was used in almost all patients. In case group, 40% (12/30) of patients received a combination of two antibiotics, 43.3% (13/30) a combination of three antibiotics and 13.3% (4/30) a combination of four antibiotics. A definitive antibiotic regimen containing colistin and/or carbapenem was the most commonly used, respectively in 80% and 73.3% of cases, followed by regimens containing tigecycline (23.3%) and aminoglycoside (20%). In control group, 8.3% (5/60) of patients received monotherapy, 31.6% (19/60) of patients received a combination of two antibiotics, 46.7% (28/60) a combination of three antibiotics and 11.7% (7/60) a combination of four antibiotics. A definitive antibiotic regimen containing carbapenem (73.3%) was the most used, followed by regimens containing colistin (55%), tigecycline (55%) and aminoglycoside (13.3%). Rifampin-containing regimens were used in 6.7% and 20% in cases and controls, respectively ($p = 0.12$). No differences were observed in the two study groups regarding the use of carbapenems, while colistin-containing regimen was used more frequently in cases than in controls ($p = 0.02$). Conversely, tigecycline-containing regimen was used more frequently in controls ($p = 0.007$) (Table 1).

Time to initiate definitive antibiotic therapy was 2.7 days for both groups. Length of antibiotic therapy was similar in the two groups, 15.1 days for cases and 12.3 days for controls ($p = 0.12$).

In the first 24 h from septic shock onset, treatment with two or more antibiotics displaying in vitro activity was reported in 16.7% of cases and in 23.3% of controls and definitive therapy with two or more antibiotics displaying in vitro activity was reported in 20% of cases and 26.7% of controls, without statistical differences. The mean ($\pm$ SD) administered NAC dosage was 1520 ± 504 mg/die, ranging from 1200 to 3000 mg/die, according to treating physicians. Mean ($\pm$ SD) duration of NAC treatment was 16.6 ± 7.1 days and no adverse events were recorded during NAC administration.

Overall 7-day (13.3% in cases, 25% in controls) and 14-day (20% in cases, 31.7% in controls) mortality rates were lower in cases than controls, without reaching the statistical significance. On the other hand, the 30-day mortality rate (48.9%) was lower in cases than controls at univariate analysis (33.3% in cases versus 56.7% in controls, $p = 0.05$). Figure 2 shows the 30-day overall survival rate in cases and controls.

In addition, mortality was higher when septic shock was caused by CR-Ab [22/36 (61.1%) versus 22/54 (40.7%) in CR-Ab and CR-Kp, respectively].

At the univariate analysis, risk factor for mortality were age ($p = 0.01$), CR-Ab infection ($p < 0.001$), not receiving NAC ($p = 0.05$), whereas time to initiate definitive therapy ($p = 0.017$) and definitive therapy with two or more antibiotics displaying in vitro activity ($p = 0.005$) were protective.

At the multivariate analysis, independent risk factors for mortality were not receiving NAC (HR: 3.6; 95% CI, 1.59 to 8.22; $p = 0.002$) and CR-Ab infection (HR: 2.8; 95% CI, 1.08 to 7.24; $p = 0.034$); whereas time to initiate definitive therapy (HR: 0.83; 95% CI, 0.70 to 0.98; $p = 0.026$) and definitive therapy with two or more antibiotics displaying in vitro activity (HR: 0.21; 95% CI, 0.06 to 0.73; $p = 0.014$) were protective, regardless of age, sex, SAPS II score, source of infection or the type of antibiotics used as definitive therapy (Table 2).

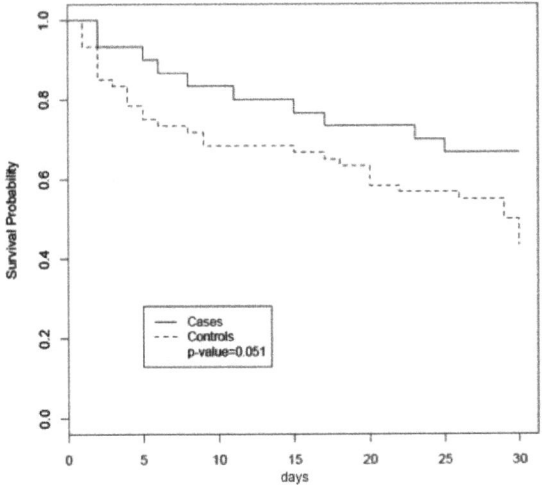

Figure 2. Overall 30-day survival rate in patients with carbapenem-resistant *K. pneumoniae* or *A. baumannii* septic shock receiving antibiotics plus intravenous NAC (cases, n = 30) or antibiotics only (controls, n = 60).

Table 2. Indipendent risk factors for 30-day mortality of patients with septic shock caused by carbapenem-resistant *Klebsiella pneumoniae* and *Acinetobacter baumannii*.

Variable	Univariate Analysis			Multivariate Analysis		
	HR	95% CI	*p*-Value	HR	95% CI	*p*-Value
Controls (not receiving NAC)	1.99	0.98–4.04	0.05	3.61	1.59–8.22	0.002
Sex	0.88	0.46–1.68	0.70	1.35	0.68–2.69	0.38
Age	1.02	1.00–1.05	0.015	1.02	0.99–1.05	0.17
SAPS II	1.01	0.99–1.03	0.30	1.01	0.98–1.05	0.25
CR-Ab	3.29	1.81–6.00	<0.001	2.79	1.07–7.24	0.03
≥2 in-vitro active antibiotics	0.22	0.08–0.63	0.005	0.21	0.06–0.73	0.014
Number of antibiotics in definitive therapy	0.69	0.47–1.03	0.07	0.65	0.39–1.09	0.10
Pneumonia	1.74	0.86–3.53	0.12	0.79	0.32–1.94	0.62
Use of colistin	0.94	0.51–1.73	0.86	0.50	0.19–1.32	0.16
Time to definitive antibiotic therapy	0.81	0.69–0.96	0.01	0.82	0.69–0.97	0.026

NAC: N-acetylcysteine; CR-Ab: Carbapenem-resistant *Acinetobacter baumannii*. SAPS II: Simplified Acute Physiology Score II. CI: Confidence interval.

3. Discussion

Septic shock is associated with high mortality rate, particularly when caused by CR Kp or CR Ab [5,6,39,40] being the latter associated to a worse prognosis [39]. To the best of our knowledge, this case-control study analyzed for the first time the effects on 30-day mortality of NAC administration in addition to antibiotic therapy in critically ill patients with septic shock due to CR-Kp or CR-Ab. With this regard, we were able to demonstrate that in patients who received NAC, 30-day mortality was significantly lower than in controls.

NAC is the N-acetyl derivative of the amino acid L-cysteine with anti-oxidant properties thanks to the increase of glutathione in the body, able to reduce free oxygen radicals and to inhibit the effect of pro-inflammatory cytokines [41]. Additionally, NAC has also a vasodilatation activity on microcirculation that improves locoregional blood flow [17]. All of the abovementioned phenomena may have important implications in the setting of a dysregulated host response to infection with a high release of pro-inflammatory cytokines, reactive oxygen species and a profound alteration of microcirculation, as it occurs in septic shock [13–16]. In animal models, it was demonstrated that NAC ameliorates endotoxin shock-induced organ damage through the reduction of free radicals and inflammatory cytokines production [31]. Of note, this effect was observed when NAC was administered either as a pre-treatment or as a post-treatment drug [31] Furthermore, several studies demonstrated in vitro activity of NAC against a large variety of microorganisms, including *K. pneumoniae* and *A. baumannii* [21–23,26]. In particular, preliminary results from our group showed that NAC was highly synergic with meropenem against clinical strains of CR-Kp and CR-Ab whereas Pollini et al. found a remarkable synergism of colistin/NAC combinations against CR-Ab [21,22,26].

However, in spite of the promising results from both in vitro and animal studies, human studies might suggest otherwise. On one side, some NAC studies in patients with sepsis showed encouraging results as far as improved tissue oxygenation and hepatosplanchnic flow, decreased oxidative damage and reduction in IL-8 blood concentrations are concerned [32–36]. On the other hand, a meta-analysis of 41 randomized clinical trials investigating the role of NAC on clinical outcomes in sepsis patients showed no benefit on mortality, length of stay, duration of mechanical ventilation, and incidence of new organ failure with early or late NAC administration [37]. Rather, the latter was associated with hemodynamic instability. As a consequence, the authors concluded that clinicians should not routinely use intravenous NAC in sepsis. The conclusion was confirmed even after subgroups analysis between studies focusing on systemic inflammatory response syndrome or sepsis/septic shock. However, when looking in depth within the meta-analysis, all studies referred to the period 1991–2009 and heterogeneity among study populations was also observed [37]. Furthermore, in almost all studies NAC was given after the sepsis syndrome had been established, potentially too late to be beneficial on outcome. Additionally, another potentially important concern was that high doses have been used in the majority of the abovementioned randomized clinical trials, namely 150 mg/kg, which may allow formation of toxic intermediate molecules interfering with potential benefits of NAC therapy [42].

Conversely, in our study NAC was administered at the very early phase of infection before the development of sepsis syndrome and the mean dosage of NAC (1520 mg/die) was lower than that used in previous study, thus reducing the risk of toxic intermediates production.

Finally, a recent randomized clinical trial investigating the effect of different antioxidants in septic shock showed that NAC was able to improve antioxidant capacity, in the absence of significant adverse reactions or side effects [38].

Early antibiotic therapy represents a cornerstone of critical care management in septic shock patients [4,40,43–46]. Accordingly, in our study a protective effect on mortality was related to the time to initiate definitive therapy, defined as the time between infection onset and initial definitive in vitro active therapy. Combination therapy was the most used treatment in our study; however, previous studies suggested that the key factor for decreasing the mortality is not the number of drugs used but rather the administration of at least two in vitro-active antibiotics, in particular for CR-Kp [6,46,47]. Treatment with two or more in vitro-active antibiotics is difficult to achieve in the presence of MDR bacteria because limited options are available to treat these infections, especially for CR-Ab. In fact, in our study only 36.7% of patients were treated with two or more antibiotics showing in vitro activity against the isolates and this probably explains the high mortality rates observed in our population, which is, however, similar to that reported in the literature [6]. Nevertheless, treatment with two or more in vitro-active antibiotics was associated with lower mortality.

Although a difference was observed in the two study groups regarding the use of regimens containing colistin and tigecycline, with the former more frequently used in cases than controls, this did not affect overall mortality.

In our study, 30-day mortality for CR-Ab was higher than that observed for CR-Kp. The impact of CR-Ab on clinical outcome was also highlighted in multivariable analysis, thus confirming the recent literature data, which showed a mortality rate of up to 60% and 40% in the presence of septic shock caused by CR-Ab and CR-Kp, respectively [5,6,48].

Our study has some limitations that should be acknowledged. First, the retrospective nature of the study is an intrinsic limitation of this analysis. Second, the sample size is relatively low and included all patients with septic shock caused by CR-Kp or CR-Ab observed in the two ICUs, without a sample size calculation. Therefore, the results of our study might be considered preliminary and further multicenter prospective studies are needed to confirm our findings. Third, cases and controls came from two distinct cohorts of patients and therefore differences could be related to intrinsic differences between populations and microorganism, despite the extensive patients' matching (age, SAPS II score, causative agent and source of infection). However, we were confident that the potential differences were minimized by the fact that both ICUs had a dedicated Infectious Diseases consultant who was in charge for the treatment of all patients and who belonged to the same well-established consultation system. Consequently, the Infectious Diseases consultants had the same diagnostic and therapeutic approach towards patients admitted to these 2 ICUs (Supplementary Figure S1). Fourth, NAC was not administered in all cases at the same dosage and timing and consequently the results need to be interpreted cautiously. Lastly, since study population included mainly patients who had pneumonia, conclusions should apply to ICU patients with pneumonia-associated septic shock caused by CR-Kp and CR-Ab. An additional limitation was the lack of oxidative markers (i.e nitrate/nitrite ratio, glutathione) measurements before and after NAC therapy.

Nevertheless, we believe that the present investigation has some important strenghts, which might have contributed to bias reduction, such as: (i) patients were matched for several variables, which might have had theirselves an influence on the primary outcome of the study (30-day mortality); (ii) each ICU had a dedicated infectious diseases consultant referring to the same well-established consultation system, thus assuring the same clinical and therapeutic approach to infections in both cases and controls. Furthermore, it represents a real-life clinical experience providing useful suggestions to clinicians about the management of a difficult-to-treat infection such as septic shock caused by CR-Kp and CR-Ab.

4. Materials and Methods

We performed a retrospective, observational case:control study (1:2) in patients with septic shock caused by CR-Kp or CR-Ab hospitalized in two different ICUs [IRCCS Neuromed for cases and Sapienza University (Rome, Italy) for controls, the latter derived from a historical cohort of patients [6]. Both ICUs have a dedicated Infectious Diseases consultant referring to a well-established consultation system at Policlinico Umberto I, Sapienza University of Rome, with the same clinical and therapeutic approach [49–51] (Supplementary Figure S1). Cases included patients with septic shock receiving intravenous NAC in combination with antimicrobials, controls included patients with septic shock not receiving NAC. For every case, two matched controls were randomly selected from patients who did not receive NAC. Cases and controls were matched for age, SAPS II score, causative agent and source of infection. Data collection for cases was blinded for the outcome. Inclusion criteria were: (i) ICU admission, (ii) presence of septic shock during ICU stay, (iii) laboratory documented and confirmed infection by CR-Kp or CR-Ab and iv) intravenous administration of NAC for cases, whereas exclusion criteria were (i) a documented infection localized to the central nervous system at admission or during hospital stay, (ii) age under 18 years old or (iii) missing key data.

The Ethical Commitees approved the study (no. 4547–2017 for Sapienza; approval 20 March 2019 for IRCCS Neuromed) whereas informed consent was waived due to the retrospective nature of the research.

4.1. Baseline Assessment

Patient data were extracted from medical records and from hospital computerized databases or clinical charts. The following information was reviewed: demographics, clinical and laboratory findings, comorbid conditions, microbiological data, duration of ICU and hospital stay, incidence of infections during hospitalization, treatments and procedures administered during hospitalization and/or in the 90 days prior to infection, classes of antibiotics received on admission and/or after admission before a positive culture of a biological sample was obtained, the simplified acute physiology score II (SAPS II) at the time of infection, source of infection, antibiotic regimens used for CR-Ab or CR-Kp infections, and 30-day mortality. According to both hospital's guidelines, colonization with CR-Kp and CR-Ab strains was routinely evaluated by rectal swab, respiratory specimens and urine culture at the time of ICU admission and every week afterwards.

4.2. Definitions

Infections were defined according to the standard definitions of the ECDC [52] and septic shock was defined according to the SEPSIS-3 criteria definition, a subset of sepsis with persisting hypotension requiring vasopressors to maintain mean arterial pressure of 65 mmHg or greater and having a serum lactate level greater than 2 mmol/L despite adequate volume resuscitation [53].

A CR-Ab or CR-Kp infection was defined as clinical signs of infection and culture of blood, urine, cerebrospinal fluid or a biological sample from skin and skin structures, lung, or abdomen yielding a CR-Ab or a CR-Kp strain.

Infection onset was defined as the date of collection of the index culture (i.e., the first blood culture that yielded the study isolate). Infections were classified as hospital acquired if the index culture had been collected > 48 h after hospital admission and no signs or symptoms of infection had been noted at admission. Primary bloodstream infection (BSI) was defined as BSI occurring in patients without a recognized source of infection.

The severity of clinical conditions was determined by using SAPS II score calculated at the time of septic shock onset. Length of hospital and ICU stay were calculated as the number of days from the date of admission to the date of discharge or death.

Depending on the number of drugs used (one or more), treatment regimens were classified as monotherapy or combination therapy. Definitive antibiotic therapy was defined as the definitive antimicrobial treatment based on in vitro CR-Ab or CR-Kp isolates susceptibilities. Antibiotic regimens were also classified according to the following: one antibiotic displaying in vitro activity, and two or more antibiotics displaying in vitro activity. Time to initial definitive therapy was the time between infection onset and initial definitive therapy.

Intravenous NAC was administered in patients with respiratory conditions characterized by excessive and/or thick mucus production as soon as signs of a possible infection developed (i.e., at the very early phase of infection) as adjunctive therapy and stopped together with antibiotic therapy. Dosages of intravenous NAC ranged from 1200 to 3000 mg/die, according to treating physicians. Intravenous NAC was administered in saline solution with 30–60 min infusion rate.

4.3. Statistical Analysis

Continuous variables were compared using Student's t test or Mann-Whitney U test and were described as mean ± standard deviation (SD) or as median and interquartile range (IQR) according to whether the distribution of the variables was normal or non-normal. Chi-squared test (χ^2) and Fisher's exact test were used to compare categorical variables. Univariate and multivariate analyses were performed to evaluate factors related to 30-days mortality. Variables with a p value two-sided <0.05 were considered statistically significant. The results obtained were analyzed using a commercially available statistical software package (version 15, STATA Corp, College Station, TX, USA: StataCorp LLC).

5. Conclusions

In conclusion, in the challenging context of increasing antimicrobial resistance and restricted therapeutic options, this study suggests that a combined use of NAC plus antibiotics might reduce the 30-day mortality rate in ICU patients with septic shock caused by CR-Kp and CR-Ab. Therefore, our preliminary data seem to encourage further clinical investigations on the role of NAC as an adjuvant therapy in ICU patients with septic shock due to multi-drug resistant Gram-negative bacilli.

Supplementary Materials: The following are available online at https://www.mdpi.com/2079-6382/10/3/271/s1, Figure S1: Treatment protocol in critically ill patients with suspected Gram-negative infection implemented by Infectious Diseases consultants at the Intensive Care Unit of IRCCS Neuromed (Pozzilli) and Sapienza University of Rome.

Author Contributions: Conceptualization, A.O. and M.V.; methodology, A.O.; formal analysis, D.A.F.; data collection: A.B., A.R., F.C., G.C., F.A.; writing—original draft preparation, A.O.; writing—review and editing, M.V., C.M.M.; supervision, C.M.M., M.V. All authors have read and agreed to the published version of the manuscript.

Funding: This research received no external funding.

Institutional Review Board Statement: The study was conducted according to the guidelines of the Declaration of Helsinki, and approved by the Institutional Review of Sapienza (no. 4547–2017) and IRCCS Neuromed (approval data 20 March 2019).

Informed Consent Statement: The study was conducted according to the guidelines of the Declaration of Helsinki, and approved by the Institutional Review Board of IRCCS Neuromed for cases and of Sapienza University of Rome for controls. Informed consent was waived due to the retrospective nature of the research.

Data Availability Statement: The data used to support the findings of this study are available from the corresponding author upon request.

Acknowledgments: The authors thank the nursing staff for their contribution.

Conflicts of Interest: The authors declare no conflict of interest.

References

1. Kang, C.-I.; Kim, S.-H.; Park, W.B.; Lee, K.-D.; Kim, H.-B.; Kim, E.-C.; Oh, M.-D.; Choe, K.-W. Bloodstream Infections Caused by Antibiotic-Resistant Gram-Negative Bacilli: Risk Factors for Mortality and Impact of Inappropriate Initial Antimicrobial Therapy on Outcome. *Antimicrob. Agents Chemother.* **2005**, *49*, 760–766. [CrossRef] [PubMed]
2. Garnacho-Montero, J.; Dimopoulos, G.; Poulakou, G.; Akova, M.; Cisneros, J.M.; de Waele, J.; Petrosillo, N.; Seifert, H.; Timsit, J.F.; Vila, J.; et al. Task force on management and prevention of *Acinetobacter baumannii* infections in the ICU. *Intensiv. Care Med.* **2015**, *41*, 2057–2075. [CrossRef] [PubMed]
3. Cassini, A.; Högberg, L.D.; Plachouras, D.; Quattrocchi, A.; Hoxha, A.; Simonsen, G.S.; Colomb-Cotinat, M.; Kretzschmar, M.E.; Devleesschauwer, B.; Cecchini, M.; et al. Attributable deaths and disability-adjusted life-years caused by infections with antibiotic-resistant bacteria in the EU and the European Economic Area in 2015: A population-level modelling analysis. *Lancet Infect. Dis.* **2019**, *19*, 56–66. [CrossRef]
4. Dickinson, J.D.; Kollef, M.H. Early and Adequate Antibiotic Therapy in the Treatment of Severe Sepsis and Septic Shock. *Curr. Infect. Dis. Rep.* **2011**, *13*, 399–405. [CrossRef] [PubMed]
5. Busani, S.; Serafini, G.; Mantovani, E.; Venturelli, C.; Giannella, M.; Viale, P.; Mussini, C.; Cossarizza, A.; Girardis, M. Mortality in Patients with Septic Shock by Multidrug Resistant Bacteria. *J. Intensiv. Care Med.* **2017**, *34*, 48–54. [CrossRef]
6. Russo, A.; Giuliano, S.; Ceccarelli, G.; Alessandri, F.; Giordano, A.; Brunetti, G.; Venditti, M. Comparison of Septic Shock Due to Multidrug-Resistant *Acinetobacter baumanniior Klebsiella pneumoniae* Carbapenemase-Producing K. pneumoniae in Intensive Care Unit Patients. *Antimicrob. Agents Chemother.* **2018**, *62*, e02562-17. [CrossRef]
7. Falcone, M.; Bassetti, M.; Tiseo, G.; Giordano, C.; Nencini, E.; Russo, A.; Graziano, E.; Tagliaferri, E.; Leonildi, A.; Barnini, S.; et al. Time to appropriate antibiotic therapy is a predictor of outcome in patients with bloodstream infection caused by KPC-producing *Klebsiella pneumoniae*. *Crit. Care* **2020**, *24*, 1–12. [CrossRef]

8. Marik, P.E.; Khangoora, V.; Rivera, R.; Hooper, M.H.; Catravas, J. Hydrocortisone, Vitamin C, and Thiamine for the Treatment of Severe Sepsis and Septic Shock. *Chest* **2017**, *151*, 1229–1238. [CrossRef]
9. Victor, V.M.; Rocha, M.; de la Fuente, M. Immune cells: Free radicals and antioxidants in sepsis. *Int. Immunopharmacol.* **2004**, *4*, 327–347. [CrossRef]
10. Heming, N.; Lamothe, L.; Ambrosi, X.; Annane, D. Emerging drugs for the treatment of sepsis. *Expert Opin. Emerg. Drugs* **2016**, *21*, 27–37. [CrossRef]
11. Pinsky, M.R. Antioxidant therapy for severe sepsis: Promise and perspective. *Crit. Care Med.* **2003**, *31*, 2697–2698. [CrossRef] [PubMed]
12. Ergin, B.; Guerci, P.; Zafrani, L.; Nocken, F.; Kandil, A.; Gurel-Gurevin, E.; Demirci-Tansel, C.; Ince, C. Effects of N-acetylcysteine (NAC) supplementation in resuscitation fluids on renal microcirculatory oxygenation, inflammation, and function in a rat model of endotoxemia. *Intensiv. Care Med. Exp.* **2016**, *4*, 29. [CrossRef]
13. Angus, D.C.; van der Poll, T. Severe Sepsis and Septic Shock. *N. Engl. J. Med.* **2013**, *369*, 840–851. [CrossRef]
14. Ait-Oufella, H.; Maury, E.; Lehoux, S.; Guidet, B.; Offenstadt, G. The endothelium: Physiological functions and role in microcirculatory failure during severe sepsis. *Intensiv. Care Med.* **2010**, *36*, 1286–1298. [CrossRef] [PubMed]
15. Ince, C.; Mayeux, P.R.; Nguyen, T.; Gomez, H.; Kellum, J.A.; Ospina-Tascón, G.A.; Hernandez, G.; Murray, P.; de Backer, D. The Endothelium in Sepsis. *Shock* **2016**, *45*, 259–270. [CrossRef] [PubMed]
16. Ince, C. The microcirculation is the motor of sepsis. *Crit. Care* **2005**, *9*, S13–S19. [CrossRef]
17. Chertoff, J. N-Acetylcysteine's Role in Sepsis and Potential Benefit in Patients with Microcirculatory Derangements. *J. Intensiv. Care Med.* **2018**, *33*, 87–96. [CrossRef]
18. Sadowska, A.M.; Verbraecken, J.; Darquennes, K.; de Backer, W.A. Role of N-acetylcysteine in the management of COPD. *Int. J. Chronic Obstr. Pulm. Dis.* **2006**, *1*, 425–434. [CrossRef]
19. Green, J.L.; Heard, K.J.; Reynolds, K.M.; Albert, D. Oral and Intravenous Acetylcysteine for Treatment of Acetaminophen Toxicity: A Systematic Review and Meta-analysis. *West. J. Emerg. Med.* **2013**, *14*, 218–226. [CrossRef] [PubMed]
20. Blasi, F.; Page, C.; Rossolini, G.M.; Pallecchi, L.; Matera, M.G.; Rogliani, P.; Cazzola, M. The effect of N-acetylcysteine on biofilms: Implications for the treatment of respiratory tract infections. *Respir. Med.* **2016**, *117*, 190–197. [CrossRef] [PubMed]
21. Pollini, S.; Boncompagni, S.; di Maggio, T.; di Pilato, V.; Spanu, T.; Fiori, B.; Blasi, F.; Aliberti, S.; Sergio, F.; Rossolini, G.M.; et al. In vitro synergism of colistin in combination with N-acetylcysteine against *Acinetobacter baumannii* grown in planktonic phase and in biofilms. *J. Antimicrob. Chemother.* **2018**, *73*, 2388–2395. [CrossRef]
22. Mascellino, M.; de Angelis, M.; Miele, M.C.; Stringaro, A.R.; Colone, M.; Oliva, A. Potential Role of N-Acetyl-Cysteine Towards Mul-ti-Drug Resistant *Acinetobacter baumannii* and *Klebsiella pneumoniae*. In Proceedings of the ASM Microbe, San Francisco, CA, USA, 20–24 June 2019; p. AAR02-637.
23. Parry, M.F.; Neu, H.C. Effect of N-acetylcysteine on antibiotic activity and bacterial growth in vitro. *J. Clin. Microbiol.* **1977**, *5*, 58–61.
24. Aslam, S.; Darouiche, R.O. Role of Antibiofilm-Antimicrobial Agents in Controlling Device-Related Infections. *Int. J. Artif. Organs* **2011**, *34*, 752–758. [CrossRef] [PubMed]
25. Marchese, A.; Bozzolasco, M.; Gualco, L.; Debbia, E.A.; Schito, G.C.; Schito, A.M. Effect of fosfomycin alone and in combination with N-acetylcysteine on E. coli biofilms. *Int. J. Antimicrob. Agents* **2003**, *22*, 95–100. [CrossRef]
26. Oliva, A.; de Angelis, M.; Costantini, S.; Mascellino, M.T.; Mastroianni, C.M.; Vullo, V. High activity of N-acetylcysteine in combination with beta-lactam antibiotics against carbapenem-resistant *Acinetobater baumannii*. In Proceedings of the ECCMID 2018, Madrid, Spain, 21–24 April 2018.
27. Rodríguez-Rosado, A.I.; Valencia, E.Y.; Rodríguez-Rojas, A.; Costas, C.; Galhardo, R.S.; Rodríguez-Beltrán, J.; Blázquez, J. N-acetylcysteine blocks SOS induction and mutagenesis produced by fluoroquinolones in *Escherichia coli*. *J. Antimicrob. Chemother.* **2019**, *74*, 2188–2196. [CrossRef] [PubMed]
28. Garozzo, A.; Tempera, G.; Ungheri, D.; Timpanaro, R.; Castro, A. N-Acetylcysteine Synergizes with Oseltamivir in Protecting Mice from Lethal Influenza Infection. *Int. J. Immunopathol. Pharmacol.* **2007**, *20*, 349–354. [CrossRef] [PubMed]
29. Geiler, J.; Michaelis, M.; Naczk, P.; Leutz, A.; Langer, K.; Doerr, H.-W.; Cinatl, J. N-acetyl-l-cysteine (NAC) inhibits virus replication and expression of pro-inflammatory molecules in A549 cells infected with highly pathogenic H5N1 influenza A virus. *Biochem. Pharmacol.* **2010**, *79*, 413–420. [CrossRef] [PubMed]
30. Ghezzi, P.; Ungheri, D. Synergistic Combination of N-Acetylcysteine and Ribavirin to Protect from Lethal Influenza Viral Infection in a Mouse Model. *Int. J. Immunopathol. Pharmacol.* **2004**, *17*, 99–102. [CrossRef]
31. Hsu, B.-G.; Lee, R.-P.; Yang, F.-L.; Harn, H.-J.; Chen, H.I. Post-treatment with N-acetylcysteine ameliorates endotoxin shock-induced organ damage in conscious rats. *Life Sci.* **2006**, *79*, 2010–2016. [CrossRef]
32. Spies, C.; Giese, C.; Meier-Hellmann, A.; Specht, M.; Hannemann, L.; Schaffartzik, W.; Reinhart, K. Einfluss der prophylaktischen Gabe von N-Azetylzystein auf klinische Indikatoren der Gewebeoxygenierung unter Hyperoxie bei kardialen Risikopatienten. *Anaesthesist* **1996**, *45*, 343–350. [CrossRef]
33. Spapen, H.; Zhang, H.; Demanet, C.; Vleminckx, W.; Vincent, J.-L.; Huyghens, L. Does N-Acetyl-L-Cysteine Influence Cytokine Response During Early Human Septic Shock? *Chest* **1998**, *113*, 1616–1624. [CrossRef] [PubMed]
34. Ortolani, O.; Conti, A.; de Gaudio, A.R.; Masoni, M.; Novelli, G. Protective Effects of N-Acetylcysteine and Rutin on the Lipid Peroxidation of the Lung Epithelium during the Adult Respiratory Distress Syndrome. *Shock* **2000**, *13*, 14–18. [CrossRef] [PubMed]

35. Rank, N.; Michel, C.; Haertel, C.; Med, C.; Lenhart, A.; Welte, M.; Meier-Hellmann, A.; Spies, C. N-acetylcysteine increases liver blood flow and improves liver function in septic shock patients: Results of a prospective, randomized, double-blind study. *Crit. Care Med.* **2000**, *28*, 3799–3807. [CrossRef]
36. Paterson, R.L.; Galley, H.F.; Webster, N.R. The effect of N-acetylcysteine on nuclear factor-κB activation, interleukin-6, interleukin-8, and intercellular adhesion molecule-1 expression in patients with sepsis. *Crit. Care Med.* **2003**, *31*, 2574–2578. [CrossRef]
37. Szakmany, T.; Hauser, B.; Radermacher, P. N-acetylcysteine for sepsis and systemic inflammatory response in adults. *Cochrane Database Syst. Rev.* **2012**, *2012*, CD006616. [CrossRef] [PubMed]
38. Aisa-Alvarez, A.; Soto, M.E.; Guarner-Lans, V.; Camarena-Alejo, G.; Franco-Granillo, J.; Martínez-Rodríguez, E.A.; Ávila, R.G.; Pech, L.M.; Pérez-Torres, I. Usefulness of Antioxidants as Adjuvant Therapy for Septic Shock: A Randomized Clinical Trial. *Medicina* **2020**, *56*, 619. [CrossRef]
39. Falcone, M.; Russo, A.; Iacovelli, A.; Restuccia, G.; Ceccarelli, G.; Giordano, A.; Farcomeni, A.; Morelli, A.; Venditti, M. Predictors of outcome in ICU patients with septic shock caused by *Klebsiella pneumoniae carbapenemase*–producing *K. pneumoniae*. *Clin. Microbiol. Infect.* **2016**, *22*, 444–450. [CrossRef]
40. Lopez-Cortes, L.E.; Cisneros, J.M.; Fernández-Cuenca, F.; Bou, G.; Tomas, M.; Garnacho-Montero, J.; Pascual, A.; Martinez-Martinez, L.; Vilá, J.; Pachón, J.; et al. Monotherapy versus combination therapy for sepsis due to multidrug-resistant *Acinetobacter baumannii*: Analysis of a multicentre prospective cohort. *J. Antimicrob. Chemother.* **2014**, *69*, 3119–3126. [CrossRef]
41. Zafarullah, M.; Li, W.Q.; Sylvester, J.; Ahmad, M. Molecular mechanisms of N-acetylcysteine actions. *Cell. Mol. Life Sci.* **2003**, *60*, 6–20. [CrossRef]
42. Harman, L.S.; Mottle, C.; Mason, R.P. Free radical metabolites of L-cysteine oxidation. *J. Biol. Chem.* **1984**, *259*, 5606–5611. [CrossRef]
43. Kumar, A.; Roberts, D.; Wood, K.E.; Light, B.; Parrillo, J.E.; Sharma, S.; Suppes, R.; Feinstein, D.; Zanotti, S.; Taiberg, L.; et al. Duration of hypotension before initiation of effective antimicrobial therapy is the critical determinant of survival in human septic shock. *Crit. Care Med.* **2006**, *34*, 1589–1596. [CrossRef]
44. Ferrer, R.; Artigas, A.; Suarez, D.; Palencia, E.; Levy, M.M.; Arenzana, A.; Pérez, X.L.; Sirvent, J.-M. Effectiveness of Treatments for Severe Sepsis. *Am. J. Respir. Crit. Care Med.* **2009**, *180*, 861–866. [CrossRef]
45. Levy, M.M.; Artigas, A.; Phillips, G.S.; Rhodes, A.; Beale, R.; Osborn, T.; Vincent, J.-L.; Townsend, S.; Lemeshow, S.; Dellinger, R.P. Outcomes of the Surviving Sepsis Campaign in intensive care units in the USA and Europe: A prospective cohort study. *Lancet Infect. Dis.* **2012**, *12*, 919–924. [CrossRef]
46. Tumbarello, M.; Viale, P.; Viscoli, C.; Trecarichi, E.M.; Tumietto, F.; Marchese, A.; Spanu, T.; Ambretti, S.; Ginocchio, F.; Cristini, F.; et al. Predictors of Mortality in Bloodstream Infections Caused by *Klebsiella pneumoniae Carbapenemase*-Producing *K. pneumoniae*: Importance of Combination Therapy. *Clin. Infect. Dis.* **2012**, *55*, 943–950. [CrossRef]
47. Tumbarello, M.; Trecarichi, E.M.; de Rosa, F.G.; Giannella, M.; Giacobbe, D.R.; Bassetti, M.; Losito, A.R.; Bartoletti, M.; del Bono, V.; Corcione, S.; et al. Infections caused by KPC-producing *Klebsiella pneumoniae*: Differences in therapy and mortality in a multicentre study. *J. Antimicrob. Chemother.* **2015**, *70*, 2133–2143. [CrossRef] [PubMed]
48. Russo, A.; Bassetti, M.; Ceccarelli, G.; Carannante, N.; Losito, A.R.; Bartoletti, M.; Corcione, S.; Granata, G.; Santoro, A.; Giacobbe, D.R.; et al. Bloodstream infections caused by carbapenem-resistant *Acinetobacter baumannii*: Clinical features, therapy and outcome from a multicenter study. *J. Infect.* **2019**, *79*, 130–138. [CrossRef]
49. Augustine, M.R.; Testerman, T.L.; Justo, J.A.; Bookstaver, P.B.; Kohn, J.; Albrecht, H.; Al-Hasan, M.N. Clinical Risk Score for Prediction of Extended-Spectrum β-Lactamase–Producing Enterobacteriaceae in Bloodstream Isolates. *Infect. Control. Hosp. Epidemiol.* **2016**, *38*, 266–272. [CrossRef]
50. Gutiérrez-Gutiérrez, B.; Salamanca, E.; de Cueto, M.; Hsueh, P.-R.; Viale, P.; Paño-Pardo, J.R.; Venditti, M.; Tumbarello, M.; Daikos, G.; Pintado, V.; et al. A Predictive Model of Mortality in Patients with Bloodstream Infections due to *Carbapenemase*-Producing Enterobacteriaceae. *Mayo Clin. Proc.* **2016**, *91*, 1362–1371. [CrossRef] [PubMed]
51. Giannella, M.; Trecarichi, E.M.; de Rosa, F.; del Bono, V.; Bassetti, M.; Lewis, R.; Losito, A.; Corcione, S.; Saffioti, C.; Bartoletti, M.; et al. Risk factors for carbapenem-resistant *Klebsiella pneumoniae* bloodstream infection among rectal carriers: A prospective observational multicentre study. *Clin. Microbiol. Infect.* **2014**, *20*, 1357–1362. [CrossRef] [PubMed]
52. European Centre for Disease Prevention and Control (ECDC). European Antimicrobial Resistance Surveillance Network (EARS-Net). Available online: https://www.ecdc.europa.eu/en/home (accessed on 20 January 2021).
53. Singer, M.; Deutschman, C.S.; Seymour, C.W.; Shankar-Hari, M.; Annane, D.; Bauer, M.; Bellomo, R.; Bernard, G.R.; Chiche, J.-D.; Coopersmith, C.M.; et al. The Third International Consensus Definitions for Sepsis and Septic Shock (Sepsis-3). *JAMA* **2016**, *315*, 801–810. [CrossRef] [PubMed]

MDPI
St. Alban-Anlage 66
4052 Basel
Switzerland
Tel. +41 61 683 77 34
Fax +41 61 302 89 18
www.mdpi.com

Antibiotics Editorial Office
E-mail: antibiotics@mdpi.com
www.mdpi.com/journal/antibiotics

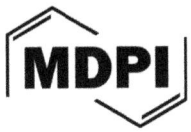

www.ingramcontent.com/pod-product-compliance
Lightning Source LLC
LaVergne TN
LVHW070729100526
838202LV00013B/1200